AF581233

Anabolic Treatments *for* Osteoporosis

Pharmacology and Toxicology: Basic and Clinical Aspects

Mannfred A. Hollinger, Series Editor
University of California, Davis

Forthcoming Titles

Basis of Toxicity Testing, Second Edition, Donald J. Ecobichon
CNS Injuries: Cellular Responses and Pharmacological Strategies, Martin Berry and Ann Logan
Lead and Public Health: Integrated Risk Assessment, Paul Mushak
Molecular Bases of Anesthesia, Eric Moody and Phil Skolnick
Receptor Characterization and Regulation, Devendra K. Agrawal

Published Titles

Anabolic Treatments for Osteoporosis, James F. Whitfield and Paul Morley
Antibody Therapeutics, 1997, William J. Harris and John R. Adair
Muscarinic Receptor Subtypes in Smooth Muscle, 1997, Richard M. Eglen
Antisense Oligodeonucleotides as Novel Pharmacological Therapeutic Agents, 1997, Benjamin Weiss
Drug Delivery Systems, 1996, Vasant V. Ranade and Mannfred A. Hollinger
Experimental Models of Mucosal Inflammation, 1996, Timothy S. Gaginella
Brain Mechanisms and Psychotropic Drugs, 1996, Andrius Baskys and Gary Remington
Receptor Dynamics in Neural Development, 1996, Christopher A. Shaw
Ryanodine Receptors, 1996, Vincenzo Sorrentino
Therapeutic Modulation of Cytokines, 1996, M.W. Bodmer and Brian Henderson
Pharmacology in Exercise and Sport, 1996, Satu M. Somani
Placental Pharmacology, 1996, B. V. Rama Sastry
Pharmacological Effects of Ethanol on the Nervous System, 1996, Richard A. Deitrich
Immunopharmaceuticals, 1996, Edward S. Kimball
Chemoattractant Ligands and Their Receptors, 1996, Richard Horuk
Pharmacological Regulation of Gene Expression in the CNS, 1996, Kalpana Merchant
Human Growth Hormone Pharmacology: Basic and Clinical Aspects, 1995, Kathleen T. Shiverick and Arlan Rosenbloom
Placental Toxicology, 1995, B. V. Rama Sastry
Stealth Liposomes, 1995, Danilo Lasic and Frank Martin
TAXOL®: Science and Applications, 1995, Matthew Suffness

Pharmacology and Toxicology: Basic and Clinical Aspects

Published Titles Continued

Endothelin Receptors: From the Gene to the Human, 1995, Robert R. Ruffolo, Jr.
Alternative Methodologies for the Safety Evaluation of Chemicals in the Cosmetic Industry, 1995, Nicola Loprieno
Phospholipase A_2 in Clinical Inflammation: Molecular Approaches to Pathophysiology, 1995, Keith B. Glaser and Peter Vadas
Serotonin and Gastrointestinal Function, 1995, Timothy S. Gaginella and James J. Galligan
Chemical and Structural Approaches to Rational Drug Design, 1994, David B. Weiner and William V. Williams
Biological Approaches to Rational Drug Design, 1994, David B. Weiner and William V. Williams
Direct Allosteric Control of Glutamate Receptors, 1994, M. Palfreyman, I. Reynolds, and P. Skolnick
Genomic and Non-Genomic Effects of Aldosterone, 1994, Martin Wehling
Peroxisome Proliferators: Unique Inducers of Drug-Metabolizing Enzymes, 1994, David E. Moody
Angiotensin II Receptors, Volume I: Molecular Biology, Biochemistry, Pharmacology, and Clinical Perspectives, 1994, Robert R. Ruffolo, Jr.
Angiotensin II Receptors, Volume II: Medicinal Chemistry, 1994, Robert R. Ruffolo, Jr.
Beneficial and Toxic Effects of Aspirin, 1993, Susan E. Feinman
Preclinical and Clinical Modulation of Anticancer Drugs, 1993, Kenneth D. Tew, Peter Houghton, and Janet Houghton
In Vitro *Methods of Toxicology*, 1992, Ronald R. Watson
Basis of Toxicity Testing, 1992, Donald J. Ecobichon
Human Drug Metabolism from Molecular Biology to Man, 1992, Elizabeth Jeffreys
Platelet Activating Factor Receptor: Signal Mechanisms and Molecular Biology, 1992, Shivendra D. Shukla
Biopharmaceutics of Ocular Drug Delivery, 1992, Peter Edman
Pharmacology of the Skin, 1991, Hasan Mukhtar
Inflammatory Cells and Mediators in Bronchial Asthma, 1990, Devendra K. Agrawal and Robert G. Townley

Anabolic Treatments *for* Osteoporosis

Edited by

James F. Whitfield, Ph.D.

Paul Morley, Ph.D.

Institute for Biological Sciences
The National Research Council of Canada
Ottawa, Ontario

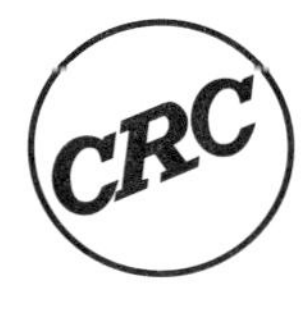

CRC Press
Boca Raton New York

Library of Congress Cataloging-in-Publication Data

Anabolic treatments for osteoporosis / edited by James F. Whitfield
and Paul Morley.
p. cm. — (Pharmacology and toxicology)
Includes bibliographical references and index.
ISBN 0-8493-8556-3 (alk. paper)
1. Osteoporosis—Hormone therapy. 2. Parathyroid hormone-
-Therapeutic use. 3. Somatomedin—Therapeutic use. I. Whitfield,
James F. II. Morley, Paul, Ph.D. III. Series: Pharmacology &
toxicology (Boca Raton, Fla.)
[DNLM: 1. Osteoporosis—drug therapy. 2. Parathyroid Hormones-
-therapeutic use. 3. Prostaglandins E—therapeutic use.
4. Fluorides—therapeutic use. WE 250 A532 1997]
RC931.073A53 1997
616.7′16—dc21
DNLM/DLC
for Library of Congress 97-15242
CIP

Direct all inquiries to CRC Press LLC, 2000 Corporate Blvd., N.W., Boca Raton, Florida 33431.

International Standard Book Number 0-8493-8556-3
Library of Congress Card Number 97-15242
Printed in the United States of America 1 2 3 4 5 6 7 8 9 0
Printed on acid-free paper

The Editors

James F. Whitfield, B.Sc. (McGill University), M.Sc. (University of Western Ontario), Ph.D. (University of Western Ontario)

After receiving his Ph.D. in 1955, Dr. Whitfield joined the Biology and Health Physics Division of Atomic Energy of Canada at Chalk River, Ontario, where he carried out pioneering research on the insertion of bacteriophageλ into its host cell's genome. But he soon joined forces with Ray Rixon to discover and characterize the potent radioprotective and radiotherapeutic actions of the parathyroid hormone. He left Chalk River in 1962 to set up a cell biology laboratory at the European Joint Research Center at Ispra in northern Italy, where he carried out some of the first studies of the mechanisms, and the role of Ca^{2+} in the mechanisms, underlying radiation-triggered apoptosis in human and rat thymocytes. Dr. Whitfield returned to Canada in 1965 to start a cell biology laboratory at the National Research Council of Canada. Since then he has participated in research that has led to the discovery of the controlling roles of Ca^{2+} and cyclic AMP in normal cell proliferation and the loss of these controls during carcinogenesis. He and his group have established the key roles of the parathyroid hormone and the parathyroid hormone-related protein (PTHrP) in the control of the proliferation and differentiation of kcratinocytes, hepatocytes in the regenerating liver, and spleen and thymic lymphocytes. As will be seen in this book, he and his colleagues have, most recently, mapped the parathyroid hormone's two signaling regions and are now applying this knowledge to the design of new parathyroid hormone fragments for stimulating bone growth in osteoporotic humans.

Paul Morley, B.Sc. (University of Waterloo), M.Sc. (University of Western Ontario), Ph.D. (University of Western Ontario)

Paul Morley trained in the field of reproductive endocrinology with David T. Armstrong and Franco Calaresu and received his Ph.D. degree in 1990. His thesis work investigated the hormonal and neural regulation of ovarian thecal cell androgen production. He then held a Medical Research Council of Canada Postdoctoral Fellowship at the Loeb Medical Research Institute in Ottawa, where he studied the roles of ions and ion channels in ovarian steroidogenesis. In 1992 he joined the National Research Council of Canada as a research associate and since then has become an Associate Research Officer. He heads the Ions & Ion Channels Laboratory, which has made important discoveries concerning the contributions of calcium ions and calcium-conducting ion channels in endocrine and neural systems. He also works as part of the group involved in the design and testing of novel parathyroid hormone fragments/analogs for treating osteoporosis.

Contributors

Kristina Åkesson, M.D., Ph.D.
Department of Medicine
Loma Linda University
Mineral Metabolism Unit
Jerry L. Pettis Memorial V.A. Medical Center
Loma Linda, California

Zafrira Avnur, Ph.D.
Osteoporosis and Endocrine Research
Roche Bioscience
Palo Alto, California

David J. Baylink, M.D.
Department of Medicine
Loma Linda University
Chief, Mineral Metabolism Unit
Jerry Pettis Memorial V.A. Medical Center
Loma Linda, California

L. J. Fraher, Ph.D.
Department of Medicine
Lawson Research Institute
St. Joseph's Health Centre
London, Ontario, Canada

Harold M. Frost, M.D., Dr.Sc.
Southern Colorado Clinic
Pueblo, Colorado

Esther Hill, Ph.D.
Osteoporosis and Endocrine Research
Roche Bioscience
Palo Alto, California

A. B. Hodsman, M.B., ERCP
Department of Medicine
Lawson Research Institute
St. Joseph's Health Centre
London, Ontario, Canada

Anna Johansson
Department of Internal Medicine
University Hospital
Uppsala, Sweden

John L. Krstenansky
Osteoporosis and Endocrine Research
Roche Bioscience
Palo Alto, California

R. M. Langille, Ph.D.
Institute for Biological Sciences
National Research Council of Canada
Ottawa, Ontario, Canada

K.-H. William Lau, Ph.D.
Department of Medicine
Loma Linda University
Mineral Metabolism Unit
Jerry L. Pettis Memorial V.A. Medical Center
Loma Linda, California

Mei Li, M.D.
Department of Physiological Sciences
College of Veterinary Medicine
University of Florida
Gainesville, Florida

Cesar R. Libanati, M.D.
Department of Medicine
Loma Linda University
Mineral Metabolism Unit
Jerry L. Pettis Memorial V.A. Medical Center
Loma Linda, California

G. Marchand, B.Comm.
Institute for Biological Sciences
National Research Council of Canada
Ottawa, Ontario, Canada

Georgia I. McRae, M.A.
Osteoporosis and Endocrine Research
Roche Bioscience
Palo Alto, California

Paul Morley, Ph.D.
Institute for Biological Sciences
National Research Council of Canada
Ottawa, Ontario, Canada

Lis Mosekilde, M.D., Ph.D.
Department of Cell Biology
Institute of Anatomy
University of Aarhus
Aarhus, Denmark

Clifford J. Rosen, M.D.
Maine Center for Osteoporosis Research and Education
St. Joseph Hospital
Bangor, Maine

Brian H. Vickery, Ph.D.
Osteoporosis and Endocrine Research
Roche Bioscience
Palo Alto, California

Ruth Waters, M.Ed.
Osteoporosis and Endocrine Research
Roche Bioscience
Palo Alto, California

P. H. Watson, Ph.D.
Department of Medicine
Lawson Research Institute
St. Joseph's Health Centre
London, Ontario, Canada

James F. Whitfield, Ph.D.
Institute for Biological Sciences
National Research Council of Canada
Ottawa, Ontario, Canada

G. E. Willick, Ph.D.
Institute for Biological Sciences
National Research Council of Canada
Ottawa, Ontario, Canada

Thomas J. Wronski, Ph.D.
Department of Physiological Sciences
College of Veterinary Medicine
University of Florida
Gainesville, Florida

Preface

Osteoporosis has become a major concern for the women who are its major targets in the aging populations of Europe, Japan, and North America, for the people who must fund their care, and a challenge for the healthcare professionals and pharmaceutical firms who are expected to do something about it. So far, attention has focused on what appears to have been the easiest strategy — the slowing or inhibition of osteoclastic bone resorption with only a limited, secondary increase of bone mass resulting from the filling-in of holes left by the inhibited osteoclasts. Until now there seemed to be little hope of finding the most desirable of drugs — a true anabolic drug that can directly, safely, and selectively stimulate bone growth and thus strengthen remaining bone and even replace lost bone.

But things are changing! There is a much-belated interest and exploitation of a discovery made in the early 1930s that, when given intermittently in small doses, the parathyroid hormone is a potent bone builder, the action of which we now believe is mediated by a cyclic AMP-induced production of growth- and function-stimulating factors such as IGF-I by osteoblasts. At the same time, there has been an increasingly effective fashioning of the fluoride ion and the parathyroid hormone into promising anabolic drugs. Clearly, we shall soon be able to build bone in osteoporotic patients with these "new" anabolic tools and then keep the new bone with a growing arsenal of antiresorptive bisphosphonates, estrogens, or calcitonin.

In these chapters we tell the exciting story of the emerging anabolic strategies for treating osteoporosis. We start with a fresh look at the intricacies of bone biology, osteopenia, and osteoporosis. We then turn to the anabolic agents and their intracellular mediators that hopefully will soon be the star players in the treatment of osteoporosis.

James F. Whitfield
Paul Morley
Ottawa
June 1997

Table of Contents

Chapter 1

Osteoporoses: Their Nature and Therapeutic Targets

(Insights from a New Paradigm)

Harold M. Frost

CONTENTS

0-8493-8556-3/98/$0.00+$.50

I. INTRODUCTION

To understand a disease requires knowing three things: 1) Its nature (the pathology); 2) which tissue-level and other mechanisms cause the pathology (its pathogenesis); and 3) what makes the mechanisms do that (control by hormones, genes, calcium, vitamins, growth factors, drugs, mechanics, etc.). For osteoporoses, understanding of 1 and 2 improved dramatically after 1964, but mainstream skeletal thought has not accounted for this improved understanding adequately, due partly to poor interdisciplinary communication,[1,2] and as others also have noted.[3-6] This chapter concerns 1 and 2, since understanding 3 requires understanding them first.

A new skeletal-biologic paradigm combines biomechanics with histomorphometric, clinical, and other evidence and ideas.[6-11] Among other things, it concerns osteoporoses, their management and research, and the potential of bone anabolic agents for preventing and curing such diseases. To work effectively, such agents must have specific biologic and mechanical effects, and must avoid or solve specific problems. This chapter reviews some of those matters. It also offers a test of one's knowledge of the cell- and molecular-biologic roots of the tissue-level bone physiology involved in osteoporoses. Readers be warned: It is nasty. I flunked it.

Some definitions appear in the Glossary at the end of the chapter. While some authorities might favor another way to classify osteoporoses, the following one fits multidisciplinary data and shows some of their relevance. It views osteoporoses as a continuum that bridges two different end states or syndromes.[2,7]

II. A CLASSIFICATION OF OSTEOPENIAS AND OSTEOPOROSES

Let a *physiologic osteopenia* mean less bone than age and sex comparable norms, but in people less physically active than others. These people have no trouble with bones unless they fall. Their bone meets the needs of their usual activities very well. The resulting fractures affect wrists and hips far more than the spine.

The inactivity can be associated with aging, an aversion to exercise, or chronic debilitating problems that cause muscle weakness and excessive fatigue. Examples include chronic cardiac, hepatic, pulmonary, and renal disease or failure, malnutrition, muscular dystrophy, paralyses, degenerative neural diseases, stroke, long-term nursing home and wheelchair residence, and severe polyarthritis. Such osteopenias are common.

Let a *true osteoporosis* mean an osteopenia, plus a bone pain syndrome and/or spontaneous fractures caused by normal physical activities, plus bone fragility increased above what the osteopenia alone can explain. Such bone does not meet the needs of these patients' usual activities. Its problems affect the spine more than the limb bones, and include spontaneous and often asymptomatic vertebral body compression fractures and wedging, as well as vertebral body end-plate "cod fishing." Of course if these patients fall, they can fracture wrists and hips too. These affections are less common than physiologic osteopenias.

The combinations or "continuum." Features of these two situations should overlap in many people. This could partly explain why it took so long to recognize them as different entities at opposite ends of a "pathogenetic–pathologic continuum." Both affect more women than men, and far more adults than children. Table 1.1 lists some tissue-level features of bone physiology that help to determine the nature and pathogenesis of

TABLE 1.1

Some Tissue-Level Bone Features[a] Involved in the Pathogenesis, Prevention, and Cure of Osteoporoses

BMU creations, general	Periosteal BMU creations
BMU creations, next to marrow	Duration of the ARF sequence
Relative numbers of 'blasts, 'clasts, rho, general	Rho, periosteal
Rho next to marrow	Periosteal formation drift
Formation drift, general	'blasts/mm^2 bone surface/drift
Formation drift, next to marrow	Resorption drift, periosteal
Resorption drift, general	'clasts/mm^2 bone surface/drift
Resorption drift, next to marrow	mm^2/formation drift
mm^2/resorption drift	Microdamage detection
Microdamage, general	Microdamage momentary burden
Microdamage repair	Microdamage threshold strain
Microdamage creation	Remodeling threshold strain
Modeling threshold strain	Metaphyseal cortical thickness
Epiphyseal cortical thickness	Endochondral ossification
The chondral modeling barrier	

[a] The mechanostat. Cell- and molecular-biologic features let each of the above features work, as the parts of a car let it work. Normally, different things then control how slowly or quickly the features work, or if they work improperly or not at all, somewhat as a car's driver can be lazy, hurried, asleep, or even drunk. In the paradigm's view, the driver of the bone "car" is mechanical usage. All else would exist to help the car obey the needs of its "driver." If those things prevent the car from obeying its driver, disease can result, and true osteoporoses are examples.

osteopenias and osteoporoses. Later, the chapter poses hard questions about its entries.

III. BIOLOGICAL MECHANISMS THAT AFFECT BONE STRENGTH

A. Endochondral Ossification

Beneath growth plates in children endochondral ossification creates our initial supplies of spongiosa that stops at skeletal maturity around 16 years of age in girls, and 18 years in boys.[12] It can increase but not decrease bone mass, mostly of spongiosa.

B. Bone Modeling Drifts

Biologically separate formation and resorption drifts create and use osteoblasts and osteoclasts, respectively, to shape and size bones and trabeculae in the cross-sectional sense, and to shape them longitudinally[12-15] (Figure 1.1) Global modeling can increase the bone bank and strength but rarely reduces them. Most active during growth, drifts

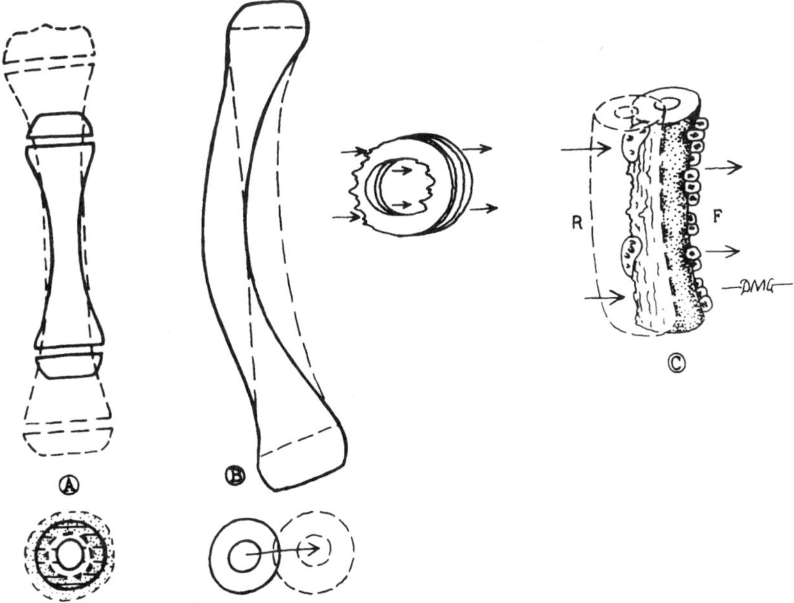

Figure 1.1
Bone modeling drifts. (A) An infant's long bone with its original size and shape in solid line. To keep this shape as it grows in length and diameter, its surfaces must move in tissue space as the dashed lines suggest. *Formation drifts* make and control osteoblasts to build some surfaces up. *Resorption drifts* make and control osteoclasts to remove material from others. (B) A different drift pattern can correct the fracture malunion in a child, shown in solid line. The cross-section to the right shows the cortical–endosteal as well as the periosteal drifts that do that. (C) Shows how the drifts in B would move the whole segment to the right. *Note:* Large forces, such as are encountered in weight lifting, make modeling strengthen bone better than smaller forces, as encountered in marathon running, no matter how frequent. (From Frost, H. M., Osteogenesis imperfecta. The setpoint proposal. *Clin. Orthop. Rel. Res.*, 216, 280, 1987. With permission.)

can affect trabeculae for life, but become inefficient on adult cortical bone. Formation drifts originally create all cortical bone. Then secondary osteons can gradually replace some of it (see Section III.C). "Global" means averaged over a whole bone or skeleton.

Formation drifts lie on smooth cement lines (arrest lines). They involve an *A*ctivation → *F*ormation or A→F cellular sequence. Resorption drifts involve an *A*ctivation → *R*esorption or A→R cellular sequence.

C. Bone Remodeling BMUs (Basic Multicellular Units)

BMUs turn bone over in small "packets" in an *A*ctivation → *R*esorption → *F*ormation or A→R→F sequence that finishes in about four months (Figure 1.2).[12,16-19] The best known BMU product is the secondary osteon. This remodeling goes on for life on all bone surfaces. Changing how much

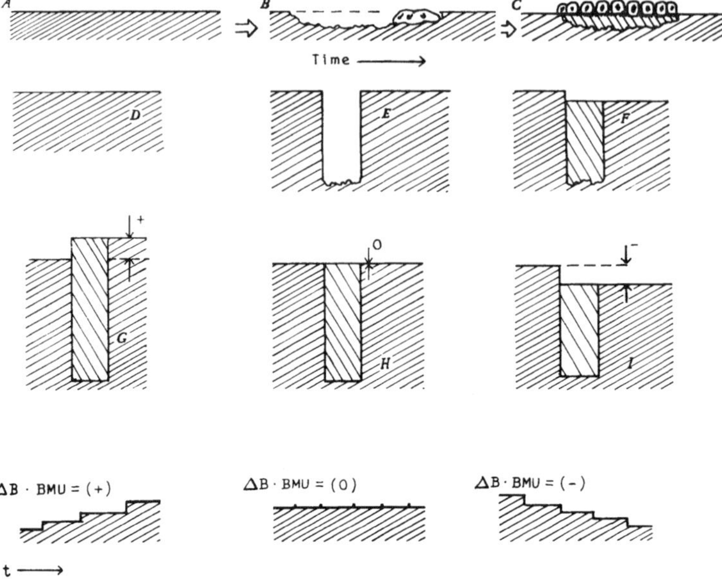

Figure 1.2
Bone remodeling BMUs. Top row: An activation event on a bone surface at (A) causes a packet of bone resorption at (B), and then replacement of the resorbed bone at (C). The BMU makes and controls the osteoclasts and osteoblasts that do this. Second row: Idealize those events to emphasize the amounts of bone resorbed (E) and formed (F) by completed BMUs. Third row: In these "BMU graphs" (after Frost), (G) shows a small excess of formation over resorption as on periosteal surfaces (that excess = rho and is positive). (H) Shows equalized resorption and formation as on haversian surfaces (rho = zero). (I) Shows a net deficit of formation, as on cortical–endosteal and trabecular surfaces (the deficit = rho and is negative). Bottom row: These "stair graphs" (after P. J. Meunier) show the effects on the local bone balance and mass of a series of BMUs of the kind immediately above. Rho means the net gain or loss of bone per typical completed BMU. Healthy adult human skeletons probably create and complete around three million BMUs annually, along with corresponding numbers of new but short-lived osteoclasts and osteoblasts. (From Frost, H. M., Osteogenesis imperfecta. The setpoint proposal. *Clin. Orthop. Rel. Res.*, 216, 280, 1987. With permission.)

bone *completed* BMUs resorb and form can affect bone losses or gains. Let any difference equal Greek lower case "rho" (Figure 1.3).[18] Completed BMUs next to marrow usually remove more bone than they form (rho is negative), to cause lifelong trabecular and cortical–endosteal bone losses. Inside cortical bone, BMUs resorb and form nearly equal amounts (rho tends toward zero). On periosteal surfaces, BMUs may resorb less than they form (rho might be positive). Global remodeling by BMUs can conserve or reduce bone mass and strength, but seldom if ever does it increase them. It also repairs the bone microdamage described below to prevent Looser's zones (pseudofractures) in osteomalacia, and spontaneous fractures of whole bones and individual trabeculae.

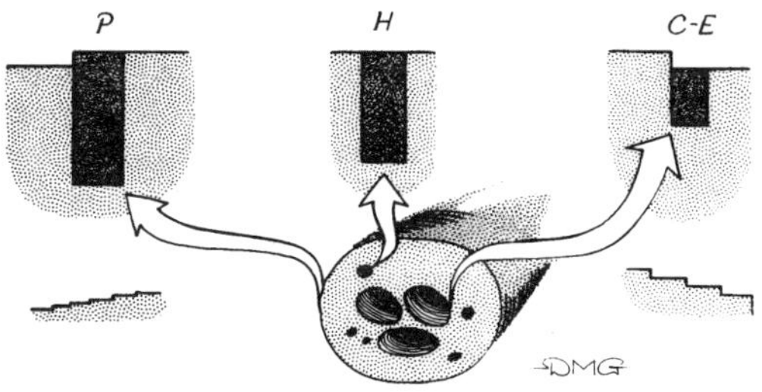

Figure 1.3
Rho. Top left: On *P*eriosteal surfaces, completed BMUs might sometimes make more bone than they resorb, so the difference, rho, would be positive. Middle top: On *H*aversian surfaces inside cortical bone, resorption and formation in completed BMUs tend to equalize so rho tends toward zero. Top right: Where bone touches marrow — cortical endosteal and trabecular surfaces (C-E) — BMUs make less bone than they resorb so rho is negative. The "stair graphs," bottom left and right, show the effect on the local bone balance of a series of completed BMUs that have the rho values shown above. (From Frost, H. M., Wolff's Law and bone's structural adaptations to mechanical usage: an overview for clinicians. *Angle Orthodont.*, 64, 187, 1994. With permission.)

Increased numbers of BMUs increase the number of temporary holes in a bone. That temporarily missing bone comprises the *remodeling space*.[19-21] It normally takes up about 5 to 10% of a bone. It can increase many times when BMU creations increase, and more in spongiosa than in cortical bone. The new bone packets made by BMUs lie on cement lines scalloped by Howship's lacunae (reversal lines).

D. Adults and Children Compared

Excluding longitudinal bone growth, an adult's bone mass and strength depend on how much bone endochondral ossification and modeling added during growth, and how much bone remodeling removed then and in adult life. All three activities affect bone mass and strength in children. Only remodeling functions effectively in adults, with the exception that trabecular modeling can go on for life. An adult can have an osteopenia because too little bone accumulated during growth, or remodeling removed too much afterward, or both.

IV. BONE STRENGTH, ARCHITECTURE, MICRODAMAGE, AND FRACTURE MECHANICS

Bone strength depends partly on its materials properties such as stiffness, ultimate strength, and yield point.[22-25] They vary little with age, bone, species, and disease when compared to the following features. A bone's strength as an organ depends partly on the bone content in a given cross-section. In general, the more bone the stronger the bone. A bone's strength depends partly on its cross-section size, shape, and cortical thickness, or architecture.[24-27] As a hollow cylinder equal amounts of bone are stronger in bending and torque than as a solid cylinder of smaller diameter. Yet both bones could have similar strengths under longitudinal compression or tension loading. Those architectural features can cause large regional differences in bone strength. Our 12th ribs and our femurs have the same material and materials properties, but huge differences in strength due to different cross-sectional architecture and bone content.

Bone can develop microscopic fatigue damage called *microdamage* that cells can detect and BMUs normally repair.[2,28-32] It weakens bone without affecting its architecture. When it overwhelms its repair, it can accumulate to cause stress and spontaneous fractures of bones and trabeculae, and pseudofractures in osteomalacia. It helps to increase bone fragility in true osteoporoses. While microdamage was recognized long ago from clinical-pathologic evidence,[19,33] mainstream skeletal thought only began to accept it in this decade.[32,34-40] Spontaneous fractures should *always* stem from increased microdamage.

Bone has an operational microdamage threshold range (the MESp, centered near 3000 microstrain), below which microdamage repair usually keeps up with the need. Above it, microdamage can begin to accumulate. As a growing bone's total loads increase over 20 times between birth and maturity, mechanically controlled modeling adjusts its architecture and strength to keep its strains and their gradients comfortably below that threshold.[2,41]

Bone strength is another continuum matter. It varies without recognizable natural steps between the opposite extremes of far stronger than normal, and exceptionally fragile.

Injuries can apply one-time loads to a bone to which it had not adapted. For example, our distal radius adapts well to the usual loads on it, so they do not break it. Yet a fall can put very large bending and torque loads on the radius to which it never had a chance to adapt, so they do break it. Likewise for hips, shoulders, and ankles. Here too the size of the loads caused by very violent and very slight injuries should be at opposite ends of a continuum.

In elderly people, extremity bone fractures from falls begin in the metaphyseal or/and epiphyseal cortex of the bone, and not in spongiosa or the bone shafts (diaphyses).[42] They include wrist and hip fractures, and fewer ankle, humeral surgical neck, tibial plateau, femoral supracondylar, pelvic, and rib fractures.[43] To minimize those fractures the epiphyseal and metaphyseal cortices need strengthening. Strengthening diaphyses and spongiosa would not suffice,[42] although strengthening vertebral spongiosa should help in the spine. Curiously, most past human and animal research on this problem focused on metaphyseal spongiosa and diaphyseal cortex,[41,42] although notable exceptions exist.[44-46] See also Sections VII and VIII.

V. SOME VITAL BIOMECHANICS

Bone can monitor its mechanical usage and signal its cell systems when and where more or less bone is needed, and if microdamage exists.[2,6-11] This lets bone mass and strength respond predictably to mechanical usage. For that reason, and given similar sex, age, height, diet, race, and weight, less-active people usually have less bone, and more fragile bone, than more vigorous people.[47] The biologic activities arrange that in the following way.

A. Modeling

When and where bone strains reach or exceed a lower threshold range (the MESm, centered near 1000 microstrain), mechanically controlled modeling drifts switch ON and begin to change local bone mass and architecture in ways that strengthen it and reduce subsequent strains toward the bottom of that range. In children this increases the cross-sectional bone bank and bone strength. In adults it has small effects on cortical modeling, but trabecular modeling can operate throughout life. The modeling threshold normally lies below the microdamage threshold. Where strains stay below the MESm, mechanically controlled modeling by drifts would stop or go OFF. Or, normally:

$$\text{Strains} <\approx 1000\,\mu E \rightarrow \text{modeling OFF}$$

$$\text{Strains} >\approx 1000\,\mu E \rightarrow \text{modeling ON} \rightarrow \text{stronger bone}$$

B. Remodeling

When and where bone strains fall and stay below a third threshold range (the MESr, probably near 50 to 100 microstrain), BMU creations increase toward their maximum, and completed BMUs next to marrow make far less bone than normal (rho goes very negative). This increases permanent bone loss next to marrow. (Why only there? Nobody knows yet.) As strains rise above that threshold, BMU creations begin to fall toward normal, and the bone they resorb and make tends to equalize. This reduces bone turnover and conserves bone and its strength.

C. Some Disuse Effects

In children, sudden disuse reduces longitudinal bone growth, modeling drifts, their additions of new bone, and strengthening of existing bone.[48-51] BMU creations increase, and next to marrow completed BMUs make less bone than they resorb (rho goes more negative). The resulting "child's disuse-pattern osteopenia" has less spongiosa, widened marrow cavities, thinned cortices, reduced outside bone diameters, and somewhat shorter, weakened bones. In adults, sudden disuse causes the same BMU responses as in children. Trabecular and cortical–endosteal bone losses increase. Again, adults lack endochondral ossification and effective cortical modeling. The resulting "adult disuse-pattern osteopenia" also has less spongiosa, widened marrow cavities, thinned cortices and weakened bones, but bone lengths and outside diameters stay normal. For chronic disuse, see below.

D. Some Hypervigorous Mechanical Usage Effects

In children, chronic hypervigorous mechanical usage, as in weight lifting, football, soccer, and hard physical labor, tends to increase longitudinal bone growth, bone modeling drifts, additions of spongiosa and compacta, and bone mass and strength. It depresses BMU creations and equalizes resorption and formation by completed BMUs (rho tends toward zero), which conserves existing bone and makes its turnover normal. In adults these same BMU responses happen, so here too bone is conserved. After some years, such adults can have more bone, and stronger bones, because they kept their original bone better than adults who lost it "normally" with aging. Sudden hypervigorous mechanical usage can temporarily increase remodeling.[52] Or, normally and approximately:

Strains $<\approx 100\ \mu E \rightarrow$ *"disuse mode" remodeling* $\rightarrow$ *loss of bone/strength*

Strains $<\approx 100\ \mu E \rightarrow$ *remodeling in the bone/strength "conservation mode"*

E. The Two-Stage, Tissue-Dynamic Remodeling Pattern in Disuse

The first stage in this pattern causes an osteopenia, and the second maintains it afterward. The stages usually overlap, which makes this another continuum matter, with different states at opposite ends of the continuum.[2]

The initial tissue dynamics: Sudden partial disuse increases BMU creations more than it decreases the bone each BMU makes (rho goes more negative), so bone turnover, formation, resorption, and net losses next to marrow all increase. Sudden total disuse increases BMU creations even more, but now BMUs make far less bone than normal next to marrow, or even none (rho goes markedly negative). This further accelerates net bone losses, but now global formation and turnover become subnormal.

The final tissue dynamics: After years of the above activities and loss of considerable bone, *surprise*: BMU creations, bone turnover, and net bone losses, all reduce toward or even below normal, and then tend to stay or plateau there. Resorption and formation in completed BMUs also tend to equalize. In cybernetic terms, the initial dynamics would represent some of this system's transients. The final dynamics would represent a steady-state adaptation to chronic disuse.[1,53]

Gradual-onset disuse: Gradual-onset disuse would still cause the above changes, but so slowly that present methods might not detect them. After years or decades, their effects on bone mass, architecture, and strength eventually become clear. This little-discussed but common situation should happen in most aging humans and mammals, and in people developing debilitating conditions like those discussed in Section II.

F. The Mechanically Adapted State

Accumulated evidence suggests that everywhere in a normal bone, except the cranial vault, ethmoids, turbinates, and surfaces covered by cartilage,[2,6] strains should range between the boundaries defined by the MESr and MESm, or between ≈50 and 1000 microstrain. So, normally, and where μE means microstrain and the adapted state defines a "comfort zone" where bone fits its mechanical usage well enough not to need major changes in architecture, strength or mass:

$$\begin{array}{llllll} |\, MESr \ldots < \ldots MESm \,| & << & MESp & <<<< & \text{Fracture strain} \\ |\approx 50\,\mu E \ldots \approx 1000\,\mu E\,| & & \approx 3000\,\mu E & & \approx 25{,}000\,\mu E \\ |\, \text{“adapted state”} \,| & & & & \end{array}$$

These strain values apply only to longitudinal tension and compression. Shear and strain gradients may help to control a bone's architectural adaptations too, but how is unknown. Until we know, the longitudinal values can provide useful indices. These biologic reactions to mechanical challenges reveal some behavioral features of the mechanostat discussed later in this chapter. Increased remodeling usually increases bone loss next to marrow, and the remodeling space too. The former can only happen when BMU creations increase. Decreased remodeling conserves bone and reduces the remodeling space and bone turnover.

At this point some readers may wonder how the foregoing material applies to this chapter's subject. The explanation follows.

VI. RELEVANCE TO OSTEOPENIAS AND TRUE OSTEOPOROSES

While osteopenias and true osteoporoses are in the process of developing in children and adults, the accompanying anatomical bone loss and bone-tissue dynamic patterns strongly copy the above two-stage mechanical disuse pattern.[2,54-56] That suggests bone's adaptive mechanisms function normally in physiologic osteopenias, since their usual physical activities would cause no bone problems. It also suggests the adaptive mechanisms malfunction in true osteoporoses, since normal physical activities do cause bone problems in these patients. This means that increasing the bone bank and strength in those two conditions, and preventing the conditions too, might require different treatments.

That would also mean the nonmechanical causes of true osteoporoses should impair modeling and remodeling responses to mechanical usage. That message seems clear in the accumulated evidence.[47,56-58] Still, some who view nonmechanical agents (hormones, vitamins, minerals, drugs, cytokines, etc.) as dominating the control of bone mass and strength might wish to contest the message. As is their right of course. Stay tuned...

The above material suggests that physiologic osteopenias are not true diseases, since people so affected have no bone problems until a fall or other injury happens. This should apply to most postmenopausal women. Injuries can cause fractures in anybody at any age. Would one cite all such fractures as proof of a bone disease? If not, what natural instead of arbitrary criteria would distinguish healthy from diseased people in this regard? Is this not another continuum problem instead of one involving two unrelated states?

Estimates that 30% or so of people over 55 years of age have "osteoporosis" depended on different definitions than those given above.[43,59-61] In my experience, physiologic osteopenias considerably outnumbered true osteoporoses in people of any age. Could most of that 30% have a physiologic osteopenia instead of a true osteoporosis? While many studies claimed to deal only with patients with a "spontaneous crush fracture syndrome" or something similar, in 50 years I have seen so few "pure," true osteoporoses that such claims seem suspect. If people with physiologic osteopenias outnumbered those with true osteoporoses in many past studies, could that explain the failure to find, in the means of group data, potentially causal abnormalities in the fewer true osteoporotics? Does a tendency exist to dismiss some data from the latter as "outliers"? If a continuum of syndromes bridges the two end states described earlier, how reliably could past studies distinguish one end state from the other in seeking their respective features and causes?

VII. THERAPEUTIC OBJECTIVES, TARGETS, PROBLEMS

To summarize: 1) Modeling can add bone, and remodeling can conserve or remove it. Equally, modeling can strengthen bones, and remodeling can conserve their strength or weaken them. 2) Modeling and remodeling cannot provide each other's effects. They are different and independent. 3) An osteopenia makes bones weaker than before, and so does microdamage. Their effects can combine and probably usually do in true osteoporoses. 4) Too little bone for someone's mechanical usage raises its strains toward the microdamage threshold, which increases microdamage, which increases bone fragility, which facilitates spontaneous fractures, fractures from low-energy injuries, and a bone pain syndrome. 5) Normally, increased microdamage always increases the remodeling that repairs it. This summary suggests the following targets for agents intended to prevent or cure osteopenias and osteoporoses, and some problems to avoid or resolve in doing so.

A. General Objectives

There are three general objectives: to prevent increased bone fragility during growth, aging, and chronic debilitating disease; to correct increased fragility after it develops; and to minimize the falls that cause the morbidity, expense, and mortality associated with extremity bone fractures in osteopenias and osteoporoses.[43,57] In principle, formation drifts, or rho made positive, or new-woven bone, could each increase bone mass and strength, but so far no known agent makes rho go positive.

B. The Ultimate Control of Bone Losses and Conservation of Bone Strength in Adults

This depends on controlling BMU creations and rho, and *not*, repeat not, on controlling the vigor of existing osteoblasts or osteoclasts.[2,5,17,48] In more detail, that control lies in controlling the mechanisms that create new BMUs with their capillaries, precursor and supporting cells, wandering cells, and osteoblasts and osteoclasts, and that apportion their numbers and activities. The controlling mechanisms also determine if, when, and where those BMUs and cells are needed, how many, and for how long. Once created, those cells do their thing, mostly under the control of the BMU they belong to.

The same ideas would apply to modeling drifts and their ability to increase bone mass and strength. While noted long ago[17,62] and repeatedly afterward, mainstream skeletal thought still seems to misunderstand those facts.[3-5,63,64]

C. To Prevent Increased Fragility

To prevent increased fragility in children, add more bone, especially to epiphyseal and metaphyseal cortices. To do that, therapeutic agents should increase or duplicate the child's normal bone responses to hypervigorous mechanical usage. That means increasing global bone modeling, depressing global BMU creations, and making rho tend toward zero.[2]

In adults who had a normal bone bank at skeletal maturity, keep bone by potentiating or duplicating the remodeling responses to chronic hypervigorous mechanical usage. That means depressing BMU creations, and making rho tend toward zero, especially in epiphyseal and metaphyseal cortices, and in vertebrae too to prevent true osteoporoses.

This should also require improving microdamage detection and repair, particularly in the spine.

D. To Correct Already Increased Fragility

To correct fragility in children and adults, add bone by increasing global bone modeling, while depressing BMU creations and making rho tend toward zero to keep the extra bone.[65-68] Some agents might add bone by creating formation modeling drifts, as intermittent injections of parathyroid hormone can do, or by creating new woven bone, as some prostaglandins can do (see Section VII.G).[49] Again, the new bone should especially thicken and strengthen epiphyseal and metaphyseal cortices, as well as vertebral bone in true osteoporoses.

In true osteoporoses this should also require improving microdamage detection and repair, particularly in the spine. Although suggested long ago,[19] the field only recently accepted improving microdamage repair as a possible way to reduce bone fragility in true osteoporoses.[32-40] Could calcitonin have such effects? Varied publications do report improved symptoms in calcitonin-treated osteoporosis patients, but without correspondingly improved bone banks.[66-71]

E. On Independent Pharmacologic Control of Osteoclastic or Osteoblastic Activity, "Antiresorption Drugs," and the "Either-Or" Idea

Many still think agents that either depress existing osteoclasts or invigorate existing osteoblasts would normalize osteopenic bone mass and strength. Yet, on the evidence, that persistent idea is no longer tenable.[1,3,5,48] The "either-or" idea ignores bone-biologic realities described long ago,[1,17] verified since,[5,16,66-89] and reviewed above (see also Section VIII).

Often cited as "antiresorption" agents, bisphosphonates primarily decrease BMU creations.[1,90] Due to the months-long A→R→F sequence in BMUs that reduces bone resorption first, and then formation, and about equally *and always*, at least so far.[1,2,4,17,90] In adults a small 3 to 9% gain in bone ensues that plateaus and does not increase further, no matter how long the treatment or how large the dose of drug. So far all so-called antiresorption agents have caused that plateau. It must reflect, at least partly, a reduced remodeling space due to decreased BMU creations and improved mineralization of bone due to decreased turnover.[1] It also demonstrates the "bone conserving" effect of reduced BMU creations and bone turnover.

These agents are really antiactivation or antiremodeling agents, not true antiresorption agents. (Histomorphometrists call BMU creations "activation"; see also Appendix 5.1 in Reference 2.) Their antiremodeling effects tend to minimize bone loss and therefore can help to retain bone added by bone-anabolic agents such as those discussed below.

Superb animal experiments support the above statements. In them, osteoblast and osteoclast activities increased in one part of a bone and decreased in another part of the same bone at the same time, nourished by the same blood carrying the same nonmechanical "messengers" including hormones to all cells.[48,83-99] Control by blood-borne hormones or other agents of existing osteoblasts and/or osteoclasts simply cannot explain such spatially and simultaneously different responses.[1] The paradigm can. It even predicts them.[2]

One should probably make sure that new antiremodeling agents do not also impair microdamage repair, fracture healing, and/or global modeling. Some older agents could cause each impairment.[90,100]

F. On Photon Absorptiometry

Osteoporosis-oriented absorptiometry should evaluate the bone features most likely to let wrists or hips fracture from falls. This means the cross-section shape and size, and cortical thickness of the epiphyseal–metaphyseal regions of the wrist and hip, plus some function of their rectangular or polar moments of inertia.[24,25] As engineering figures of merit, those moments of inertia describe how cross-sectional architecture can affect a bone's strength in bending and torque, respectively.

Single- and dual-beam absorptiometry, including DEXA (dual-energy X-ray absorptiometry), and quantitative computed tomography (QCT), can evaluate those features. With suitable software, QCT can measure and calculate the bone features that most affect the susceptibility to extremity bone fractures from falls.[42,101-103] Current DEXA software does not do that very well. To show the need for it, keep the cross-sectional amount of bone the same while doubling a bone's diameter, and thus thinning its cortex. That would increase its bending strength eight times.[22-25] QCT would detect that and provide a correspondingly larger BSI (bone strength index),[101-103] but DEXA would find decreased bone "density," suggesting the larger bone was weaker, not stronger.[25,43]

Still, any noninvasive method that accounted for both bone mass and the above architectural features should provide reliable BSIs. Magnetic resonance imaging, ultrasound,[104] and better DEXA software[105] might each be adapted to this purpose.

G. The Promising "Bone-Anabolic" Effects of Parathyroid Hormone and Prostaglandins

Intermittent administration of parathyroid hormone can increase bone mass well over 30%, mostly by creating new formation drifts of lamellar bone instead of by making rho go positive in BMUs.[63,72-80] This thickens and strengthens cortices and existing trabeculae without increasing the number of trabeculae.

Some prostaglandins can also add large amounts of new woven bone on cortices and trabeculae.[81-96] These agents make bone's "backup mechanisms" and cells create new formation drifts with their capillaries, supporting and precursor cells, and osteoblasts. They do not act merely by stimulating existing osteoblasts. (Recall the "ultimate control" discussed in Section VII.B.) The cell and molecular biology upon which those effects depend deserves intense research and seems to offer the promise of extremely useful drugs. In seeking them, cell- and molecular-biologic research should find the cells that first respond to the hormone or prostaglandin "message," and then trace the intracellular and cellular-event sequences that eventually produce histologically visible new bone formation. At varied places along those sequences, there should be opportunities for "designer" drugs to duplicate the final bone anabolic effects. This would seem to be an important project for future cell- and molecular-biologic research to study.

Other things being equal, the above anabolic effects would prevent and cure osteopenias and solve the problem. But, other things are not equal in this complex, sophisticated system. As the mechanostat idea predicted,[85] when those treatments stop, remodeling begins to remove the extra bone by increasing BMU creations and making rho more negative. This is one of the mechanostat's ways of removing unneeded bone. Investigators now seek ways to retain the extra bone by using antiremodeling agents such as those mentioned above to depress the BMU creations that help to remove it.[65,66,77-80,86,87] To repeat, future research should especially study how such treatments affect the strength of epiphyseal and metaphyseal cortices, and vertebral spongiosa.

The paradigm suggests three general ways in which agents might cause the bone-anabolic effects.

1. The agents might lower the strain ranges that normally make the mechanostat switch new bone formation ON. Or, where mechanical usage means the loads applied to bone, and the resulting signals passed on by bone to the biologic mechanisms and "formation drifts" mean new lamellar or woven-bone formation drifts:

$$\begin{array}{c}\textit{Mechanical usage} \rightarrow \textit{mechanostat} \rightarrow \textit{precursor cells} \rightarrow \textit{formation drifts}\\ \uparrow \\ \textit{agent}\end{array}$$

2. Or, the agents might bypass the mechanostat and directly switch ON the precursor cell mechanisms that normally create new lamellar or woven bone formation drifts, somewhat like this:

$$\begin{array}{c}\textit{Mechanical usage} \rightarrow \textit{mechanostat} \rightarrow \textit{precursor cells} \rightarrow \textit{formation drifts}\\ \uparrow \\ \textit{agent}\end{array}$$

3. Or a combination of both might explain the effect, like this:

$$\begin{array}{c}\textit{Mechanical usage} \rightarrow \textit{mechanostat} \rightarrow \textit{precursor cells} \rightarrow \textit{formation drifts}\\ \uparrow \qquad\qquad \uparrow \\ \ldots\textit{agent}\ldots\end{array}$$

While available evidence hints that explanation number 2 may explain the above bone anabolic effects, the "mechanostat" and "precursor cell" functions each probably depend on an internal series of cellular, biochemical, gene activation, and other events. While that could make it hard to understand each function, it also means some "designer" drug acting on one or more of the many steps in that "message traffic" might control the whole function for medical purposes. The matter remains open, and is perhaps something to elaborate on at another time.

H. The Mechanostat: The Main Pharmacologic Target?

It becomes clear that lasting and safe preventions and cures for osteopenias and osteoporoses should make a patient's mechanostat "sense" a need for more bone.[2,10,85] Indeed, may I suggest that learning how to control the mechanostat may provide the most important single target facing today's osteoporosis research? Consider these points.

1. The mechanism seems to fit bone mass, architecture, and strength to its own "natural" criteria of what serves mechanical needs adequately and what does not.

2. The threshold strain values cited earlier would correspond to those criteria.
3. The mechanism would control the vital biomechanics already described.
4. By the earlier definitions, it would function normally in "pure" physiologic osteopenias in response to partial disuse.
5. It would function abnormally in "pure" true osteoporoses, regardless of the patient's mechanical usage. In a real sense, a mechanostat disease should cause true osteoporoses.
6. The mechanostat probably explains the failure so far of all efforts to normalize bone mass and strength with agents supposed to affect only osteoblasts or only osteoclasts.
7. Exactly its hypervigorous mechanical usage effects on bone mass and strength would prevent and cure osteopenias.
8. Exactly its disuse effects cause the medically important osteopenias and, in part, osteoporoses too.
9. Exactly its disuse effects remove the bone added by the bone-anabolic agents described above.

One possible way to control the mechanostat with drugs would be to change the MESm and MESr strain ranges that control its effects on modeling drifts and remodeling BMUs, respectively. The strain values in the Glossary at the end of this chapter suggest the centers of those ranges, their "set points."[2,6,10,85] Another way to control the mechanostat would lie in retarding the rate at which it could decrease bone mass and strength.[2,6] The bisphosphonate effects on remodeling described above might act in such ways. Set point changes would have easily predicted effects on bone mass, strength, and architecture.[2,6]

VIII. GENERAL COMMENTS

A. On the Role of Muscle Strength in Bone Architecture and Strength

The largest mechanical loads on bone come from muscle forces.[22,106] In the paradigm's view, bone mass, architecture, strength, and turnover adapt more to those forces than to most nonmechanical influences.[2,15,18] Elegant tests of that old idea[107] in humans and laboratory animals strongly support it. The tests used QCT-derived BSIs (bone strength indices) that account for the effect of bone architecture on bending strength, plus bone content. When compared to measured breaking strengths of bones in animals and to measured muscle strengths in humans, these BSIs predicted bone and muscle strength much more reliably than DEXA data.[27,42,101-103] Duplications of those studies by others continue to support the paradigm. Such BSIs might supplant other noninvasive indices for evaluating and following patients, and in live-animal research.

While this emphasizes the known importance of vigorous physical activity in promoting bone accumulation during growth and in keeping bone in adult life,[43,47] some misunderstanding about the meaning of "vigorous" persists in mainstream skeletal thought. As noted originally, the modeling activity that can strengthen bones and increase bone mass responds to the typical *largest* loads on bone and to the typical *largest* bone strains, and it seems little affected by smaller loads and strains no matter how frequent.[14,62] That idea now has strong experimental support.[23,47,58,108-120] It explains why activities like walking, swimming, jogging, and sit-ups, even when done to exhaustion, prove far less effective at adding bone than weight lifting, even though they do help to keep existing bone.

B. Bone-Strength-Index (BSI) Standards, Mechanical Usage, Muscle Strength

Clearly, future norms for noninvasive BSIs should account for a subject's past and present mechanical usage and muscle strength, besides features accounted for in the past. Past features include, in part, age, sex, menopausal status in women, diet, height, body weight, calcium and vitamin D intake, and race.[56] Absorptiometrists are beginning to accept this need.

C. On Treatment Modes

The idea that one should take medications continuously goes back over 2000 years, and in treating many diseases it is exactly right. Still, features of bone drifts and BMUs suggested other ways to give drugs might have useful effects[121] that began to show up afterward.

Some of these ways involve giving drugs for brief times repeated at intervals of days to weeks (*intermittent treatment*);[73,121] or giving two or more drugs in special sequences (*sequential treatment*);[49,66] or combining these two (*intermittent-sequential treatment*);[86,87,121-124] or combining one of those methods with smaller drug doses than customary;[76] or giving an agent at a special time during the activity of a biologic mechanism, such as a BMU or fracture healing (*staged treatment*);[119,121-125] or *cotreatment*.[78] Future osteoporosis treatments may well depend on such modes. The anabolic effects of parathyroid hormone and prostaglandins, combined with the bone-conserving effects of antiremodeling agents, are examples.[49,80-82]

A caveat: In seeking therapeutic agents for this system, and when interpreting their effects, one might keep in mind that an agent that depresses bone remodeling need not depress modeling too, or affect it at all, and conversely.[55,77] Some agent might even increase one activity and decrease the other.

D. On Differences in Vertebral Body and Long-Bone Metaphyseal Spongiosas

Many authors note apparent differences in responsiveness, architecture, and turnover in vertebral body and long-bone metaphyseal spongiosas.[55,56] Furthermore, vertebral spongiosa in true osteoporoses is clearly more fragile than in physiologic osteopenias, and than extremity-bone metaphyseal spongiosa where spontaneous and traumatic fractures rarely if ever begin.

While some have postulated genetic, hormonal, and local influences as causes of those differences, recently understood vital-biomechanical considerations plausibly explain at least most of them.[6,126]

E. On the Cell- and Molecular-Biologic "Faces" of Osteoporoses

Current texts and reviews provide much information about the cell- and molecular-biologic features and roots of osteoporoses.[5,47,56,121,124,125,127-129] That kind of knowledge grew explosively, it should continue, it is relevant, and yet this chapter virtually ignores it. Why?

Currently the bone roles of those things in people and other intact subjects present more enigmas than understanding. While cell- and molecular-biologic things do help the tissue-level mechanisms described above to function properly, they cannot duplicate or replace those functions. Otherwise they could make bones that are growing in paralyzed limbs, muscular dystrophy patients, or in patients with juvenile rheumatoid arthritis, develop normal architecture, strength, and mass. Since scientists and clinicians still have not studied how cell and molecular biology enable these tissue-level mechanisms or affect their responses to mechanical challenges, this chapter could not discuss them. Like its sources,[2,6-10] it reviews tissue-level functions and responses to mechanical influences that help to cause osteopenias and osteoporoses, but that need the cell- and molecular-level understanding that only further basic research can provide.

For readers who believe they do understand the cell and molecular biology beneath those tissue-level functions, why not test the belief?

F. A Self-Test

Many osteoporosis authorities assured me they account properly for bone's tissue-level functions in their work, but most of them have erred. Merely saying so would not prove it (it's one way to make "unfriends" too), so Table 1.1 offers a test of the belief. To take the test, try to answer three questions about each entry in the table.

1. What cell- and molecular-biologic features make this tissue-level function work?

2. How do those features affect this function's responses to mechanical usage challenges in intact subjects?
3. In intact subjects how do systemic agents affect those mechanical usage responses?

Systemic agents belong in category number 3 in this chapter's first paragraph. You need not reveal your test results, but if you do as miserably as I did, you now know some things future osteoporosis research *must* try to understand. Also you need not feel bad if you did poorly. Research has not found the answers yet. This test only tries to make that point without making "unfriends."

IX. CONCLUSION

Should we discourage or fear controversy? Resolving controversies has always improved knowledge and understanding in science and medicine. Most good ideas began as controversial ones, and a field without controversies usually makes little fundamental progress. Ergo, the new paradigm's advocates welcome any debate it may incite. It will survive if it is as valid as the evidence suggests — we believe it now amounts to proof[130] — and as Copernicus' solar system ideas did (*after* he died of course).

These things deserve emphasis: Other views of the above matters do not harm skeletal science in any way, or reflect adversely on people who favored and favor them. As tides arise in the affairs of men, they arise in the evolution of thought in a science too. All past and present views, those above included, are more tides that rise and pass as this science seeks and finds better understanding. The paradigm merely adds to its predecessors belatedly perceived but essential tissue-level roles in skeletal physiology and disease. Its season has begun, but another will follow.

Until then, this chapter sketches some of the ground on which future and better understanding of osteopenias and osteoporoses, their treatment with bone-anabolic and other agents, the criteria used to define them, how we monitor and diagnose them, and research on those things, should play and stand.

ACKNOWLEDGMENTS

I want to thank the staffs of the Southern Colorado Clinic, Parkview Episcopal Hospital, and St. Mary Corwin Hospital for the time to produce this and related articles and texts, and David Gavin for the drawings. I also thank the outstanding orthopedic surgeons trained at Henry Ford Hospital, Detroit, Michigan, between 1957 and 1973. Their spontaneous aid in a time of troubles made this work one of their contributions to orthopedic surgery. Some colleagues were asked to review preliminary drafts of this article, and their time and effort are greatly appreciated (Profs. L. V. Avioli, D. B. Burr, J. L. Ferretti, H. Fleisch, W. B. High, T. J. Gasser, W. S. S. Jee, L. Mosekilde, A. M. Parfitt, R. R. Recker, M. B. Schaffler, L. Sokoloff, H. E. Takahashi, and T. J. Wronski).

REFERENCES

1. Frost, H. M., *Intermediary Organization of the Skeleton*, Vols. I, II, CRC Press, Boca Raton, 1986.
2. Frost, H. M., *Introduction to a New Skeletal Physiology. I: Bone and Bones*, The Pajaro Group, Inc., Pueblo, Colorado, 1995.
3. Brown, W. and Haglund, K., Landmarks, *J. NIH Res.*, 7, 54, 1995.
4. Heaney, R. P., The bone-remodeling transient: implications for the interpretation of clinical studies of bone mass change, *J. Bone Min. Res.*, 9, 1515, 1994.
5. Parfitt, A. M., Mundy, G. R., Roodman, G. D., Hughes, D. E., and Boyce, B., A new model for the regulation of bone resorption, with particular reference to the effects of bisphosphonates, *J. Bone Min. Res.*, 11, 150, 1996.
6. Frost, H. M., *Introduction to a New Skeletal Physiology. II: Fibrous Tissue, Cartilage And Synovial Joints*, The Pajaro Group, Inc., Pueblo, Colorado, 1995.
7. Frost, H. M., *Osteoporoses: An Owner's Manual*, The Pajaro Group, Inc., Pueblo, Colorado, 1995.
8. Frost, H. M., Perspectives: on a "paradigm shift" developing in skeletal science, *Calcif. Tissue Int.*, 56, 1, 1995.
9. Frost, H. M., Spinal tissue vital biomechanics for clinicians, in *Spinal Disorders in Growth and Aging*, Takahashi, H. E., Ed., Springer-Verlag, Tokyo, 1995, 95.
10. Frost, H. M., Perspectives: A proposed general model of the mechanostat (suggestions from a new paradigm), *Anat. Rec.*, 244, 139, 1996.
11. Frost, H. M., Bone development during childhood: insights from a new paradigm, in *Paediatric Osteology*, Schönau, E., Ed., Elsevier Science Publishers, Amsterdam, 1996, 3.
12. Jee, W. S. S., The skeletal tissues, in *Cell and Tissue Biology. A Textbook of Histology*, Weiss, L., Ed., Urban and Schwartzenberg, Baltimore, 1989, 211.
13. Enlow, D. H., *Principles of Bone Remodeling*. Charles C. Thomas, Springfield, 1963.
14. Frost, H. M., *Bone Modeling and Skeletal Modeling Errors*, Charles C. Thomas, Springfield, 1973.
15. Frost, H. M., Structural adaptations to mechanical usage (SATMU):1. Redefining Wolff's Law: The bone modeling problem, *Anat. Rec.*, 226, 403, 1990.
16. Eriksen, E. F., Steiniche, T., Mosekilde, L., and Melsen, F., Histomorphometric analysis of bone in metabolic bone disease, *Endocrinol. Metab. Clin. N. Am.*, 18, 919, 1989.
17. Frost, H. M., *Mathematical Elements of Lamellar Bone Remodelling*, Charles C. Thomas, Springfield, 1964.
18. Frost, H. M., Structural adaptations to mechanical usage (SATMU):2. Redefining Wolff's Law: The bone remodeling problem, *Anat. Rec.*, 226, 414, 1990.
19. Frost, H. M., *Bone Dynamics in Osteoporosis and Osteomalacia*, Charles C. Thomas, Springfield, 1966.
20. Jaworski, Z. F. G., Lamellar bone turnover system and its effector organ. *Calcif. Tissue Int.* (Suppl) 36, 46, 1984.

21. Wronski, T.J., Walsh, C.C., and Iganaszewski, L.A., Histologic evidence for osteopenia and increased bone turnover in ovariectomized rats, *Bone*, 7, 119, 1986.
22. Currey, J. D., *The Mechanical Adaptations of Bones*, Princeton University Press, Princeton, 1984.
23. Martin, R. B. and Burr, D. B., *Structure, Function and Adaptation of Compact Bone*, Raven Press, New York, 1989.
24. Nordin, M. and Frankel, V. H., *Basic Biomechanics of the Musculoskeletal System*, 2nd. ed., Lea and Febiger, Philadelphia, 1989.
25. Cochran, G. van B., *A Primer of Orthopaedic Biomechanics*, Churchill-Livingstone, Edinburgh, 1982.
26. Compston, J. E., Bone density: BMC, BMD, or corrected BMD? *Bone*, 16, 5, 1995.
27. Ferretti, J. L., Perspectives of pQCT technology associated to biomechanical studies in skeletal research employing rat models, *Bone*, 17 (Suppl 1), 353, 1995.
28. Burr, D. B., Martin R. B., and Radin E. L., Threshold values for the production of fatigue microdamage in bone in vivo, *ORS Abs*, 69, 1983.
29. Frost, H. M., Presence of microscopic cracks in vivo in bone, *Henry Ford Hosp. Med. Bull.*, 8, 27, 1960.
30. Pattin, C. A. and Carter, D. R., Bone mechanical energy dissipation during cyclic loading, *Trans. Orthop. Res. Soc.*, 16, 129, 1991.
31. Pattin, C. A., Caler, W. E., and Carter, D. R., Cyclic mechanical property degradation during fatigue loading of cortical bone, *J. Biomech.*, 29, 69, 1996.
32. Schaffler, M. B., Choi, K., and Milgrom, C., Microcracks and aging in human femoral compact bone, *Trans. Orthop. Res. Soc.*, 19, 190, 1994.
33. Arnold, J. S., Bartley, M. H., and Tont, S. A., Jenkins, D. P., Skeletal changes in aging and disease, *Clin. Orthop.*, 49, 7, 1966.
34. Biewener, A. A., Safety factors in bone strength, *Calcif. Tissue Int.*, 53 (Suppl 1), 68, 1993.
35. Burr, D. B., Remodeling and the repair of fatigue damage, *Calcif. Tissue Int.*, 53 (Suppl 1), 75, 1993.
36. Cooper, C., The epidemiology of fragility fractures: is there a role for bone quality? *Calcif. Tissue Int.*, 53 (Suppl 1), 23, 1993.
37. Heaney, R. P., Is there a role for bone quality in fragility fractures? *Calcif. Tissue Int.*, 53 (Suppl 1), 3, 1993.
38. Parfitt, A. M., Bone age, mineral density, and fatigue damage, *Calcif. Tissue Int.*, 53 (Suppl 1), 82, 1993.
39. Schnitzler, C. M., Bone quality: a determinant for certain risk factors for bone fragility, *Calcif. Tissue Int.*, 53 (Suppl), 27, 1993.
40. Wenzel, T. E., Schaffler, M. B., and Fyrhie, D. P., In vivo trabecular microcracks in human vertebral bone, *Trans. Orthop. Res. Soc.*, 19, 57, 1994.
41. Frost, H. M., Perspectives: Applications of a biomechanical model of the endochondral ossification mechanism, *Anat. Rec.*, 240, 447, 1994.
42. Ferretti, J. L., Frost, H. M., Gasser, J. A., High, W. B., Jee, W. S. S., Jerome, C., Mosekilde, L., and Thompson, D. D., Perspectives: On osteoporosis research: Its focus and some insights of a new paradigm, *Calcif. Tissue Int.*, 57, 399. 1995.
43. Riggs, B. L. and Melton, L. J., Eds., *Osteoporosis. Etiology, Diagnosis and Treatment*, 2nd Ed., Lippincott-Raven Publishers, Hagerstown, MD, 1995.
44. Søgaard, C. H., Danielson, C. C., Thorling, E. B., and Mosekilde, L., Long term exercise of young and adult female rats: Effect on femoral neck biomechanical competence, *J. Bone Min. Res.*, 9, 409, 1994.
45. Søgaard, C. H., Wronski, T. J., McOsker, J. E., and Mosekilde, L., The positive effect of parathyroid hormone on femoral neck strength in ovariectomized rats is more pronounced than that of estrogen and bisphosphonates, *Endocrinology*, 134, 650, 1994.
46. Li, M. and Wronski T.J., Response of femoral neck to estrogen depletion and parathyroid hormone in aged rats, *Bone*, 16, 551, 1995.

47. Smith, E. L. and Gilligan, C., Mechanical forces and bone. *J. Bone Min. Res.*, 6, 139, 1989.
48. Frost, H. M., Wolff's Law and bone's structural adaptations to mechanical usage: an overview for clinicians, *Angle Orthodont.*, 64, 187, 1994.
49. Jee, W. S. S., Ed., Proceedings of the International Conference on Animal Models in the Prevention and Treatment of Osteopenia, *Bone*, Suppl., 1995.
50. Schönau, E., Ed., *Paediatric Osteology. New Trends and Diagnostic Possibilities*, Elsevier Science, Amsterdam, 1996.
51. Takahashi, H. E., Ed., *Spinal Disorders and Growth and Aging*, Springer-Verlag, Tokyo, 1995.
52. Raab-Cullen, D. M., Kimmel, D. B., Akhter, M. P., and Recker, R. R., Transient increase in bone formation after external mechanical loading, *Trans. Orthop. Res. Soc.*, 19, 276, 1994.
53. Wiener, N., *Cybernetics*, MIT Press, Cambridge, 1964.
54. Frost, H. M., Perspectives: The role of changes in mechanical usage setpoints in the pathogenesis of osteoporosis, *J. Bone Min. Res.*, 7, 253, 1992.
55. Qi, H., Li, M., and Wronski, T.J., A comparison of the anabolic effects of parathyroid hormone at skeletal sites with moderate and severe osteopenia in aged ovariectomized rats, *J. Bone Min. Res.*, 10, 948, 1995.
56. Avioli, L. V., Ed., *The Osteoporotic Syndrome*, 3rd Ed., Wiley-Liss, New York, 1993.
57. Greenspan, S. L., Myers, E. R., Maitland, L. A., Resnick, N. M., and Hayes, W. C., Fall severity and bone mineral density as risk factors for hip fracture in ambulatory elderly, *J. Am. Med. Assn.*, 271, 128, 1994.
58. Kannus, P., Sievanen, H., and Vuori, L., Physical loading, exercise and bone, *Bone*, 18 (Suppl 1), 1, 1996.
59. Babbitt, A. M., Osteoporosis, *Orthopedics*, 17, 935, 1994.
60. Bronner, F., Calcium and osteoporosis, *Am. J. Clin. Nutr.*, 60, 831, 1994.
61. Gallagher, J. C., The pathogenesis of osteoporosis, *Bone Min.*, 9, 215, 1990.
62. Frost, H. M., *Laws of Bone Structure*, Charles C. Thomas, Springfield, 1964.
63. Favus, M. J., Ed., *Primer on the Metabolic Bone Diseases and Disorders of Mineral Metabolism*, Raven Press, New York, 1993.
64. O. R. S. Abstracts, Orthopaedic Research Society, American Academy of Orthopaedic Surgeons, Chicago, 1976–1996.
65. Wronski, T. J., Dann, L. M., Qi, H., and Yen, C.-F., Skeletal effects of withdrawal of estrogen and diphosphonate treatment in ovariectomized rats, *Calcif. Tissue Int.*, 53, 210, 1993.
66. Ma, Y. F., Ferretti, J. L., Capozza, R. F., Cointry, G., Alippi, R., Zanchetta, J., and Jee, W. S. S., Effects of ON/OFF anabolic hPTH and remodeling inhibitors on metaphyseal bone of immobilized rat femurs. Tomographical (pQCT) description and correlation with histomorphometric changes in tibial cancellous bone, *Bone*, 17 (Suppl), 321, 1995.
67. Civitelli, R., Gonnelli, S., Zacchei, F., Bigazzi, S., Vattimo, A., Avioli, L. V., and Gennari, C., Bone turnover in postmenopausal osteoporosis. Effect of calcitonin treatment, *J. Clin. Invest.*, 82, 1268, 1988.
68. Eriksen, E. F., Axelrod, D. W., and Melsen, F., *Bone Histomorphometry*, Raven Press, New York, 1994.
69. Hodsman, A. B. and Fraher, L. J., Biochemical responses to sequential parathyroid hormone (1-38) and calcitonin in osteoporotic patients, *Bone Miner.*, 9, 137, 1990.
70. Mosekilde, L., Danielson, C. C., and Gasser, J. A., The effect on vertebral bone mass and strength of long term treatment with antiresorptive agents (estrogen and calcitonin), human parathyroid hormone-(1-38) and combination therapy, assessed in ovariectomized rats, *Endocrinology*, 135, 2126, 1994.
71. Tanizawa, T., Nishida, S., Yamamoto, T., Asai, S., and Takahashi, H. E., Changes of bone mineral content of lumbar spine in osteoporosis patients treated with vitamin D and calcitonin, in *Spinal Disorders in Growth and Aging*, Takahashi, H. E., Ed., Springer-Verlag, Tokyo, 1995, 215.

72. Jerome, C. P., Johnson, C. S., and Lees, C. J., Effect of treatment for 3 months with human parathyroid hormone 1-34 peptide in ovariectomized cynomolgus monkeys (Macaca fascicularis). *Bone*, 17 (Suppl), 415, 1995.
73. Hori, M., Uzawa, T., Morita, L., Noda, T., Takahashi, H., and Inoue, J., Effect of human parathyroid hormone (PTH(1-34)) on experimental osteopenia of rats induced by ovariectomy, *Bone Miner.*, 3, 193, 1988.
74. Mosekilde, L., Søgaard, C. H., Danielson, C. C., Torring, O., and Nilsson, M.H. L., The anabolic effects of PTH on rat vertebral body mass are also reflected in the quality of bone, assessed by biomechanical testing: A comparison study between hPTH(1-34) and hPTH(1-84), *Endocrinology*, 129, 421, 1991.
75. Slovic, D. M., Rosenthal, D. I., Doppelt, D. H., Potts, J. T. Jr., Daly, M. A., Campbell, J. A., and Neer, R. M., Restoration of spinal bone in osteoporotic men by treatment with human parathyroid hormone (1-34) and 1,25-dihydroxyvitamin D, *J. Bone Min. Res.*, 1, 377, 1986.
76. Takahashi, H., Ed., *Bone Morphometry*, Nishimura Ltd., Niigata, Japan, 1990.
77. Baumann, B. D. and Wronski, T. J., Response of cortical bone to antiresorptive agents and parathyroid hormone in aged ovariectomized rats, *Bone*, 16, 247, 1995.
78. Li, M., Mosekilde, L., Søgaard, C. H., Thomsen, J. S., and Wronski, T. J., Parathyroid hormone monotherapy and cotherapy with antiresorptive agents restore vertebral bone mass and strength in aged ovariectomized rats, *Bone*, 16, 629, 1995.
79. Wronski, T. J., Yen, C.-F., Qi, H., and Dann, L. M., Parathyroid hormone is more effective than estrogen or bisphosphonates for restoration of lost bone mass in ovariectomized rats, *Endocrinology*, 132, 823, 1993.
80. Wronski, T. J. and Yen, C. F., Anabolic effects of parathyroid hormone on cortical bone in ovariectomized rats, *Bone*, 15, 51, 1994.
81. High, W. B., Effects of orally administered prostaglandin on cortical bone turnover in dogs: A histomorphometric study, *Bone*, 8, 363, 1988.
82. Jee, W. S. S., Mori, X., Li, X., and Chan, S., Prostaglandin E2 enhances cortical bone mass and activates intracortical bone remodeling in intact and ovariectomized female rats, *Bone*, 11, 253, 1990.
83. Ma, Y. F., Ke, H. Z., and Jee, W. S. S., Prostaglandin E_2 adds bone to a cancellous bone site with a closed growth plate and low bone turnover in ovariectomized rats, *Bone*, 15, 137, 1994.
84. Norrdin, R. W., Jee, W. S. S., and High, W. B., The role of prostaglandins in bone *in vivo*, *Prostaglandins, Leukotrienes and Essential Fatty Acids*, 41, 139, 1990.
85. Frost, H. M., The mechanostat: A proposed pathogenetic mechanism of osteoporoses and the bone mass effects of mechanical and nonmechanical agents, *Bone Miner.*, 2, 73, 1987.
86. Jee, W. S. S., Tang, L., Ke, H. Z., Setterberg, R. B., and Kimmel, D. B., Maintaining restored bone with bisphosphonate in the ovariectomized rat skeleton: Dynamic histomorphometry of changes in bone mass, *Bone*, 14, 493, 1993.
87. Li, Q. N., Jee, W. S. S., Ma, Y. F., Ke, H. Z., Xie, H., Huang, L. F., and Liang, N. C., Risedronate pretreatment does not hamper the anabolic effects of prostaglandin E-2 in OVX rats, in *Proceedings of the International Conference on Animal Models in the Prevention and Treatment of Osteopenia*, Jee, W. S. S., Ed., *Bone* (Suppl), 17, 261, 1995.
88. Parfitt, A. M., Drezner, M. K., Glorieux, F. H., Kanis, J. A., Malluche, H., Meunier, P. J., Ott, S. M., and Recker, R. R., Bone histomorphometry: standardization of nomenclature, symbols and units, *J. Bone Min. Res.*, 2, 595, 1987.
89. Recker, R. R., Ed., *Bone Histomorphometry. Techniques and Interpretation*, CRC Press, Boca Raton, 1983.
90. Fleisch, H., *Bisphosphonates in Bone Disease. From the Laboratory to the Patient*, The Parthenon Publishing Group, London, 1995.
91. Chen, M.-M., Yeh, J. K., and Aloia, J. F., Skeletal alterations in hypophysectomized rats: II. A histomorphometric study on tibial cortical bone, *Anat. Rec.*, 241, 513, 1995.

92. Jee, W. S. S., Ed., *The Aged Rat Model for Bone Biology Studies*, Scanning Microscopy International, Chicago, 1991.
93. Jee, W. S. S. and Li, X. J., Adaptation of cancellous bone to overloading in the adult rat: A single photon absorptiometry and histomorphometry study, *Anat. Rec.*, 227, 418, 1990.
94. Jee, W. S. S., Li, X. J., and Schaffler, M. B., Adaptation of diaphyseal structure with aging and increased mechanical usage in the adult rat. A histomorphometrical and biomechanical study, *Anat. Rec.*, 230, 332, 1991.
95. Jee, W. S. S., Li, X. J., and Ke, H. Z., The skeletal adaptation to mechanical usage in the rat, *Cells and Mater.* (Suppl 1), 131, 1991.
96. Jee, W. S. S., Ke, H. Z., and Li, X. J., Long-term anabolic effects of prostaglandin-E_2 on tibial diaphyseal bone in male rats, *Bone Miner.*, 15, 33, 1991.
97. Li, X. J. and Jee, W. S. S., Adaptation of diaphyseal structure to aging and decreased mechanical loading in the adult rat. A densitometric and histomorphometric study, *Anat. Rec.*, 229, 291, 1991.
98. Li, X. J., Jee, W. S. S., and Chow, S.-Y., Woodbury, D. M., Adaptation of cancellous bone to aging and immobilization in the rat. A single photon absorptiometry and histomorphometry study, *Anat. Rec.*, 227, 12, 1990.
99. Yeh, J. K., Chen, M. M., and Aloia, J. F., Skeletal alterations in hypophysectomizd rats: I. A histomorphometric study in tibial cancellous bone, *Anat. Rec.*, 241, 505, 1995.
100. Flora, L., Hassing, G. S. D., Parfitt, A. M., and Villanueva, A. R., Comparative skeletal effects of two diphosphonates in dogs, *Metab. Bone Dis. Rel. Res.*, 2, 389, 1980.
101. Ferretti, J. L., Capozza, R. F., Tysarczyk-Niemeyer, G., Schiessl, H., and Steffens, M., Tomographic determination of stability parameters allows noninvasive estimation of bending or torsion strength, *Osteopor. Int.*, 5, 298, 1995.
102. Ferretti, J. L., Capozza, R. F., and Zanchetta, J. R., Mechanical validation of a tomographic (pQCT) index for noninvasive estimation of rat femur bending strength, *Bone*, 18, 1, 1996.
103. Schiessl, H., Personal communications. He compared a pQCT-derived bone strength index in the human radius and ulna to the measured strength of muscles that load those bones in people of both sexes, varied ages, varied body types and varied states of health. The correlation coefficient between the BSIs and muscle strengths for the whole group: $r > 0.93$, 1993.
104. Van Der Perre, G. and Lowet, G., In vivo assessment of bone mineral properties by vibration and ultrasonic wave propagation analysis, *Bone* (Suppl 1), 18, 29, 1996.
105. Yoshikawa, T., Turner, D. H., Peacock, M., Slemenda, C. W., Weaver, C. M., Teegarden, D., Markwardt, P., and Burr, D. B., Geometric structure of the femoral neck measured during dual-energy X-ray absorptiometry, *J. Bone Min. Res.*, 9, 1053, 1994.
106. Pauwels, F., *Atlas zur Biomechanik der gesunden und kranken Hufte*, Springer-Verlag, Berlin, 1973.
107. Thompson, D'Arcy W., *On Growth and Form*, University of Cambridge Press, Cambridge, 1942.
108. Snow-Harter, C., Bouxsein, M. L., and Lewis, B. T., Muscle strength as a predictor of bone mineral density in young women, *J. Bone Min. Res.*, 5, 589, 1990.
109. Bassey, E. J. and Ramsdale, S. J., Increase in femoral bone density in young women following high-impact exercise, *Osteoporosis Int.*, 4, 72, 1994.
110. Aniansson, A., Zetterberg, C., Hedberg, M., and Henriksson, K., Impaired muscle function with aging, *Clin. Orthop. Rel. Res.*, 191, 193, 1994.
111. Boonen, S., Broos, P., and Dequecker, J., Age-related factors in the pathogenesis of senile (Type II) femoral neck fractures, *Orthopedics*, 19, 198, 1996.
112. Colletti, L. A., Edwards, J., and Gordon, L., The effects of muscle-building exercise on bone mineral density of the radius, spine and hip in young women, *Calcif. Tissue Int.*, 45, 12, 1989.

113. Doyle, F., Brown, J., and Lachance, C., Relation between bone mass and muscle weight, *Lancet*, 1, 391, 1970.
114. Kritz-Silverstein, M. and Barrett-Connor, E., Grip strength and bone mineral density in older women, *J. Bone Min. Res.*, 9, 45, 1004.
115. Madsen, O., Schaadt, O., and Bliddal, H., Relationship between quadriceps strength and bone mineral density of the proximal tibia and distal forearm in women, *J. Bone Min. Res.*, 8, 1439, 1993.
116. Murray, M., Gardner, G., Mollinger, L., and Sepic, S., Strength of isometric and isokinetic contractions: Knee muscles of men aged 20 to 86, *Phys. Ther.*, 60, 412, 1980.
117. Robinson, T. L., Snow-Harter, C., Taaffe, D. R., Gillis, D., Shaw J., and Marcus, R., Gymnasts exhibit higher bone mass than runners despite similar prevalence of amenorrhea and oligomenorrhea, *J. Bone Min. Res.*, 10, 26, 1995.
118. Taafe, D. R., Snow-Harter, C., Connoly, D. A., Robinson, T. L., Brown, M. D., and Marcus, R., Differential effects of swimming versus weight-bearing activity on bone mineral status of eumenorrheic athletes. *J. Bone Min. Res.*, 10, 586, 1995.
119. Torrance, A. G., Mosley, J. R., Suswillo, R. F. L., and Lanyon, L. E., Noninvasive loading of the rat ulna *in vivo* induces a strain-related modeling response uncomplicated by trauma or periosteal pressure, *Calcif. Tissue Int.*, 54, 241, 1994.
120. Turner, C. H., Forwood, M. R., Rho, J., and Yoshikawa, T., Mechanical loading thresholds for lamellar and woven bone formation, *J. Bone Min. Res.*, 9, 87, 1994.
121. Frost, H. M., Treatment of osteoporoses by manipulation of coherent bone cell populations, *Clin. Orthop. Rel. Res.*, 143, 227, 1979.
122. Miller, P. D., Neal, B. J., and McIntyre, D. O., The effect of coherence (ADFR) therapy with phosphate and etidronate on axial bone mineral density in postmenopausal osteoporosis, in *Osteoporosis 1987. Cyclical Etidronate for Osteoporosis*, Osteoporosis ApS, Copenhagen, 1989, 41.
123. Anderson, C., Cape, R. D. T., Crilly, R. G., Hodsman, A. B., and Wolfe B. M. J., Preliminary observations of a form of coherence therapy for osteoporosis, *Calcif. Tissue Int.*, 36, 341 1984.
124. Rasmussen, H. and Bordier, P., *The Physiological and Cellular Basis of Metabolic Bone Disease*, Williams and Wilkins, Baltimore, 1974.
125. Bak, B., Jorgensen, P. H., and Andreassen, T. T., The stimulating effect of growth hormone on fracture healing is dependent on onset and duration of administration, *Clin. Orthop. Rel. Res.*, 264, 295, 1991.
126. Frost, H. M. and Jee, W. S. S., Perspectives: Applications of a biomechanical model of the endochondral ossification mechanism, *Anat. Rec.*, 240, 447, 1994.
127. Duncan, R. L. and Turner, C. H., Mechanostransduction and the functional response of bone to mechanical strain, *Calcif. Tissue Int.*, 57, 344, 1995.
128. Reddi, A. H., Bone morphogenetic proteins, bone marrow stromal cells, and mesenchymal cells. Maureen Owen revisited, *Clin. Orthop. Rel. Res.*, 313, 115, 1995.
129. Turner, R. T., Riggs, B. L., and Spelsberg, T. C., Skeletal effects of estrogen, *Endocrin. Rev.*, 15, 275, 1994.
130. Jee, W. S. S., Since 1965 this Professor of Anatomy at the University of Utah School of Medicine organized uniquely seminal, annual, multidisciplinary Hard Tissue Workshops. Worldwide, they probably influenced how people think about and study skeletal disease more than any other meetings held in this century. The paradigm mentioned in this text had its genesis there, with input and critique from hundreds of international authorities on skeletal physiology, pathology, disease, research, biology, and biomechanics.

GLOSSARY

Architecture: the size, shape, and orientation of a bone, the amount of bone tissue in it, and the disposition of that tissue in anatomical space

Bone bank and bone mass: the amount of bone tissue in a bone or skeleton, preferably viewed as a volume

BMU: Basic Multicellular Unit of bone remodeling. In ≈4 months, and in an *activation → resorption → formation* sequence, it turns over ≈0.05 mm^3 of bone. When it makes less bone than it resorbs, this tends to remove bone permanently. How much it removes is called "rho" (see below). See Figure 1.2. Adult humans may create about 3 million new BMUs annually

Fragility, increased: more easily fractured by normal activities or an injury

Mechanical usage: all the forces or loads applied to bones during our usual physical activities. The largest loads come from muscles. For the femur, and during vigorous sports, they can briefly exceed five times body weight. Weight lifters have more bone and stronger bones than marathon runners, joggers, and swimmers, who put far more numerous but smaller loads on their bones

MESm: minimum effective strain threshold for switching mechanically controlled bone modeling drifts ON. A range centered near ≈1000 μE

MESp: the operational bone microdamage threshold. As a strain, it is a range centered near ≈3000 μE. As a clue to its nature, when cycled at 2000 microstrain bone's fatigue life ≈10 million cycles, the equivalent of 40 years of normal human physical activities. At 4000 μE its fatigue life falls below 20,000 cycles, the equivalent of two months of such activities. As strains only double in that range, microdamage increases over 400 times[29,30]

MESr: the minimum effective strain for mechanically controlled BMU-based remodeling, above which BMU creations begin to decrease and rho becomes less negative. A range centered near ≈50–100 μE

Microdamage: microscopic physical damage in a structural material due to materials fatigue. It increases as the number of load–deload or strain–destrain cycles increases, and as the size of the loads or strains increases. It weakens a bone without affecting its size, shape, content of material, or appearance in any way

Modeling: the biologic processes that produce functionally purposeful sizes and shapes to skeletal organs. Mostly modeling drifts do it in bones. See Figure 1.1. An important function lies in adjusting skeletal architecture to keep peak strains below the operational microdamage thresholds of all skeletal organs

Osteopenia: less bone than usual for most healthy people of the same age, height, weight, sex, and race. It need not represent a disease

Remodeling: turnover of bone in small packets by BMUs (see above). Pre-1964 literature did not distinguish between modeling and remodeling and lumped them together as remodeling. That can be confusing. However, while drifts and BMUs create and use the same kinds of osteoblasts and osteoclasts to do their work, in the same bone at the same time the 'blasts and 'clasts in drifts and BMUs can act and respond differently and independently to age, mechanical usage, hormones, vitamins, drugs, calcium, in different parts of the same bone, etc.

Resorption: this term has different meanings in the literature, which causes some confusion. Some authors use it to mean net bone loss, and in that sense they discuss "antiresorption agents," of which few true ones exist. Others use it in the sense of bone resorption by osteoclasts, and refer to net losses of bone as such separately. It has the latter meaning in this text

Rho: (lower case Greek): the difference between the amount of bone resorbed by a typical completed BMU, and that formed. In healthy adults and next to marrow a ballpark value ≈ -0.003 mm^3 of bone permanently removed per BMU.[2] See Figure 1.3.

Strain: The deformation or change in dimensions and/or shape caused by a load on any structure or structural material. Special gages can measure bone strains in the laboratory and *in vivo*.[33] Loads *always* cause strains, even if very small ones (see *ultimate strength* below).

Stress: the elastic resistance of the intermolecular bonds in a material to being stretched by strains. Loads cause strains, which then cause stresses. Three "principal" strains and stresses include tension, compression, and shear. We cannot measure stress directly. One must calculate it from other information that often includes strain.

Turnover: the amount of older bone replaced by new bone, usually in annual terms.

Ultimate strength: the load or strain that, when applied once, fractures a bone, ruptures a tendon or ligament, or fractures an articular cartilage. Normal lamellar bone's fracture strength expressed as a strain ≈25,000 (c.v. ≈0.25) microstrain, which corresponds to a change in length of 2.5%, i.e., from 100% of its original length to 97.5% of that length under compression, or 102.5% of it under tension. A 25,000 microstrain of normal bone also corresponds to an ultimate or fracture stress of ≈16,000 pounds per square inch, or ≈130 megapascals.

Chapter **2**

Osteoporosis — Mechanisms and Models

Lis Mosekilde

CONTENTS

0-8493-8556-3/98/$0.00+$.50

I. INTRODUCTION

In order to develop optimum animal models for osteoporosis research, an extensive knowledge of human bone quality is needed. Bone quality is a combination of bone mass, architecture, and material strength. And all these factors change during aging, the menopause, development of osteoporosis, and also during different treatment regimens. In the following sections, normal age-related changes in human vertebral bodies will be described. Particular attention has been paid to the vertebral bodies, because vertebral fractures are the first and also the most common osteoporotic fractures. Thereafter, the need to develop animal models for osteoporosis research is described. Finally, the anabolic effects of PTH on bone quality in animal models is discussed in detail.

II. HUMAN BONE — VERTEBRAE

A. Peak Bone Mass and Strength

The vertebral body is the load-bearing part of the vertebra. When peak bone mass has been attained (at the age of 25 to 30 years), the vertebral body consists of a central trabecular network encased in a bony shell approximately 400 to 500 μm thick. The central trabecular network is isotropic in the horizontal plane but anisotropic in all other directions (Figure 2.1a). This special architecture provides maximum strength with minimum bone mass. In young individuals the load-bearing capacity of a lumbar vertebral body is 1000 kg, or more (Table 2.1).[1] Peak bone mass is 25 to 30% higher in men than in women, mainly because the size (cross-sectional area) is larger in men than in women.

(a)

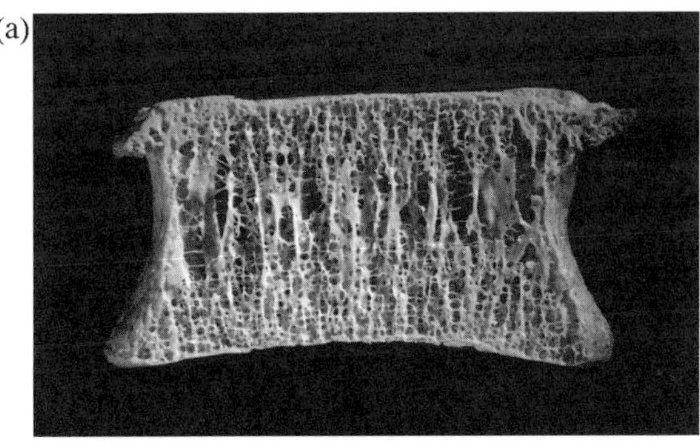

(b)

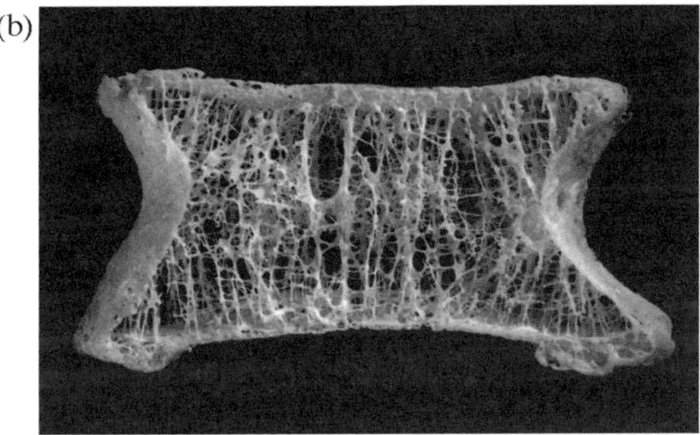

Figure 2.1
Age-related changes in human vertebral bodies. (a) Frontal section of vertebral body from young individual. (b) Frontal section of vertebral body from an old individual. (From Mosekilde, Lis, Assessing bone quality in animal models, *Bone*, 17, S343, 1995. With permission.)

B. Normal Age-Related Changes

With age, internal trabecular bone mass and architecture change due to the remodeling process. These changes start in the center of the verte-

TABLE 2.1
In Vitro Data Concerning Human Vertebral Body Characteristics in Relation to Age

Age, Years	20–40	70–80	Osteoporotic
Trabecular bone volume, BV/TV, %	15–20	8–12	4–8
Ash-density, g/cm^3	0.20–0.25	0.10–0.15	0.060–0.090
Cortical thickness, μm	400–500	200–300	120–150
Load-bearing capacity, kg	1000–1200	150–250	60–150
Load-bearing capacity of cortical rim as % of total	25–30	70–80	80–90

bral body (the vascular region) and progress superiorly and inferiorly from there. There is also an age-related thinning of the endplates and of the "cortical" shell due to endosteal bone resorption (Figure 2.1b). Concomitantly, there is a change in cross-sectional area, partly due to periosteal bone formation (modeling)[1] and partly due to osteophyte formation.[2] This changes the strong vertebral body of a young individual to one with a load-bearing capacity of only 150 to 250 kg in an elderly individual (Table 2.1).[1] These are all normal, age-related changes but will, if they become pronounced, cause fragility fractures of the vertebral bodies. In order to determine the importance for vertebral bone strength of these age-related changes, it is vital to know which factors influence bone biomechanical competence *in vitro* and *in vivo.*

C. Structural Determinants of Vertebral Strength and Mechanisms Responsible for Loss of Strength

The strength of the vertebral body is determined by several key factors of which: 1) vertebral body cross-sectional area; 2) thickness of the cortical rim; 3) thickness of the endplates; and 4) density, combined with connectivity of the central trabecular network, are the most important. The exact roles of each of these factors have never been determined, due partly to the complexity of the structure and partly to the fact that each factor changes independently with age, immobilization, metabolic bone diseases, and other conditions such as disc degeneration or osteophyte formation.

1. Cross-Sectional Area

The cross-sectional area of the vertebral body is directly correlated with the load-bearing capacity of the vertebral body both during pure compression and bending loads, which are the two dominating forces on the vertebral body during normal, daily activity. The cross-sectional area of the vertebral bodies is 20 to 30% larger in young men than in women of corresponding ages.[1] Vigorous exercise directly affects the vertebral body cross-sectional area,[3] an effect that might be caused by direct periosteal stimulation, as shown by Pead et al.[4] The 20 to 30% greater cross-sectional area of the male vertebral bodies (being genetic, hormonal, or mechanically induced) will, of itself, result in a 20 to 30% higher load-bearing capacity than seen in female vertebral bodies. However, in many *in vivo* bone density measurements, this important size factor has been neglected (see Section III.A).

The cross-sectional area of vertebral bodies seems to increase with age in men but not in women.[1] This age-related increase, seen solely in male vertebral bodies, can partly offset the concomitant decline in material properties (that is seen in both sexes), and it is therefore an important compensatory mechanism for the age-related decline in bone density. At other skeletal sites, for example the long bones, an age-related increase in cross-sectional area has been demonstrated for men, but not for women, and a direct stimulatory effect of loading on periosteal expansion has been suggested.[5]

2. *Thickness of the Cortical Shell*

The thickness of the cortical shell and the importance of this for the load-bearing capacity of the vertebral body is a matter of debate. The normally held view has been that the vertebral body consists of approximately 70% trabecular bone and 30% cortical bone.[6] However, Nottestad et al.[7] showed the opposite: 30 to 40% trabecular bone and 60 to 70% cortical bone. Both viewpoints could be correct, because the trabecular bone mass in the central part of the vertebral body declines with age much faster than cortical bone.[8] Therefore, a shift in trabecular/cortical bone mass ratio with age should be expected. While the central trabecular bone mass dominates in the vertebral bodies of younger individuals, cortical bone seems to dominate in the very old. The relative importance of the cortical shell therefore increases with age in biomechanical terms.[9,10]

In young individuals, the load-bearing capacity of the cortical rim is only 20 to 25% of the total capacity of the vertebral body. With age, the cortical ring becomes thinner in both men and women, and at the age of 80 to 90 years has a thickness of only 200 to 300 μm (i.e., the same as a single trabecula). Despite the thinness of the cortical shell in elderly individuals, it might at this age contribute some 70 to 80% of the load-bearing capacity of the vertebral body, as the trabecular network has become degraded (Table 2.1).[8]

Thinning of the cortical shell is caused by endosteal resorption in both men and women, but in men there is also a significant modeling of the cortical shell caused by slow periosteal apposition, as mentioned above.[11-13]

The thickness of the cortical ring has been directly measured in only a very few human studies.[14] However, even in young persons, the cortical ring is very thin and merely consists of condensed trabecular bone, rather than real cortical bone with Haversian systems. This is an important point that is often overlooked due to the fact that most *in vivo* studies are conducted on animals (e.g., rats, minipigs, dogs) that not only have thick cortical rims surrounding their vertebral bodies but also have typical Haversian systems.

3. *Endplates*

The endplates have a thickness of 200 to 400 μm. They are thin, perforated structures (perforated by vessels entering the fibrocartilage of the discs from the vertebral bodies). The endplates too can be described as condensed trabecular bone. Direct measurements of age-related changes have never been performed. On their external side, the endplates have fibrocartilaginous tissue and discs, but on the internal face they are supported directly by the trabecular network. In young individuals, the discs can absorb and distribute stresses and strains applied to the vertebrae,[15] but with age the intervertebral discs lose elasticity and height and thereby their capacity to absorb and distribute loads.[15] Forces, even trivial, therefore tend to reach extremely high values at small, localized areas and can thereby cause endplate depressions or biconcave vertebrae. This is further facilitated in elderly individuals, where the endplate lacks support because of little remaining trabecular connectivity.

4. *Vertebral Trabecular Network*

The vertebral trabecular network in younger individuals is dense and well connected. On a vertical section through a vertebral body, three zones can be identified in this network: 1) An upper, sub-endplate zone with an anisotropic trabecular network consisting of 200 to 220 μm-thick vertical columns and slightly thinner (180 to 200 μm) horizontal struts. This network is regular and dense. 2) In the middle of the vertebral body is a zone with irregular, vertical columns and plates supported by thin, horizontal struts. The irregularity of this zone is mainly caused by the large basivertebral veins that pass through the vertebral body in an anterior–posterior direction. 3) The third zone, toward the lower endplate, is again regular with a dense network, as described for the upper zone (Figure 2.1a). The volumetric density of the whole trabecular network is identical for young men and young women: the ash-density is approximately 0.2 g/cm^3 and the trabecular bone volume 12 to 15% (Table 2.1).[16]

Hemopoietic marrow fills the space between the trabeculae and has an internal hydraulic effect.[17] The marrow remains hemopoietic throughout life, although with age there is a slight increase in fat cells. Several of the bone cells involved in the remodeling process are directly recruited from the hemopoietic bone marrow or from the abundant sinusoidal capillaries in the marrow. Therefore, the close connection between red marrow and bone tissue in the vertebral bodies seems to be responsible for the high turnover (remodeling) at this site. At other skeletal sites where there has been a shift from hemopoietic to fatty marrow in young adulthood (e.g., the diaphyses of the long bones), the bone turnover (remodeling activity) is much lower.

The remodeling process, having a slightly negative balance of 1 to 3 μm, primarily causes thinning of the horizontal struts in the load-bearing vertebral trabecular network and, secondarily, osteoclastic perforations (Figure 2.2). As resorption lacunae normally reach a depth of 45 to 50 μm,[18,19] one resorption cavity covering more than half the circumference of a thin trabecula, or two resorption cavities, one on each side of a trabecular structure, would easily perforate a 90 to 110 μm-thick horizontal trabecula.[1,16]

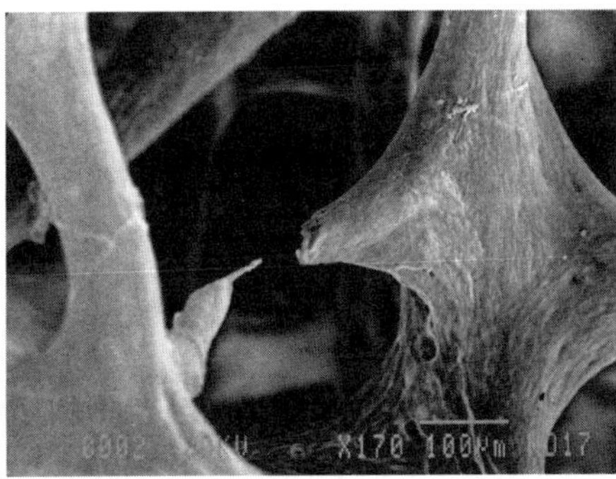

Figure 2.2
Deterioration of the human vertebral network. Osteoclastic perforation of horizontal strut. (SEM photograph). (From Mosekilde, Lis, Assessing bone quality in animal models, *Bone,* 17, S343, 1995. With permission.)

The decline in trabecular bone mass, the decline in trabecular thickness, and the perforations in the network are all caused by the remodeling process — and are, therefore, normal, age-related changes. The described pattern, with selective thinning and perforation of horizontal struts, is seen in both men and women during normal aging.[16,20] Around the menopause, the activation frequency increases,[21] and at the same time resorption depth might increase.[18] These two factors accelerate the age-related changes and increase the number of trabecular perforations in the network.[22] Furthermore, once trabecular structures have been perforated they are no longer loaded and will, therefore, be resorbed rapidly by osteoclasts (Figure 2.3).

The biomechanical consequences of the disruption of the load-bearing vertebral network are far reaching. As the strength of a trabecula is proportional to its radius squared, thinning of the vertical structures has a tremendous influence on their strength. The situation is similar concerning the length between supporting, horizontal struts: the compressive strength of the network is inversely proportional to the square of the distance between the supporting struts.[23] Furthermore, at a certain stage, when several supporting struts have disappeared, the slenderness ratio of the long, unsupported, vertical trabeculae reaches a critical value, and the structure fails because of buckling rather than compression. When this stage is reached, there is a dramatic loss of strength.[23] The loss of bone mass during aging is therefore accompanied by a disproportionate loss of strength.[24]

It should be recognized that not only is bone strength highly dependent on bone architecture and on connectivity, but also that loss of connectivity in the load-bearing network seems irreversible. Remodeling sites on disconnected, unloaded structures show no sign of bone formation (uncoupling).[25] Strain or stress applied to bone seems essential to enable osteoblasts to form new bone on existing surfaces.[26,27] The osteoblasts will

(a)

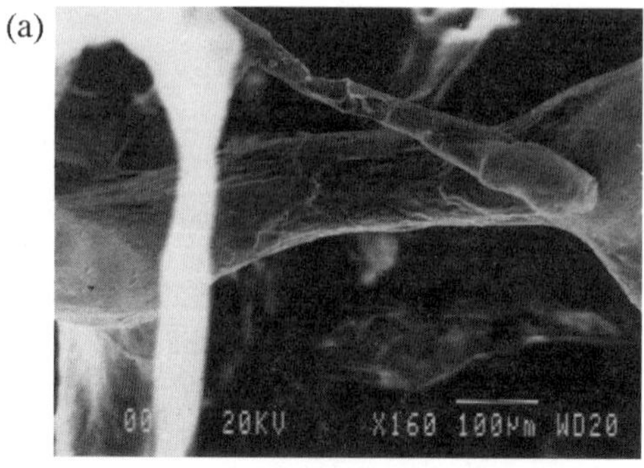

(b)

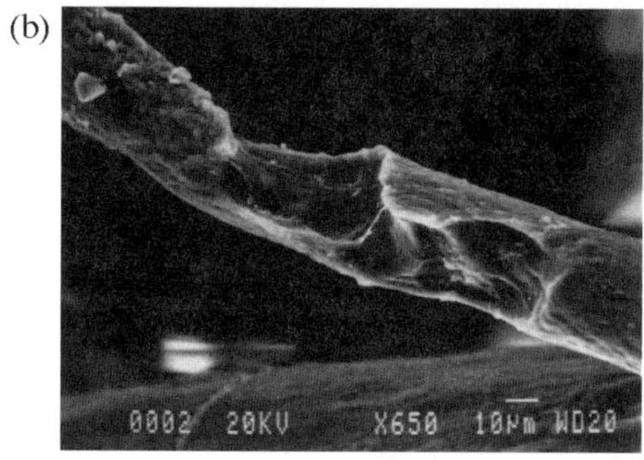

Figure 2.3
Deterioration of the human vertebral network. Previously perforated horizontal strut is resorbed by osteoclasts (SEM). (From Mosekilde, Lis, Consequences of the remodelling process for vertebral trabecular bone structure — A scanning electron microscopy study (uncoupling of unloaded structures), *Bone Miner.*, 10, 13, 1990. With permission.)

therefore be unable to refill the gaps in the network under normal circumstances. Most therapeutic regimens, since they are primarily antiresorptive, cannot facilitate this process either, but whether powerful anabolic agents like PTH will be able to do so still remains unresolved.

Consequently, a description of the mechanism by which the structures are perforated, the extent of perforations, and how different therapeutic regimens affect loss of connectivity is important. However, *in vivo* measurements can measure changes in bone mass and bone density only, but they cannot detect the important architectural changes during aging, the menopause, or different therapeutic regimens.

D. Osteoporosis

In osteoporosis, the described normal age-related changes in cortical thickness, trabecular bone density, and connectivity become even more pronounced. The sum of these changes causes a pronounced weakening of the vertebral bodies. The load-bearing capacity of whole lumbar vertebrae will often decline to values around 60 to 150 kg.

In osteoporotic patients, the cortical thickness (endplate and rim) will decline to values around 120 to 150 μm; the trabecular network ash-densities will be as low as 0.06 to 0.09 g/cm^3; and the trabecular bone volume (BV/TV) will be less than 5% (Table 2.1). At the same time, most of the horizontal struts in the network will be very thin and often perforated. These changes in trabecular bone density and architecture cause a pronounced decline (with a factor of 4 to 8) in the strength of the central trabecular bone. This disproportional decline in bone strength is caused by the trabecular structures now failing because of buckling instead of compression.[23]

The vertical trabeculae that break during daily loading will heal by normal fracture healing (woven bone formation) and form microcalluses, but this normal healing process seems to occur only if the two ends of the fracture remain in contact. These microcalluses are typically found just beneath the endplates, sometimes several hundred in one vertebral body (Figure 2.4).[28] Later, the microcalluses will be smoothed by the remodeling process (Figure 2.5). It should be noted that the remodeling process is active only in the removal of old microcalluses and is not involved in the actual microfracture healing as such. Therefore, antiresorptive agents like bisphosphonates should not impair the healing of the microfractures.

The vertebral bone strength in osteoporotic patients, too, is determined by both trabecular and cortical bone, but as the trabecular network at this stage has almost totally disappeared, the cortical shell becomes relatively more important (80 to 90% of load-bearing capacity). As in normal individuals, the size of the vertebral body (cross-sectional area) is

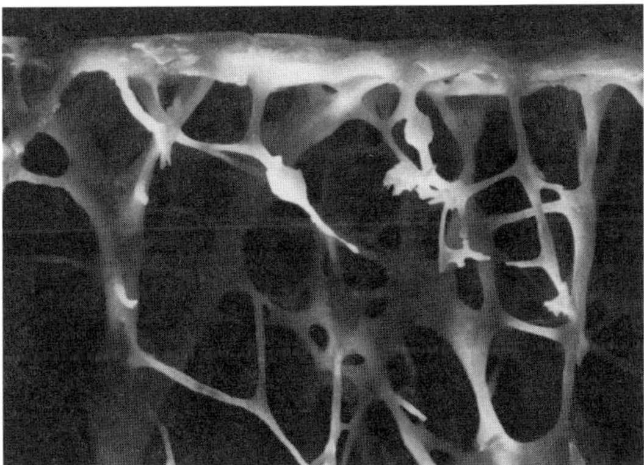

Figure 2.4
Vertebral body from elderly individual. Two microcalluses are seen just under the endplate. There are also several osteoclastic perforations in the network.

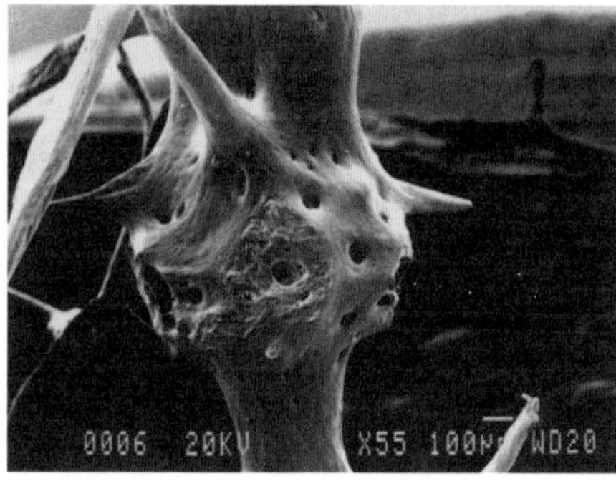

Figure 2.5
Microcallus on a vertical, load-bearing trabecula. The microcallus is being smoothed by the remodeling process. (SEM).

important for its load-bearing capacity, and some studies have shown that osteoporotic women typically have small vertebral bodies.[29,30]

III. MEASUREMENT OF VERTEBRAL BONE MASS AND QUALITY *IN VIVO* AND *IN VITRO*

A. Vertebral Bone Mass Measurements *In Vivo*

Vertebral strength cannot be measured directly *in vivo*, which is why many noninvasive density measurements have been developed as a surrogate: Quantitative computed tomography (QCT), dual photon absorptiometry (DPA), and dual energy X-ray absorptiometry (DEXA). All these techniques measure bone mass, and although they correlate highly with bone strength, they cannot account for more than 75 to 85% of the variation in bone strength in normal individuals. Furthermore, it has been shown that the age-related decline in bone strength (quality) is much more pronounced than the decline in bone mass.[23,24,31,32]

Normal noninvasive (A–P) bone-density measurements, with either DPA or DEXA, measure total vertebral mass and density (which involves the vertebral body and the posterior elements). The two techniques cannot separate trabecular and cortical elements in the vertebral body. Nor can they measure cross-sectional area. The two methods therefore provide only rough measures of changes in bone quality or strength during aging.

By using density measurements (BMD) *in vivo* (with mass corrected for vertebral body frontal area) instead of BMC measurements, the separation between individuals with high and low fracture liability might become even more difficult, as the influence of skeletal size is reduced.[29,23] As bone size is an important and independent determinant of bone strength, mathematical manipulation of areal bone density values to remove any contribution of bone size will reduce, rather than enhance, the information about fracture risk obtained from bone density measurements.[34] Furthermore, neither DPA nor DEXA gives true volumetric densities. Their densities (corrected for frontal area) will vary with the size of the vertebral body. Two vertebral bodies with the same volumetric density but different sizes would therefore have different area BMD when measured with DPA or DEXA. For an identical volumetric density, a larger vertebra would typically yield higher BMD results than a small vertebra.[35] Since the increase in bone width with aging overestimates BMD in older patients, the phenomenon causes an underestimation of the rate of bone loss.[36] As an age-related increase in bone width is seen only in men, this could explain the underestimation of bone loss in men. The greater tendency of males to osteophyte formation would further aggravate this.

QCT techniques measure true volumetric density and have the advantage of being able to measure the vertebral body alone, separate trabecular and cortical bone,[37-39] and also measure endplate area.[40,41] Recently, the ability to measure trabecular architecture *in vivo* has been described.[42] In daily routine, DEXA techniques have their advantages in that they are quicker and give a smaller radiation dose. But as a tool to aid understanding of the specific age-related changes, the changes in osteoporosis, and the specific tissue reaction to therapeutic regimens, QCT scanning seems superior to the other techniques.

However, changes in cortical shell thickness with age cannot be measured exactly *in vivo* with any of the techniques mentioned above. QCT can give only a rough estimate because the thick cortical shell seen with QCT is an artifact caused by the beam-hardening effect. Neither DPA nor DEXA can provide any data concerning cortical thickness.

B. Vertebral Bone Mass Measurements *In Vitro*

DPA, DEXA, and QCT can all be used to measure bone mass and density in *in vitro* studies. Some small *in vitro* studies have been performed,[40,41,43-45] but very large *in vitro* studies based upon autopsy specimens are needed in order to provide useful data concerning differences between measurements and in order to optimize measurement techniques.

Only such extensive studies would be able to compare density measurements with bone quality or strength and provide an indication as to whether or not bone mass should be normalized and, if it should be, to optimize the normalization procedure. Additionally, ash-density measurements and histomorphometry involving measurement of BV/TV, connectivity, cortical thickness, and endplate thickness are needed.

C. Vertebral Bone Quality Measurements *In Vivo*

Lateral spine radiographs for determination of vertebral fractures is a possible *in vivo* avenue for estimating bone quality. But this involves several problems: first of all, normal vertebral dimensions vary from vertebra to vertebra. In order to avoid misdiagnosis, it is therefore necessary for criteria of deformity to allow for this variation.[46] Definitions of fractures, classification of fractures, and determination of the severity of vertebral fragility fractures are issues that have not been generally agreed upon.[47-49] Furthermore, techniques for summarizing spinal fractures and thereby providing a spinal deformity index are still under development.[47,50] All these techniques are still an indirect way of assessing bone quality and are, more correctly, the summation of vertebral strength, intravertebral disc properties (degeneration), and actual trauma. Despite these problems, vertebral fracture incidence is generally accepted as the final end point in therapeutic trials. Recently, guidelines have been suggested for the assessment of prevalent as well as incident fractures on radiographs, using both quantitative (morphometric) and semiquantitative (visual) techniques.[51]

Another avenue for estimation of bone quality *in vivo* is detection of structural parameters important for strength by use of iliac crest bone biopsies. However, this technique also is only an indirect measurement of vertebral bone quality. Kleerekoper et al.[52] have shown that the biomechanical competence of cancellous bone is dependent not only upon the absolute amount of bone present, but also on the trabecular microstructure. Many studies have focused on the relationship between bone mass, structure, and quality. As iliac crest bone biopsies are the only available *in vivo* specimens for histomorphometric and stereological assessment, most clinical studies have been conducted on specimens from this site.[53-55] Other studies have assessed bone strength from iliac crest bone biopsies directly in order to determine the effect of aging,[56] of different treatment regimens (fluoride),[57] and of different metabolic bone diseases (hyperparathyroidism).[58] In order to use such data, it is important to show that iliac crest bone strength correlates to vertebral body strength and that changes in the iliac crest bone biopsy actually reflect changes in the spine.[55]

D. Vertebral Bone Quality Measurements *In Vitro*

Human vertebral body strength can be measured *in vitro* by use of compression tests. Different test situations have been used: Test of whole spinal segments;[59] of vertebral bodies with molded ends;[60] and of vertebral bodies with the endplates removed and with plano-parallel, sawed surfaces.[1]

The different techniques reflect the fact that it is difficult to imitate the naturally occurring load situations and normal bone biology in all respects. In normal life, the compressive load is repetitive, varies in intensity, localization, and direction, and is influenced by the often irregular endplates and the elasticity of the intervertebral discs.[8]

Despite these limitations, biomechanical tests performed on human vertebral bodies have provided useful information concerning: age-related changes in load values; discrepancy between decline in bone mass and decline in strength; and the importance of cross-sectional area for vertebral body strength. The studies have also pinpointed the very pronounced decline in bone mass and strength in males during aging which is very often overlooked in *in vivo* studies.

However, in order to give a detailed description of age-related and menopause-related changes, very extensive *in vitro* studies of human bone quality are still needed, as are studies to increase understanding of the pathophysiology and pathogenesis of osteoporosis. Concomitantly, as noninvasive techniques for clinically assessing bone strength have not yet been adequately validated, animal models providing an opportunity directly to examine bone mass, architecture, and strength are being developed and tested.

IV. RATIONALE FOR USING ANIMAL MODELS

As new agents are developed for osteoporosis prevention and intervention, the need for reliable animal models becomes more and more pressing. At the same time, the necessity of not focusing on bone mass as the sole efficacy parameter has become apparent. Before accepting any agent for clinical osteoporosis trials, the U.S. Food and Drug Administration (FDA) requires that the agent has proven its efficacy in a small animal model (screening) and also in a nonrodent animal model with known intracortical bone remodeling. The efficacy of the agent should be proven concerning both bone mass and also bone biomechanical competence.

The reason for these requirements might be that several human studies have shown a discrepancy between changes in bone mass and bone strength during aging, in osteoporotics, and during different treatment regimens. Thus, the primary objective of these animal studies is to demonstrate that long-term treatment with a specific agent will not have deleterious effects on bone quality.

V. ANIMAL MODELS AS PRECLINICAL OSTEOPOROSIS MODELS

Large and small animal models in preclinical osteoporosis research should be able to mirror most of the described normal changes in human bone. Consequently, the assessment of quality of bone in animal models requires the same investigations as are used in human bone research.[61] Additionally, prevention and intervention studies in the animal models should closely reflect human clinical studies, not only concerning changes in bone mass, architecture, and size during treatment regimens, but also concerning changes in bone structural and material quality. The end point in preclinical studies, biomechanical competence, should therefore be comparable with the fracture rate measured as the end point for bone quality in clinical studies. And to ensure the best basis for this, two preclinical models are required: the rat model, for screening; and a large animal model with intracortical bone remodeling, for verification of screening results.

A. The Rat Model

For screening different therapeutic agents, the ovariectomized rat model has now been generally accepted.[62,63] The advantages of the rat model for screening are numerous: The study can be conducted under very standardized conditions, and it is relatively cheap and short term. Rats have cancellous bone remodeling with sites very similar to those seen in human cancellous bone (Figure 2.6a and 2.6b), and it is easy to perform biomechanical tests on rat bones under standardized conditions. Ovariectomy can produce alterations in the cancellous network identical to those seen in the human skeleton during aging and the menopause (Figure 2.7).

The rat model also has some disadvantages. Rats have a different loading pattern. They have open epiphyses to the age of 12 to 24 months (depending on skeletal sites). They have very little intracortical bone remodeling, but they have pronounced bone modeling throughout life. They have hemopoietic marrow at most skeletal sites throughout life and therefore have higher bone turnover at many skeletal sites (e.g., proximal tibial end) than humans.

If one takes the disadvantages into consideration when interpreting data, the rat model seems excellent for testing differences in bone quality during screening of new agents for osteoporosis.

B. The Large Animal Model

In the event of promising screening results, the agent should be tested in a standardized large animal model with proven intracortical bone remodeling. The most efficient large animal model has yet to be determined. Primates,[64] minipigs,[65,66] dogs,[67] sheep,[68] and ferrets[69] are all being investigated.

(a)

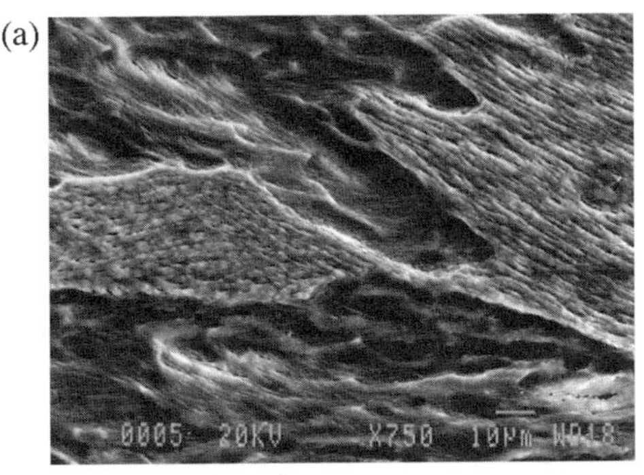

(b)

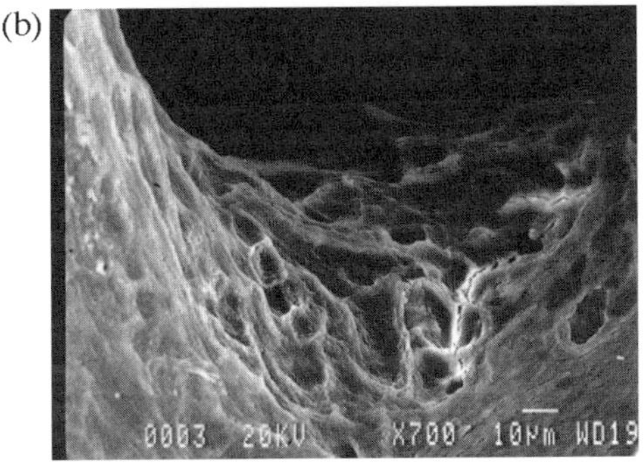

Figure 2.6
Remodeling sites (resorption) in (a) a human vertebral body and (b) a rat vertebral body. (SEM). (From Mosekilde, Lis, Assessing bone quality in animal models, *Bone*, 17, S343, 1995. With permission.)

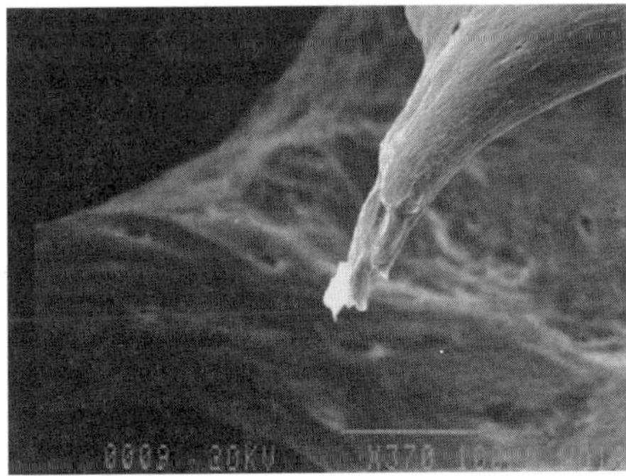

Figure 2.7
Ovariectomy-induced deterioration of a rat vertebral network. Osteoclastic perforation of the trabecular structure (SEM). (From Mosekilde, Lis, Assessing bone quality in animal models, *Bone*, 17, S343, 1995. With permission.)

The most important requirements for a large animal model are: that the animal has proven intracortical bone remodeling; that the animal has proven osteopenic response to mechanical, hormonal, or nutritional manipulation; and that the model can be standardized. However, it should be borne in mind that none of the large animal models is comparable to humans. The cancellous networks are very dense in both vertebrae and femoral necks compared with humans, and it is difficult to induce osteoclastic perforations in this network. Therefore, it is difficult to create the disproportionate loss of bone strength that is characteristic for humans in many of the large animal models. Furthermore, in most large animals vertebrae have distinct cortical shells with Haversian systems. The thickness is 1500 to 3000 μm. In human vertebrae, there is no real cortical shell — the shell is merely condensed trabecular bone. The thickness of the human vertebral "cortical shell" is 200 to 400 μm. It should also be acknowledged that neither the small nor the large animal models develop spontaneous or artificially induced osteoporotic fractures.[70] However, strict immobilization as seen in some modern farming methods seems able to induce osteoporotic fractures in large animals (pigs, cattle).

VI. RATIONALE FOR TESTING ANABOLIC AGENTS IN ANIMAL MODELS

In clinical studies, postmenopausal and age-related osteoporosis have been characterized by loss of trabecular bone mass and trabecular connectivity, thinning of cortical bone, and also a lack of capability for periosteal apposition (and thereby also a lack of compensatory increase in bone size).[30,33]

Antiresorptive agents such as estrogen, bisphosphonates, and calcitonin have shown themselves capable of increasing spinal bone mass slightly (3 to 8%).[71-73] Some studies have also indicated an increase in bone quality (reduction of fracture rate) during treatment with antiresorptive agents.[73,74] These effects seem mainly attributable to the effect of antiresorptive agents on decreasing bone remodeling activity and thereby reducing remodeling space. Therefore, it seems likely that the optimum treatment for osteoporosis would not be an antiresorptive agent but a powerful anabolic agent that could increase bone mass, maintain structural connectivity (or even improve it), increase cortical thickness, and also add bone on the periosteal surface (periosteal apposition).

Two bone anabolic agents, PTH and fluoride, are currently being tested intensively.

VII. EFFECTS OF PTH MONOTHERAPY ON BONE BIOMECHANICAL COMPETENCE IN ANIMAL MODELS

Many studies have clearly demonstrated the anabolic effect of PTH on bone mass in rat models.[75-80] This anabolic effect has been demonstrated concerning both trabecular bone and cortical bone.

Recently, several biomechanical studies have been performed concerning the effect of PTH on bone quality in young, intact male rats, in sexually mature, ovariectomized and slightly osteopenic rats, and also in aged, ovariectomized, osteopenic rats.[81-87] These studies have elucidated the effect of PTH on bone strength at different skeletal sites: vertebral bodies, femoral necks, and femoral cortical bone.

A. Vertebral Body

Measurement of vertebral body strength or biomechanical competence in rats is very relevant, as the vertebral bodies, like those in humans, consist of a dominant central trabecular core and a cortical rim. The trabecular network is structurally aligned and of the same dimensions as the human vertebral trabecular network. Furthermore, vertebral fractures are the first and also the most common osteoporotic fractures to occur in humans. The very first biomechanical study performed with PTH on rat vertebral bodies was conducted in young male rats.[81] Therefore, they had very intact and well-connected trabecular networks. The study clearly showed that PTH given intermittently caused a dose-dependent increase in bone strength after normalization for bone mass or cross-sectional area. This clearly demonstrated that PTH had no negative effect on bone material strength. A more clinically relevant study was carried out on sexually mature, ovariectomized rats.[83] This study confirmed the findings from the first study that PTH given intermittently had a clear, positive effect on bone mass and material strength. Finally, the study on aged, ovariectomized, and osteopenic rats confirmed yet again the positive effect of PTH on vertebral bone mass and strength.[86] In this study, where connections and whole trabecular structures had been lost in the vertebral cancellous bone core, the effect of PTH was still very positive (Figure 2.8).

B. Femoral Neck

In humans, the femoral neck is clinically the most important site for osteoporotic fractures. It was therefore natural also to test this site in rat models with regard to PTH. The rat femoral necks, like human femoral necks, are load-bearing. They are placed inside the hip joint and are

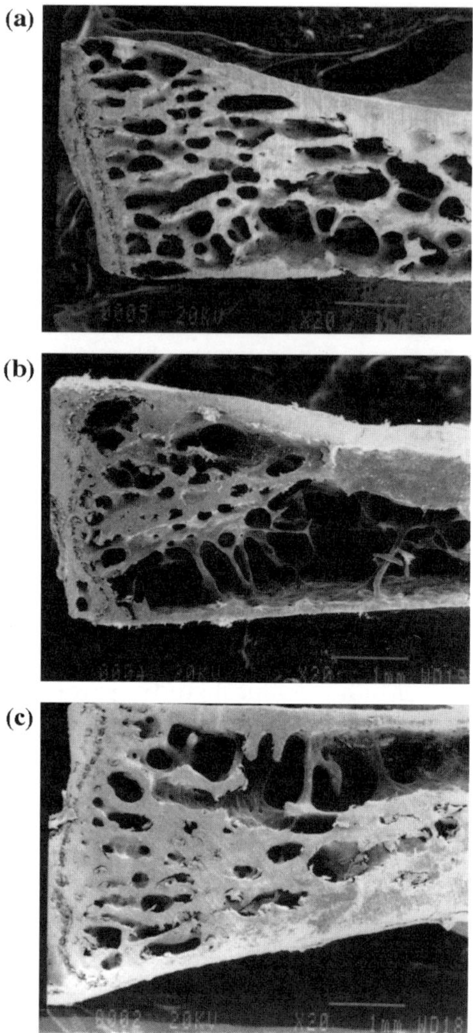

Figure 2.8
Rat vertebral bodies. (a) sham-operated. (b) Ovariectomized. (c) Ovariectomized for 8 weeks and then treated with PTH (SEM). (From Mosekilde, Lis, Assessing bone quality in animal models, *Bone*, 17, S343, 1995. With permission.)

therefore not covered with periosteal tissue; and, finally, they consist of equal proportions of cortical and trabecular bone.

With respect to PTH treatment, the femoral necks have been tested in both sexually mature ovariectomized rats[85] and aged osteopenic rats.[87] These studies clearly showed a very positive effect of PTH on rat femoral neck strength (load). No normalization procedures were performed in these studies, so changes in material strength as such could not be assessed.

C. Femoral Cortical Bone

Osteoporotic fractures do not affect the diaphyses of the long bones, and there should therefore be no reason to test long bones.[70] However, since it has been suggested several times that the pronounced anabolic effect of intermittent PTH treatment on trabecular bone mass was achieved at the expense of cortical bone ("cortical steal" phenomenon), studies on cortical bone strength would still be relevant, especially in the preclinical testing of anabolic agents. Concerning PTH, one study was performed by the use of 3-point bending of femora from young intact male rats,[82] and two further studies used a compression test on pure cortical, femoral bone from sexually mature, ovariectomized rats or from aged osteopenic rats.[84,87] All these studies clearly showed that intermittent treatment with PTH in rat models did not induce cortical steal phenomenon. On the contrary, PTH increased cortical bone strength in all studies.

The effect of PTH on biomechanical competence in these different rat models and at different skeletal sites has been very positive: an increase in bone structural and material strength has been shown in all studies and at all skeletal sites investigated (Table 2.2).

VIII. EFFECTS OF PTH IN COTHERAPY WITH ANTIRESORPTIVE AGENTS

It has previously been proven that the anabolic effect of PTH is not dependent on initial bone resorption.[88,89] Furthermore, as PTH for some years has been thought to exert its anabolic effect on trabecular bone at the expense of cortical bone, several studies have been conducted to find out whether combining PTH with an antiresorptive agent (estrogen, bisphosphonate, or calcitonin) would be superior to PTH alone.

These studies have again been conducted in sexually mature, ovariectomized rats[83-85,90] and also in aged, osteopenic ovariectomized rats.[86,87] In them, histomorphometry on tibial, metaphyseal trabecular bone[91] and tibial cortical bone[92] was combined with biomechanical testing of vertebral bodies,[83] femoral necks,[85] and femoral cortical bone.[84] All these investigations showed unequivocally that PTH alone was as effective as PTH in combination therapy concerning bone mass, structure, and strength. However, a study by Shen et al.[93] has recently shown PTH in combination with estrogen to be slightly more effective than PTH monotherapy, particularly for restoring structural connectivity.

In all these studies, the antiresorptive agents have also been tested on their own. Although they have been capable of maintaining bone mass and strength, none of these agents has been capable of increasing bone strength over the level of control (sham-operated) animals.

TABLE 2.2

Biomechanical Effects (Load Values) of PTH Given Intermittently to Rats. Different Rat Models and Different Skeletal Sites are Presented

Skeletal Site	Study Design	Control Load Value (N)	Treatment Load Value (N)	% Change	p Value
Vertebral bodies	Young, male, 5W (81)	254 ± 10	392 ± 23	54	<0.001
	Mature, OVX, 15W (83)	250 ± 15	470 ± 23	88	<0.001
	Aged, OVX, 24W (86)	342 ± 33	588 ± 25	59	<0.001
Femoral neck	Mature, OVX, 15W (85)	189 ± 4	130 ± 6	45	<0.001
	Aged, OVX, 24W (87)	116 ± 5	167 ± 5	44	<0.001
Femoral cortical bone	Young, male, 5W* (82)	144 ± 4	169 ± 5	17	<0.01
	Mature, OVX, 15W (84)	1025 ± 33	1218 ± 30	20	<0.01
	Aged, OVX, 24W (87)	915 ± 45	1531 ± 57	67	<0.001

Note: Load values are given in newtons (N). * Is from the three-point bending test, all other data are from compression tests. Means ± SEM. The number in parentheses refers to the study in the reference list.

In summary, PTH monotherapy seems as effective as PTH cotherapy in maintaining or restoring bone mass and strength in different rat models.

The effect of PTH on biomechanical competence in large animal models (primates,[94] ferrets[95]) has recently been determined concerning both vertebrae and femoral necks. Data from these studies look very promising, but have not yet been published.

IX. COMPARISON BETWEEN PTH AND OTHER BONE ANABOLIC AGENTS

For several years, fluoride has been used in human clinical trials and has proved itself capable of increasing vertebral bone mass.[96] However, some studies have indicated that this positive effect was not accompanied by a positive effect on bone quality, i.e., it did not decrease the incidence of fracture.[96,97]

Studies in pigs[98] and recently in humans[99] have both confirmed this discrepancy between bone mass and bone strength during fluoride therapy. Additionally, a study on mature, intact female rats (performed with the same techniques as several of the PTH studies) has shown a clear, dose-dependent increase in bone mass that was not followed by a similar increase in structural strength. This indicates that the bone quality had declined during fluoride therapy.[100]

Therefore, PTH and fluoride seem to act totally differently on bone: although they both have an anabolic effect on bone mass, only PTH has a positive effect on bone material and structural strength. In contrast to fluoride, PTH does not have a negative effect on the material quality of bone. An alternative explanation could be that the "therapeutic window" for fluoride is much narrower than for PTH and that the beneficial effects of fluoride on bone strength are critically dose-dependent.

X. SUMMARY

Human vertebral bone strength is determined by several factors: bone size (cross-sectional area); cortical thickness; trabecular bone density; and architecture. All these factors change with age as a result of the remodeling process. When the changes become pronounced, osteoporotic fractures occur. There is a different aging pattern for men and women: men achieve a higher peak bone mass than women (mainly because of a larger cross-sectional area of their bones); they have no accelerated bone loss in middle age; and they seem to be able to compensate for their loss of bone material strength by increasing their vertebral cross-sectional area with age. Focusing solely on the central trabecular bone, men seem to have less tendency for trabecular perforation than women. The general pattern, for both men and women is, however, an extreme (70 to 80%) decline in vertebral bone strength during normal aging. The accompanying decline in bone density is much less pronounced (35 to 45%) and may, especially in men, be partly offset by osteophyte formation.

Loading plays an important role in the maintenance of trabecular connectivity (through the remodeling process), in the orientation of the trabeculae, and the periosteal apposition (through the modeling process). Loading is therefore important for the maintenance of bone strength during normal aging.

Concerning osteoporosis treatment, a powerful anabolic agent that can add new bone of normal material quality on trabecular surfaces and on the periosteal surface is needed.

From the rat studies performed to date, PTH has proved itself capable of increasing trabecular bone mass at all skeletal sites,[75-81] and of maintaining[86] or improving[93] trabecular connectivity. At the same time, PTH has proven itself capable of increasing cortical thickness by adding bone both at the endocortical surface and also at the biomechanically more important envelope: the periosteal surface.[92] Concomitantly, PTH has been able to increase bone structural strength and maintain material strength at all skeletal sites tested.[81-90] Furthermore, in large animal models (primates and ferrets),[94,95] PTH has been shown to increase bone mass with a concomitant increase in bone strength.

Assessed on the basis of these preclinical studies, intermittently administered PTH seems to satisfy all the requirements for a powerful anabolic agent in the treatment of osteoporosis. However, before extensive clinical trials are conducted, several issues concerning PTH should be addressed in preclinical trials:

1. PTH needs to be tested more extensively in larger animal models with intracortical bone remodeling.
2. Further studies are required to assess the frequency at which PTH should be administered (are daily intervals needed, or will less frequent therapy suffice?).
3. Studies concerning more user-friendly dosing regimens are needed.

Based on preclinical studies performed mainly in rats, but also in ferrets and primates, it is concluded that intermittent PTH therapy seems promising in osteoporosis management. PTH is capable of increasing bone mass at all four envelopes: cancellous, endocortical, intracortical, and periosteal. Concomitantly, bone structural strength is increased during PTH therapy. All skeletal sites (vertebrae, tibial metaphyseal and cortical bone, femoral cortical bone, and femoral necks) are affected equally positively during treatment. Furthermore, all animal models: young, growing intact rats; mature ovariectomized rats; orchidectomized rats; aged, osteopenic rats; primates; and ferrets have responded in an equally positive manner.

REFERENCES

1. Mosekilde, Li., Sex differences in age-related loss of vertebral trabecular bone mass and structure — biomechanical consequences, *Bone*, 10, 425, 1989.
2. Schmorl, G. and Junghanns H., Development, growth, anatomy and function of the spine, in *The Human Spine in Health and Disease II*, Besemann, E. F., Ed., Grune and Stratton, New York and London, 1971.
3. Block, J. E., Genant, H. K., and Black, D., Greater vertebral bone mineral mass in exercising young men, *West. J. Med.*, 145, 39, 1986.
4. Pead, M. J., Skerry, T. M., and Lanyon, L. E., Direct transformation from quiescence to bone formation in the adult periosteum following a single brief period of bone loading, *J. Bone Min. Res.*, 3, 647, 1988.
5. Ruff, C. B. and Hayes, W. C., Sex differences in age-related remodeling of the femur and tibia, *J. Orthop. Res.*, 6, 886, 1988.
6. Eastell, R., Mosekilde, Li., Hodgson, S. F., and Riggs, B. L., Proportion of human vertebral body bone that is cancellous, *J. Bone Min. Res.*, 5, 1237, 1990.
7. Nottestad, S. Y., Baumel, J. J., Kimmel, D. B., Recker, R. R., and Heaney, R. P., The properties of trabecular bone in human vertebrae, *J. Bone Min. Res.*, 2, 221, 1987.
8. Mosekilde, Li. and Mosekilde, Le., Normal vertebral body size and compressive strength: Relations to age and to vertebral and iliac trabecular bone compressive strength, *Bone*, 7, 207, 1986.
9. Rockoff, S. D., Sweet, E., and Bleustein J., The relative contribution of trabecular and cortical bone to the strength of human lumbar vertebrae, *Calcif. Tissue Res.*, 3, 163, 1969.
10. Mosekilde, Li., Normal age-related changes in bone mass, structure and strength — consequences of the remodeling process. Thesis, Aarhus 1992, *Dan. Med. B.*, 1, 65, 1993.
11. Frost, H. M., The spinal osteoporoses. Mechanisms of pathogenesis and pathophysiology, *Clin. Endocrin. Metab.*, 2, 257, 1973.
12. Frost, H. M., A determinant of bone architecture. The minimum effective strain. *Clin. Orthop. Rel. Res.*, 175, 286, 1983.
13. Frost, H. M., Editorial: The mechanostat: a proposed pathogenic mechanism of osteoporosis and the bone mass effects of mechanical and nonmechanical agents, *Bone Miner.*, 2, 73, 1987.
14. Vesterby, A., Mosekilde, Li., Gundersen, H. J. G., Melsen, F., Mosekilde, Le., Holme, K., and Sørensen, L., Biologically meaningful determinants of the in vitro strength of lumbar vertebra, *Bone*, 12, 219, 1991.
15. Hansson, T. and Roos, B., The relation between bone mineral content, experimental compression fractures, and disc degeneration in lumbar vertebrae, *Spine*, 6, 147, 1981.
16. Mosekilde, Li., Age-related changes in vertebral trabecular bone architecture — Assessed by a new method, *Bone*, 9, 247, 1988.
17. Kazarian, L. and Graves, G. A., Compressive strength characteristics of the human vertebral centrum, *Spine*, 2, 1, 1977.
18. Eriksen, E. F., Mosekilde, Le., and Melsen F., Trabecular bone resorption depth decreases with age: Differences between normal males and females, *Bone*, 6, 141, 1985.
19. Eriksen, E. F., Normal and pathological remodeling of human trabecular bone: Three dimensional reconstruction of the remodeling sequence in normals and in metabolic bone disease, *Endocrine Reviews*, 7, 379, 1986.
20. Mosekilde, Li. and Mosekilde, Le., Sex differences in age-related changes in vertebral body size, density and biomechanical competence in normal individuals, *Bone*, 11, 67, 1990.
21. Steiniche, T., Hasling, C., Charles, P., Eriksen, E. F., Mosekilde, Le., and Melsen, F., A randomized study on the effects of estrogen/gestagen or high dose oral calcium on trabecular bone remodeling in postmenopausal osteoporosis, *Bone*, 10, 313, 1989.
22. Thomsen, J. S., Mosekilde, Li., Boyce, R. W., and Mosekilde, E., Stochastic simulation of vertebral trabecular bone remodeling, *Bone*, 15, 655, 1994.

23. Bell, G. H., Dunbar, O., Beck, J. S., and Gibb, A., Variations in strength of vertebrae with age and their relation to osteoporosis, *Calcif. Tissue Res.*, 1, 75, 1967.
24. Mosekilde, Li., Mosekilde, Le., and Danielsen, C. C., Biomechanical competence of vertebral trabecular bone in relation to ash density and age in normal individuals, *Bone*, 8, 79, 1987.
25. Mosekilde, Li., Consequences of the remodelling process for vertebral trabecular bone structure — A scanning electron microscopy study (uncoupling of unloaded structures), *Bone Miner.*, 10, 13, 1990.
26. Parfitt, A. M., Trabecular bone architecture in the pathogenesis and prevention of fracture, *Am. J. Med.*, 82, 68, 1987.
27. Parfitt., A. M., Bone remodeling: Relationship to the amount and structure of bone, and the pathogenesis and prevention of fractures, in *Osteoporosis: Etiology, Diagnosis and Management*, Riggs, B. L. and Melton L. J. III, Eds., Raven Press, New York, 1988, 45.
28. Vernon-Roberts, B. and Pirie, C. J., Healing trabecular microfractures in the bodies of lumbar vertebrae, *Ann. Rheum. Dis.*, 32, 406, 1973.
29. Krølner, B., Osteoporosis and normality: how to express the bone mineral content of lumbar vertebrae, *Clin. Physiol.*, 2, 139, 1982.
30. Gilsanz, V., Loro, M. L., Roe, T. F., Sayre, J., Gilsanz, R., and Schulz, E. E., Vertebral size in elderly women with osteoporosis: Mechanical implications and relationship to fractures, *J. Clin. Invest.*, 95, 2332, 1995.
31. Chalmers, J. and Weaver, J. K., Cancellous bone: Its strength and changes with aging and an evaluation of some methods for measuring its mineral content, *J. Bone Jt. Surg.*, 48-A, 299, 1966.
32. Weaver, J. K. and Chalmers J., Cancellous bone: Its strength and changes with aging and an evaluation of some methods for measuring its mineral content, *J. Bone Jt. Surg.*, 48-A, 289, 1966.
33. Krølner, B., Lumbar spine bone mineral content by dual photon beam absorptiometry, methodology and application in osteoporosis. Thesis, *Dan. Med. B.*, 32, 152, 1985.
34. Compston, J. E., Editorial: Bone density: BMC, BMD, or corrected BMD?, *Bone*, 16, 5, 1995
35. Jergas, M., Breitenseher, M., Gluër, C.-C., Yu, W., and Genant, H. K., Estimates of volumetric bone density from projectional measurements improve the discriminatory capability of dual X-ray absorptiometry, *J. Bone Min. Res.*, 10, 1101, 1995.
36. Adami, S. and Kanis, J. A., Perspectives: Assessment of involutional bone loss: Methodological and conceptual problems, *J. Bone Min. Res.*, 10, 511, 1995.
37. Cann, C. E., Quantitative CT for determination of bone mineral density: A review, *Radiology*, 166, 509, 1988.
38. Jones, C. D., Laval-Jeantet, A.-M., Laval-Jeantet, M. H., and Genant, H. K., Importance of measurement of spongious vertebral bone mineral density in the assessment of osteoporosis, *Bone*, 8, 201, 1987.
39. Kalendar, W. A., Felsenberg, D., Louis, O., Lopez, P., Klotz, E., Osteaux, M., and Fraga, J., Reference values for trabecular and cortical vertebral bone density in single and dual-energy quantitative computed tomography, *Europ. J. Rad.*, 9, 75, 1989.
40. Biggemann, M., Hilweg, D., and Brinkmann, P., Prediction of the compressive strength of vertebral bodies of the lumbar spine by quantitative computed tomography, *Skeletal Radiol.*, 17, 264, 1988.
41. Brinkmann P., Biggemann, M., and Hilweg, D., Prediction of the compressive strength of human lumbar vertebrae, *Spine*, 14, 606, 1989.
42. Chevalier, F., Laval-Jeantet, A. M., Laval-Jeantet, M., and Bergot, C., CT image analysis of the vertebral trabecular network in vivo, *Calcif. Tissue Int.*, 51, 8, 1992.
43. McBroom, R.J., Hayes, W.C., Edwards, W.T., Goldberg, W. P., and White, A.A., Prediction of vertebral body compressive fracture using quantitative computed tomography, *J. Bone Joint Surg.*, 67A, 1206, 1985.

44. Ørtoft, G., Mosekilde, Li., Hasling, C., and Mosekilde, Le., Estimation of vertebral body strength by dual photon absorptiometry in elderly individuals: Comparison between measurements of total vertebral and vertebral body mineral, *Bone*, 14, 667, 1993.
45. Mosekilde, Li., Bentzen, S., Ørtoft, G., and Jørgensen, J., The predictive value of quantitative computed tomography for vertebral body compressive strength and ash density, *Bone*, 10, 465, 1989.
46. Davies, K. M., Recker, R. R., and Heaney, R. P., Normal vertebral dimensions and normal variation in serial measurements of vertebrae, *J. Bone Min. Res.*, 4, 341, 1989.
47. Kleerekoper, M., Parfitt, A. M., and Ellis, B. I., Measurement of the vertebral fracture rate in osteoporosis, in *Osteoporosis I*, Christiansen, C., Arnaud, C. D., Nordin, B. E. C., Parfitt, A. M., Peck, W. A., and Riggs, B. L. Eds., Aalborg Stiftsbogtrykkeri, Denmark, 1984, p. 103.
48. Melton, L. J. III, Kan, S. H., Frye, M. A., Wahner, H. W., O'Fallon, M., and Riggs, B. L., Epidemiology of vertebral fractures in pathological rarefaction of bone, *Clin. Endocrin. Metab.*, 2, 239, 1989.
49. Hedlund, L. R. and Gallagher, J. C., Vertebral morphometry in diagnosis of spinal fractures, *Bone Miner.*, 5, 59, 1988.
50. Sauer, P., Leidig, G., Minne, H. W., Duckeck, G., Schwartz, W., Siromachkostov, L., and Ziegler, R., Spine deformity index (SDI) versus other objective procedures of vertebral fracture identification in patients with osteoporosis: A comparative study, *J. Bone Min. Res.*, 6, 227, 1991.
51. National Osteoporosis Foundation Working Group on Vertebral Fractures. Report — Assessing vertebral fractures, *J. Bone Min. Res.*, 10, 518, 1995.
52. Kleerekoper, M., Villanueva, A. R., Stanciu, J., Rao, D. S., and Parfitt, A. M., The role of three dimensional trabecular microstructure in the pathogenesis of vertebral compression fractures, *Calcif. Tissue Int.*, 37, 594, 1985.
53. Compston, J. E., Mellish, R. W. E., and Garrahan, N. J., Age-related changes in the iliac crest trabecular microanatomic bone structure in man, *Bone*, 8, 289, 1987.
54. Garrahan, N. J., Croucher, P. I., Wright, C., and Compston, J. E., A computerised technique for the quantitative assessment of resorption cavities in trabecular bone, *Bone*, 11, 241, 1990.
55. Thomsen, J. S., Barlach, J., and Mosekilde, Li., Determination of connectivity density in human iliac crest bone biopsies assessed by a computerized method, *Bone*, 18, 459, 1996.
56. Mosekilde, Li., Viidik, A., and Mosekilde, Le., Correlation between the compressive strength of iliac and vertebral trabecular bone in normal individuals, *Bone*, 6, 291, 1985.
57. Søgaard, C. H., Mosekilde, Li., Richards, A., and Mosekilde, Le., Marked decrease in trabecular bone quality after five years of sodium fluoride therapy — Assessed by biomechanical testing of iliac crest bone biopsies in osteoporotic patients, *Bone*, 15, 393, 1994.
58. Mosekilde, Le. and Mosekilde, Li., Iliac crest trabecular bone compressive strength and ash weight is increased in moderate hyperparathyroidism. Abstract. Niigata, Japan, 1988.
59. Granhed, A., Jonson, R., and Hansson, T., Mineral content and strength of lumbar vertebrae, *Acta Orthop. Scand.*, 60, 105, 1989.
60. Eriksson, S. A. V., Isberg, B. O., and Lindgren, J. U., Prediction of vertebral strength by dual photon absorptiometry and quantitative computed tomography, *Calcif. Tissue Int.*, 44, 243, 1989.
61. Mosekilde, Li., Assessing bone quality in animal models, *Bone*, 17, S343, 1995.
62. Kalu, D. N., The ovariectomized rat model of postmenopausal bone loss, *Bone Miner.*, 15, 175, 1991.
63. Frost, H. M. and Jee, W. S. S., On the rat model of human osteoporoses, *Bone Miner.*, 18, 227, 1992.

64. Jerome, C. P., Carlson, C. S., Register, T. C., Bain, F. T., Jayo, M. J., Weaver, D. S., and Adams, M. R., Bone functional changes in intact, ovariectomized, and ovariectomized, hormone-supplemented adult cynomolgus monkeys (*Macaca fascicularis*) evaluated by serum markers and dynamic histomorphometry, *J. Bone Min. Res.*, 9, 527, 1994.
65. Mosekilde, Li., Weisbrode, S. E., Safron, J. A., Stills, H F., Jankowsky, M. L., Ebert, D. C., Danielsen, C. C., Søgaard, C. H., Franks, A. F., Stevens, M. L., Paddock, C. L., and Boyce, R. W., Evaluation of the skeletal effects of combined mild dietary calcium restriction and ovariectomy in Sinclair S-1 Minipigs: a pilot study, *J. Bone Min. Res.*, 8, 1311, 1993.
66. Boyce, R. W., Ebert, D. C., Youngs, T. L., Paddock, C. L., Mosekilde, Li., Stevens, M., L., and Gundersen, H. J., Unbiased estimation of vertebral trabecular connectivity or trabecular number in calcium-restricted ovariectomized Sinclair S-1 minipigs, *Bone*, 16, 637, 1995.
67. Podbesek, R., Edouard, C., Meunier, P. J., Parsons, J. A., Reeve, J., Stevenson, R. W., and Zanelli, J. M., Effects of two treatment regimes with synthetic human parathyroid hormone fragment on bone formation and the tissue balance of trabecular bone in greyhounds, *Endocrinology*, 112, 1000, 1983.
68. Turner, A. S., Mallinckrodt, C. H., Alvis, M. R., and Bryant, H. U., Dose-response effects of estradiol implants om bone mineral density in ovariectomized ewes, *Bone*, 17, 421S, 1995.
69. McOsker, J. E., Mackey, M. S., Tressler, D. L., Depew, C. S., and Ebert, D. C., Efficacy of risedronate for prevention of bone loss in the ovariectomized ferret, *Calcif. Tissue Int.*, 56, 492, 1995.
70. Frost, H. M., Gasser, J. A., High, W. B., Jee, W. S. S., Jerome, C., Mosekilde, Li., and Thompson, D. D., Editorial: Perspectives on osteoporosis research: Its focus and some insights from a new paradigm, *Calcif. Tissue Int.*, 57, 399, 1995.
71. Harris, S. T., Genant, H. K., Baylink, D. J., Gallagher, J. C., Karp, S. K., McConnell, M. A., Green, E. M., and Stoll, R. W., The effects of estrogen on spinal bone density of postmenopausal women, *Arch. Intern. Med.*, 151, 1980. 1991.
72. Reginster, J.- Y., Management of high turnover osteoporosis with calcitonin, *Bone*, 13, S37, 1992.
73. Thamsborg, G., Storm, T. L., Sykluski, R., Nielsen, H. K., and Sørensen, O. H., Effect of different doses of nasal salmon calcitonin on bone mass, *Calcif. Tissue Int.*, 48, 302, 1991.
74. Overgaard, K., Hansen, M. A., Jensen, S. B., and Christiansen, C., Effect of calcitonin given intranasally on bone mass and fracture rates in established osteoporosis: a dose-response study, *Br. Med. J.*, 305, 556, 1992.
75. Hefti, E., Trechsel, U., Bonjour, J. P., Fleisch, H., and Schenk, R., Increase of whole body calcium and skeletal mass in normal and osteoporotic adult rats treated with parathyroid hormone, *Clinical Science*, 62, 389, 1982.
76. Gunness-Hey, M. and Hock, J. M., Increased trabecular bone mass in rats treated with human synthetic parathyroid hormone, *Metab. Bone Dis. & Rel. Res.*, 5, 177, 1984.
77. Liu, C. C and Kalu, D. N., Human parathyroid hormone — (1-34) prevents bone loss and augments bone formation in sexually mature ovariectomized rats, *J. Bone Min. Res.*, 5, 973, 1990.
78. Liu, C. C., Kalu, D. N., Salerno, E., Echon, R., Hollis, B. W., and Ray, M., Pre-existing bone loss associated with ovariectomy in rats is reversed by parathyroid hormone, *J. Bone Min. Res.*, 6, 1071, 1991.
79. Hock, J. M., Gera, I., Fonseca, J., and Raisz, L. G., Human parathyroid hormone-(1-34) increases bone mass in ovariectomized and orchidectomized rats, *Endocrinology*, 122, 2899, 1988.
80. Kalu, D. N., Echon, R., and Hollis, B. V., Modulation of ovariectomy-related bone loss by parathyroid hormone in rats, *Mech. Ageing Dev.*, 56, 49, 1990.

81. Mosekilde, Li., Søgaard, C. H., Danielsen, C. C., Tørring, O., and Nilsson, M. H. L., The anabolic effect of human parathyroid hormone (hPTH) on rat vertebral body mass are also reflected in the quality of bone, assessed by biomechanical testing: A comparison study between hPTH(1-34) and hPTH(1-84), *Endocrinology*, 129, 421, 1991.
82. Ejersted, C., Andreassen, T. T., Oxlund, H., Jørgensen, P. H., Bak, B., Häggblad, J., Tørring, O., and Nilsson, M. H. L., Human parathyroid hormone (1-34) and (1-84) increase the mechanical strength and thickness of cortical bone in rats, *J. Bone Min. Res.*, 9, 1097, 1993.
83. Mosekilde, Li., Søgaard, C. H., McOsker, J. E., and Wronski, T. J., PTH has a more pronounced effect on vertebral bone mass and biomechanical competence than antiresorptive agents (estrogen and bisphosphonate) — assessed in sexually mature, ovariectomized rats, Bone, 15, 401, 1994.
84. Mosekilde, Li., Danielsen, C. C., Søgaard, C. H., McOsker, J. E., and Wronski, T. J., The anabolic effects of parathyroid hormone on cortical bone mass and strength — Assessed in a sexually mature, ovariectomized rat model, *Bone*, 16, 223, 1995.
85. Søgaard, C. H., Wronski, T. J., McOsker, J. E., and Mosekilde, Li., The positive effect of parathyroid hormone on femoral neck bone strength in ovariectomized rats is more pronounced than that of estrogen or bisphosphonates, *Endocrinology*, 134, 650, 1994.
86. Mosekilde, Li., Danielsen, C. C., and Gasser, J. A., The effect on vertebral bone mass and strength of long term treatment with antiresorptive agents (Estrogen and Calcitonin), human parathyroid hormone-(1-38), and combination therapy, assessed in aged ovariectomized rats, *Endocrinology*, 135, 2126, 1994.
87. Mosekilde, Li., Danielsen, C. C., and Gasser J. A., Unpublished data, 1994.
88. Tam, C. S., Heersche, J. N. M., Murray, T. M., and Parsons, J. A., Parathyroid hormone stimulates the bone apposition rate independently of its resorptive action: Differential effects of intermittent and continuous administration, *Endocrinology*, 110, 506, 1982.
89. Hock, J. M., Hummert, J. R., Boyce, R., Fonseca, J., and Raisz, L. G., Resorption is not essential for the stimulation of bone growth by hPTH-(1-34) in rats in vivo, *J. Bone Min. Res.*, 449, 1989.
90. Li, M., Mosekilde, Li., Søgaard, C H., Thomsen, J. S., and Wronski, T. J., Parathyroid hormone monotherapy and cotherapy with antiresorptive agents restore vertebral bone mass and strength in aged ovariectomized rats, *Bone*, 16, 629, 1995.
91. Wronski, T. J., Yen, C.-F., Qi, H., and Dann, L. M., Parathyroid hormone is more effective than estrogen or bisphosphonates for restoration of lost bone mass in ovariectomized rats. *Endocrinology*, 132, 823, 1993.
92. Wronski, T. J. and Yen C.-F., Anabolic effects of parathyroid hormone on cortical bone in ovariectomized rats, *Bone*, 15, 51, 1994.
93. Shen, V., Dempster, D. W., Birchman, R., Xu, R., and Lindsay, R., Loss of cancellous bone mass and connectivity in ovariectomized rats can be restored by combined treatment with parathyroid hormone and estradiol, *J. Clin. Invest.*, 91, 2479, 1993.
94. Jerome, C., Mosekilde, Li., and Thomsen, J. S., Unpublished data, 1996.
95. Mosekilde, Li., Thomsen, J. S., and McOsker, J. E., Unpublished data, 1996.
96. Riggs, B. L., Hodgson, S. F., O'Fallon, W.M., Chao, E. Y. S., Wahner, H. W., Muhs, J. M., Cedel, S. L., and Melton, L. J., Effect of fluoride treatment on the fracture rate in postmenopausal women with osteoporosis, *N. Engl. J. Med.*, 322, 802, 1990.
97. Kleerekoper, M., Peterson, E., Philips, E., Nelson, D., Tilley, B., and Parfitt, A. M., Continuous sodium fluoride therapy does not reduce vertebral fracture rate in postmenopausal osteoporosis, *J. Bone Min. Res.*, 4 (Suppl. 1), S376, 1989.
98. Mosekilde, Li., Kragstrup, J., and Richards, A., Compressive strength, ash weight, and volume of vertebral trabecular bone in experimental fluorosis in pigs, *Calcif. Tissue Int.*, 40, 318, 1987.

99. Søgaard, C. H., Mosekilde, Li., Richards, A., and Mosekilde, Le., Marked decrease in trabecular bone quality after five years of sodium fluoride therapy — assessed by biomechanical testing of iliac crest bone biopsies in osteoporotic patients, *Bone*, 15, 393, 1994.
100. Søgaard, C. H., Mosekilde, Li., Schwartz, W., Leidig, G., Minne, H. W., and Ziegler, R., Effects of fluoride on rat vertebral body biomechanical competence and bone mass, *Bone*, 16, 163, 1995.

Chapter 3

PTH: Skeletal Effects in the Ovariectomized Rat Model for Postmenopausal Bone Loss

Thomas J. Wronski and Mei Li

CONTENTS

0-8493-8556-3/98/$0.00+$.50

I. INTRODUCTION

PTH has traditionally been considered a bone catabolic hormone due to its well-known role in calcium homeostasis of increasing serum calcium through a stimulatory effect on bone resorption.[1] PTH was also hypothesized to be involved in the pathogenesis of postmenopausal osteoporosis in that the skeleton was thought to be more sensitive to the catabolic actions of PTH in the estrogen-deplete state.[2,3] In view of these concepts, it is somewhat surprising that PTH is currently being investigated as a therapy for postmenopausal osteoporosis. However, in contrast to its more widely known bone catabolic effects, PTH has also been reported to have anabolic effects on the skeleton. The first such report was published in 1932 by Selye.[4] His initial findings in intact rats have since been confirmed by many investigators who detected substantial increases in bone mass in rats treated intermittently with PTH.[5-12] Since agents with an anabolic effect on bone are rare, it is important to evaluate the therapeutic potential of PTH for osteoporosis. As an essential step in this process, the skeletal effects of PTH should be thoroughly characterized in the ovariectomized (OVX) rat, a widely used animal model for postmenopausal bone loss.[13,14] The results of these studies are summarized below.

II. TREATMENT PROTOCOLS

An investigator has a choice of the PTH holoprotein or several of its fragments in performing preclinical studies with the hormone. Experimental animals are treated most frequently and effectively with the 1-34 fragment of synthetic hPTH.[5-12] However, the holoproteins hPTH (1-84) and bPTH (1-84) as well as the fragment hPTH (1-38) also have strong skeletal effects.[5,6,9,11] PTH-related protein (PTHrP) 1-34 was found to increase cancellous bone mass somewhat in intact rats,[15] but this anabolic response was less pronounced than that of hPTH (1-34). On the other hand, an analog of PTHrP (1-34), RS-23581, has been reported to increase osteoblast numbers and cancellous bone mass to the same extent as hPTH (1-34) in OVX rats.[16] (See Chapter 6.) Another PTH analog with outstanding potential is hPTH (1-31)NH_2, which stimulates adenylate cyclase but not protein kinase C or phospholipase Cβ. This analog markedly increased cancellous bone mass in the distal femur of OVX rats to the same extent as hPTH (1-34).[17] (See Chapter 5.) Other analogs of hPTH (1-34) that may be bone selective are being developed and tested in an effort to maintain the bone anabolic effects of the hormone while minimizing the potential for side effects.[18]

It is well established that augmentation of bone mass by PTH is dependent on an intermittent mode of administration. Both continuous and intermittent treatment of intact rats with PTH increase bone formation.[6,19] However, continuous PTH treatment increases bone resorption to the same or a greater extent so that bone mass is either unchanged or even decreased.[6,19] In contrast, intermittent treatment with the hormone via sc injections markedly stimulates bone formation to a greater extent than bone resorption and augments bone mass.[5-12] This phenomenon is not specific to the rat because it has also been observed in intact dogs treated with PTH.[20] Regarding frequency of administration, the bone anabolic effects of PTH reported by Hock and colleagues in intact and OVX rats were induced by daily sc injections of the hormone.[7,8,15,19,21] However, such frequent treatment does not appear to be necessary because subsequent studies have detected strong skeletal effects in rats treated for 3 or 5 days per week with PTH.[22-28]

Regarding dose, rats have been treated with hPTH (1-34) at doses ranging from 0.5 to 1000 μg/kg body weight. The most commonly used dose that certainly induces a powerful bone anabolic effect is 80 μg/kg,[7-9,16,21,25,29-31] but similar effects have been observed in cancellous bone of rats treated with 30 to 60 μg/kg of PTH.[24,26-28,32,33] Shen et al.[34] used a low dose of PTH (2.5 μg/kg) in OVX rats to be consistent with the dose used in clinical trials in osteoporotic patients. Although this low dose of the hormone stimulated bone formation somewhat and partially restored lost bone in OVX rats, the observed skeletal effects were not nearly as strong as those in OVX rats treated with moderate doses of PTH. High doses of the hormone (400 to 1000 μg/kg) also have a strong bone anabolic effect, but some of the newly formed bone is woven rather than lamellar in nature.[11,23] Marrow fibrosis is another potential undesirable side effect of treatment with high doses of PTH.[23] In any case, the proper dose of hPTH (1-34) for treatment of intact or OVX rats appears to be 30 to 80 μg/kg. This dose should be administered intermittently by sc injections at least 3 times per week. Of course, the recommended dose and regimen of PTH are dependent on the use of a peptide of high purity and potency.

III. EFFECTS OF PTH ON CANCELLOUS BONE IN OVX RATS

During the early stages of estrogen depletion, OVX rats exhibit rapid cancellous bone loss associated with increased bone turnover (i.e., a generalized increase in both bone resorption and formation).[13,14] These skeletal events are consistent with bone changes in oophorectomized and early postmenopausal women.[35,36] The first studies with PTH in OVX rats focused on the ability of the hormone to prevent bone loss in these estrogen-deplete animals. Treatment with PTH soon after ovariectomy was found to provide at least complete protection against the development of osteopenia.[21,29,37] In fact, the hormone was capable of increasing cancellous bone mass in OVX rats to a level greater than that of sham-operated control rats.[29] The mechanism for the observed bone-protective effect of PTH obviously involved a stimulation of bone formation as both osteoblast numbers and fluorochrome-based variables were found to be markedly increased in PTH-treated OVX rats.[29] Somewhat surprisingly, the hormone was also found to decrease osteoclast numbers and tartrate-resistant acid phosphatase (TRAP) positive, multinucleated cells in OVX rats.[29,38] These findings suggest that PTH inhibited bone resorption as well as stimulated bone formation in OVX rats. In view of these desirable effects on bone resorption and formation, it is small wonder that PTH-treated OVX rats exhibited a positive bone balance without loss of cancellous bone.

Despite these encouraging findings, there is little reason to develop PTH as a preventive measure for early postmenopausal bone loss. The antiresorptive agents estrogen and bisphosphonates are capable of depressing bone turnover and maintaining normal bone mass in postmenopausal women at a fraction of the cost of PTH and with a more convenient route of administration (oral vs. sc injection). For these reasons, the great majority of the more recent studies have focused on the ability of PTH to restore lost cancellous bone in osteopenic OVX rats. These studies as well as the prevention studies referred to above are summarized in Table 3.1. OVX rats were allowed to develop cancellous osteopenia in their long bones for at least 2 weeks postovariectomy before initiating PTH treatment. The hormone was found by many investigators to restore lost cancellous bone completely in the osteopenic long bones and vertebrae of OVX rats.[17,22-28,30-33,39-43] The only studies that failed to confirm this finding involved use of a very low dose of PTH or a short treatment period. Although there is some evidence for a plateau in the augmentation of cancellous bone mass by PTH,[31,44] such a plateau is not evident in OVX rats until their cancellous bone mass well exceeds that of age-matched control rats. The ability of PTH to completely restore lost cancellous bone in osteopenic OVX rats is seen in Figure 3.1.

Regarding the effects of PTH on trabecular microarchitecture, the hormone is consistently found to increase trabecular thickness and decrease trabecular separation in osteopenic OVX rats to at least the levels of sham-operated control rats.[18,26,32,33,43] Some investigators have also reported trabecular number to be increased somewhat in PTH-treated OVX rats,[28,34] but this has not been a consistent finding.[18,26,33,41,43] Furthermore, trabecular number, in contrast to trabecular thickness, has never been reported to be restored to control levels in osteopenic OVX rats treated with PTH.[28,34] Therefore, the major process by which PTH restores lost cancellous bone in OVX rats appears to be a widening of existing trabeculae (Figure 3.1). This beneficial skeletal effect of the hormone may result in some improvement in trabecular connectivity in osteopenic OVX rats.[32] However, Lane et al.[26] reported that PTH failed to improve trabecular connectivity in OVX rats that had lost more than 50% of their cancellous

TABLE 3.1

Effects of PTH 1-34 on Cancellous Bone in OVX Rats

Age at OVX (mo)	Age at Sacrifice (mo)	PTH Dose (μg/kg)	Treatment Duration	Treatment Frequency	Bone Mass[a]	Bone Resorption[b]	Bone Formation[c]	Reference
1	1.5	80	12 d	daily	↑	NM	NM	21
2.5	9	1.5	25 wk	3×/wk	NC	NC	NC	22
		6			↑	↑	↑	
3	6	30	8 wk	3×/wk	↑	NC	↑	28
3	6	30	12 wk	3×/wk	↑	NC	↑	24
3	5	80	5 wk	6×/wk	↑	NC	↑	31
	6.5		10 wk		↑	↓	↑	
	7.5		15 wk		↑	↑	↑	
3	5	80	3 wk	daily	↑	↓	↑	30
3	17.5	80	10 wk	5×/wk	↑	NC	↑	25, 50
3	4	80, 160	5 wk	daily	↑	↓	↑	29
3	4	80	19 d	daily	↑	NM	↑	16
3	4.5	50	4 wk	5×/wk	↑	NM	↑	27
4	6	2.5	4 wk	daily	↑	NC	↑	34
4	5.5–6	20	1, 2 wk	6×/wk	NC	NC	↑	41
	6–7		3, 4, 6 wk		↑	NC	↑	
	7.5		8 wk		↑	↓	NC	
5	7	40	4 wk	daily	↑	NC	↑	32
5	12	8.3, 25, 75, 225	15 wk	daily	↑	NM	NM	42[d]

TABLE 3.1 *(continued)*

Effects of PTH 1-34 on Cancellous Bone in OVX Rats

Age at OVX (mo)	Age at Sacrifice (mo)	PTH Dose (μg/kg)	Treatment Duration	Treatment Frequency	Bone Mass[a]	Bone Resorption[b]	Bone Formation[c]	Reference
6	9	4	1 mo	5×/wk	NC	NC	↑	18, 26
		40, 400			↑	↓	↑	
6	8.5	0.55	4 wk	daily	NC	NC	NC	33
		5.5, 55			↑	NC	↑	
6	10	20	3 wk	5×/wk	↑	↑	↑	49
12	20	100	6 mo	5×/wk	↑	NM	NM	40[e]
12	24.5	160	2 wk	daily	↑	NC	↑	39
16	16–17	80	1 wk	daily	NC	NM	↑	45

Abbreviations: NC, no change; NM, not measured.

[a] Bone mass: cancellous bone volume, trabecular bone calcium content, or bone mineral density of vertebra or cancellous bone-enriched regions of long bones.

[b] Bone resorption: osteoclast or eroded surface.

[c] Bone formation: osteoblast surface, osteoid surface, or bone formation rate (tissue or surface referent).

[d] Rats were treated with hPTH 1-84 rather than hPTH (1-34).

[e] Rats were treated with hPTH 1-38 rather than hPTH (1-34).

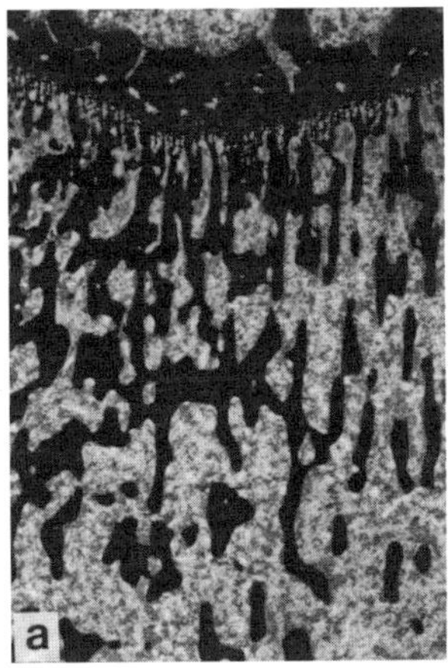

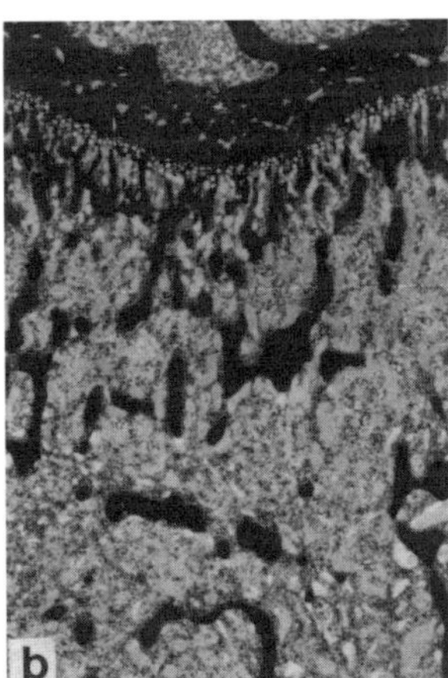

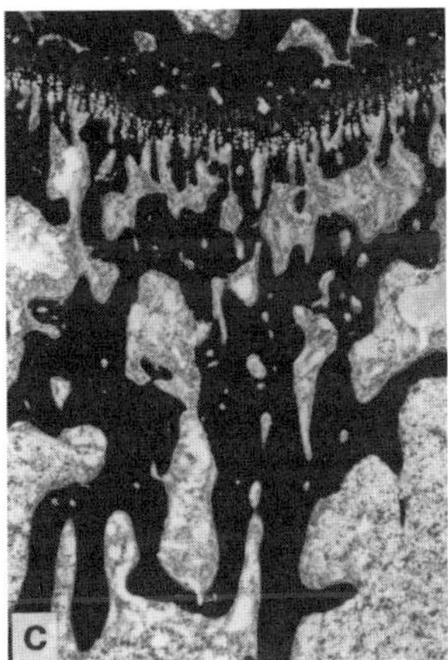

Figure 3.1
Proximal tibial metaphyses from a sham-operated control rat (a) and an osteopenic OVX rat (b) prior to the beginning of PTH treatment. Note the reduced mass of darkly stained cancellous bone indicative of moderate cancellous osteopenia in the OVX animal. In the proximal tibial metaphysis from an OVX rat treated for 5 weeks with PTH (c), the hormone completely restored lost cancellous bone as the greatly thickened bone spicules are obvious. (From Wronski, T. J., Yen, C.-F., Qi, H., and Dann, L. M., Parathyroid hormone is more effective than estrogen or bisphosphonates for restoration of lost bone mass in ovariectomized rats, *Endocrinology*, 132, 823, 1993. With permission.)

bone mass. Therefore, the ability of PTH to restore trabecular connectivity may be limited by the severity of the osteopenia that develops before treatment.

The obvious increase in cancellous bone mass in PTH-treated OVX rats suggests that the hormone markedly stimulates bone formation. Histomorphometric analyses confirmed this impression. Cellular indices of bone formation, such as osteoblast number and surface, were found to be increased several-fold by PTH treatment.[16,22,25,27,30,31,33,41,45] In addition, marked increases in dynamic, fluorochrome-based indices of bone formation such as mineralizing surface, mineral apposition rate, and bone formation rate were detected in OVX rats treated with PTH.[22,25,27,28,30-34,39,41,45] This combination of cellular and fluorochrome-based data provides unequivocal evidence that PTH increases both the number and activity of osteoblasts. The PTH-induced increase in osteoblast numbers occurs within 5 to 7 days of the beginning of treatment.[16,45] This rapid response strongly implies that PTH induces bone formation on quiescent bone surfaces in OVX rats without the need for prior bone resorption, as was previously demonstrated by Hock et al. in intact rats.[46] Hodsman and Steer[47] reached a similar conclusion in their clinical study of PTH-treated osteoporotic patients. The powerful stimulatory effect of PTH on cancellous bone formation can be seen in Figure 3.2.

The cellular origin of the increased osteoblast numbers observed in PTH-treated rats is unclear. Nishida et al.[48] proposed that the osteoblast population of young intact rats treated with PTH increased due to enhanced proliferation and differentiation of osteoprogenitor cells in the bone marrow. In contrast, Dobnig and Turner[45] concluded from [^{3}H] thymidine labeling of aged intact and OVX rats that the PTH-induced osteoblasts originate from bone lining cells rather than osteoprogenitor cells. Their finding was confirmed by ultrastructural studies in younger OVX rats treated with two analogs of PTH, with the added observation that the PTH-induced osteoblasts revert to bone lining cells after cessation of PTH treatment.[16] It is important to resolve whether osteoprogenitor and/or bone lining cells contribute to the osteoblast pool in PTH-treated OVX rats since the two cell populations in question have very different proliferative potentials. For example, if bone lining cells with little or no proliferative ability are the primary source for PTH-induced osteoblasts, the anabolic effect of PTH would be limited by the number of pre-existing bone lining cells.[45] A plausible sequence of events in the bone microenvironment after exposure to PTH may involve an initial rapid conversion of bone lining cells to osteoblasts followed later by differentiation of marrow-derived osteoprogenitor cells into osteoblasts (see also Chapter 5).

In contrast to the well-established stimulatory effect of PTH on bone formation, the effects of the hormone on bone resorption in OVX rats are less clear. One of the weaknesses of bone histomorphometry is that, unlike bone formation rate, bone resorption rate is difficult to measure directly. Therefore, one must rely primarily on measurements of eroded surface or osteoclast number and surface as indices of bone resorption. As mentioned above, several studies on the prevention of bone loss in OVX rats have shown that PTH treatment decreases osteoclast number.[29,38] In studies designed to restore lost bone in osteopenic OVX rats, the consensus is that PTH has no effect on osteoclast variables (Table 3.1). However, the hormone has been reported to increase[22,31,49] and decrease[30,41] indices of

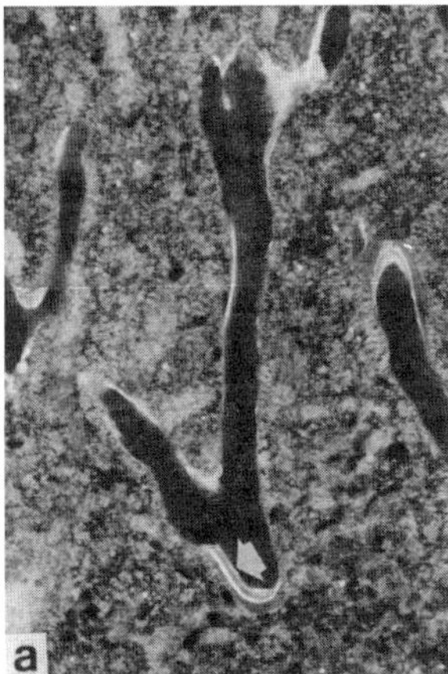

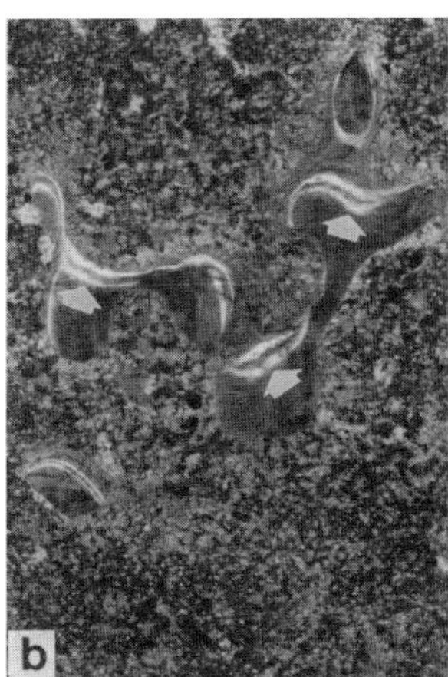

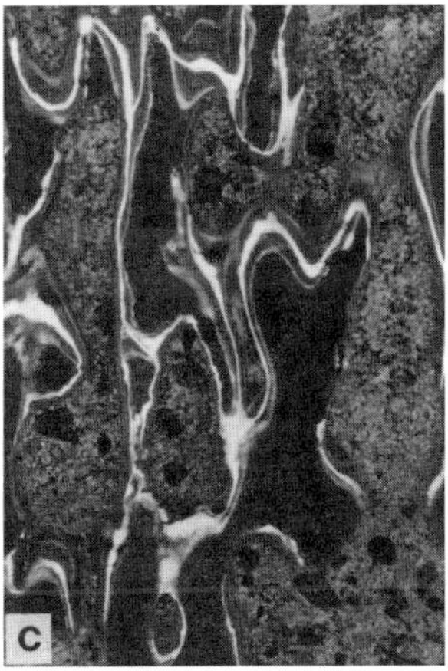

Figure 3.2
Cancellous bone tissue located 1 to 2 mm from the growth-plate metaphyseal junction in proximal tibial metaphyses from a sham-operated control rat (a) and an OVX rat (b) before PTH treatment. Note the increased incidence of double fluorochrome labels (arrows) indicative of increased bone formation in the untreated OVX rat compared to the control rat. In cancellous bone from a PTH-treated OVX rat (c), an even higher proportion of bone surfaces have double fluorochrome labels as the hormone markedly stimulated bone formation. (From Wronski, T. J., Yen, C.-F., Qi, H., and Dann, L. M., Parathyroid hormone is more effective than estrogen or bisphosphonates for restoration of lost bone mass in ovariectomized rats, *Endocrinology*, 132, 823, 1993. With permission.)

bone resorption in OVX rats. These conflicting results may be explained on the basis of temporal variations in the response of osteoclast surface to PTH. For example, PTH-treated OVX rats were found to have normal, decreased, and increased values for osteoclast surface at 5, 10, and 15 weeks of treatment with the hormone, respectively.[31] It is noteworthy that increased osteoclast variables were detected in PTH-treated OVX rats in studies involving long-term treatment (15 to 25 weeks) with the hormone.[22,31] Therefore, increased bone resorption may be a consequence of prolonged PTH treatment. In any case, the marked increase in cancellous bone mass in PTH-treated OVX rats indicates that bone formation far exceeds bone resorption to produce a positive bone balance during the early stages of PTH treatment.

Most of the above studies were performed in OVX rats that were 3 to 6 months of age at surgery. Furthermore, PTH treatment was initiated at relatively early times postovariectomy. The question arises whether the observed bone anabolic effects of PTH would be as pronounced when aged OVX rats are treated at later times postovariectomy. This important question was addressed by several investigators. Ibbotson et al.[39] reported that PTH stimulated bone formation and increased cancellous bone mass in the osteopenic lumbar vertebrae of OVX rats that were 2 years of age and one year postovariectomy at the beginning of treatment. PTH had a similar bone anabolic effect in OVX rats with vertebral osteopenia that were 15 months of age and one year postovariectomy at the beginning of treatment.[25] These findings suggest that the bone anabolic response to PTH in OVX rats is not dependent on age or stage of estrogen depletion.

A factor that does affect the ability of PTH to restore lost bone in OVX rats is the degree of cancellous osteopenia at the beginning of treatment. In aged OVX rats at one year postovariectomy, the proximal tibia is severely osteopenic with a cancellous bone volume of less than 5%.[25] In these same animals, the lumbar vertebral body and femoral neck are only moderately osteopenic with cancellous bone volumes of 20 to 25%.[25,50] Although PTH failed to restore lost cancellous bone completely in the severely osteopenic proximal tibia of aged OVX rats, the hormone was found to completely reverse cancellous bone loss in the moderately osteopenic lumbar vertebra and femoral neck.[25,50] The consensus of studies in both young and aged OVX rats is that PTH increases trabecular thickness considerably but does not have a major effect on trabecular number.[18,26,33,41,43,49] Therefore, the efficacy of PTH treatment may be compromised at a severely osteopenic skeletal site that lacks adequate numbers of cancellous bone spicules (with pre-existing bone surfaces) to serve as a template for new bone formation. In support of this contention, Zerwekh et al.[51] recently reported that osteoporotic patients with severe osteopenia do not respond as well as moderately osteopenic patients to another bone anabolic agent, sodium fluoride.

In summary, numerous investigators have found that PTH has a powerful anabolic effect on cancellous bone in OVX rats. The hormone completely protects against cancellous bone loss in the early estrogen-deplete state. More important, PTH can fully restore lost cancellous bone in osteopenic OVX rats, provided that the osteopenia is not too severe at the beginning of PTH treatment. The positive bone balance in PTH-treated

OVX rats is due primarily to a marked stimulatory effect on bone formation. These findings in an animal model of estrogen depletion, which are generally consistent with the results of clinical trials,[47,52-54] provide strong support for PTH as a promising therapy for postmenopausal osteoporosis.

IV. EFFECTS OF PTH ON CORTICAL BONE IN OVX RATS

In view of some reports from clinical studies that PTH augments cancellous bone at the expense of cortical bone,[55,56] an understanding of the effects of PTH on cortical bone is critical to the development of the hormone as an osteoporosis therapy. Unfortunately, the rat is not an optimal animal model for studies of the effects of a therapeutic agent on cortical bone since it normally lacks Haversian systems (osteons). Consequently, the rat cannot be used to determine whether PTH treatment increases intracortical porosity, as was recently reported to occur in intact dogs treated with PTH.[57] Furthermore, cortical bone loss develops slowly in OVX rats and is much less pronounced than cancellous bone loss. Therefore, it is difficult to perform studies in OVX rats with established cortical osteopenia. Nevertheless, the OVX rat can provide some insight into the responses of the periosteal and endocortical surfaces to PTH and the resulting changes in cortical bone mass. Studies of the effects of PTH on cortical bone in OVX rats are summarized in Table 3.2.

Similar to cancellous bone, PTH has been consistently found to augment cortical bone in OVX rats.[21,29,32,50,58-60] This finding is due primarily to a stimulatory effect of PTH on both periosteal and endocortical bone formation, as evidenced by highly significant increases in fluorochrome-based variables such as mineralizing surface and mineral apposition rate.[28,29,50,58,60] The osteoblast population along the endocortical surface as well as the size of individual endocortical osteoblasts have also been reported to increase in PTH-treated OVX rats.[29] In fact, the anabolic response to PTH is at least twofold greater at the endocortical surface of OVX rats compared to the periosteal surface.[29,58,60] Although the effects of PTH on cortical osteoclasts have not been studied extensively, Liu et al.[29] did report a marked decrease in endocortical osteoclast numbers in OVX rats treated with PTH. This finding, in combination with increased endocortical bone formation, is consistent with the PTH-induced decrease in medullary area of the tibial shaft.[29,58,60] In these studies that achieved a positive effect of PTH on cortical bone, OVX rats were treated with PTH at a dose of 80 μg/kg at least 5 times per week. In contrast, Takano et al.[28] reported that treatment of OVX rats with PTH 3 times per week at a dose of 30 μg/kg did not have a substantial anabolic effect on cortical bone as it did on cancellous bone. Therefore, the ability of PTH to augment cortical bone in OVX rats appears to be more dependent on dose and frequency of administration than is its ability to augment cancellous bone. Never-

TABLE 3.2

Effects of PTH 1-34 on Cortical Bone in OVX Rats

Age at OVX (mo)	Age at Sacrifice (mo)	PTH Dose (μg/kg)	Treatment Duration	Treatment Frequency	Bone Mass[a]	Bone Resorption[b]	Bone Formation[c]	Reference
1	1.5	80	12 d	daily	↑	NM	NM	21
3	6	30	8 wk	3×/wk	NC	NM	↑	28
3	5, 6.5, 7.5	80	5, 10, 15 wk	6×/wk	↑	NM	↑	58, 59
3	5	80	3 wk	daily	NC	↓	↑	30
3	17.5	80	10 wk	5×/wk	↑	NM	↑	50, 60
3	4	80, 160	5 wk	daily	↑	↓	↑	29
4	6	2.5	4 wk	daily	NC	NM	NM	34
5	7	40	4 wk	daily	↑	NM	NM	32
12	24.5	160	2 wk	daily	NC	NM	↑	39

Abbreviations: NC, no change; NM, not measured.

[a] Bone mass: cortical bone area, or bone mineral density at cortical bone-enriched regions of long bone.

[b] Bone resorption: endocortical osteoclast surface.

[c] Bone formation: periosteal and/or endocortical bone formation rate.

theless, it is important to emphasize that cortical bone loss has never been reported in PTH-treated OVX rats.

Most of the above studies were performed in relatively young OVX rats at early times postovariectomy. Therefore, at the beginning of PTH treatment, these animals had normal or even increased cortical bone mass compared to age-matched control rats. However, some studies were performed in aged OVX rats with established cortical osteopenia, as indicated by decreased cortical thickness of the tibial shaft and femoral neck.[50,60] Despite the advanced age (15 months) and late stage of estrogen depletion (one year postovariectomy) of these animals, PTH was still found to stimulate both periosteal and endocortical bone formation and augment cortical bone mass. In fact, PTH increased cortical bone mass in these aged OVX rats to at least the same extent as that observed in younger OVX rats.[58] This finding indicates that, much like cancellous bone, the anabolic response of cortical bone to PTH does not decline with age or stage of estrogen depletion in OVX rats.

V. EFFECTS OF PTH ON BONE STRENGTH IN OVX RATS

The evidence that PTH stimulates bone formation and augments both cortical and cancellous bone mass in OVX rats is unequivocal. However, it is essential to determine whether the newly formed bone induced by PTH treatment is structurally sound. This question is especially important in view of findings that new bone formed in response to another anabolic agent, sodium fluoride, may, depending on dose and formulation, be primarily woven in nature, poorly calcified, and biomechanically weak.[61-63] Consequently, some clinical studies have shown that fluoride-treated osteoporotic patients have unchanged or even increased fracture rates despite increased cancellous bone mass.[64,65] It is important to evaluate this potential weakness in other bone anabolic agents.

Fortunately, several lines of evidence indicate that the new bone formed in OVX rats in response to PTH treatment is of high quality. The presence of discrete fluorochrome labels along bone surfaces in PTH-treated OVX rats indicates that the new bone is lamellar in nature rather than woven, which would label diffusely with fluorochromes. Furthermore, the well-documented formation of wider trabeculae composed of structurally superior lamellar bone in response to PTH treatment suggests that the hormone improves bone strength. This impression has been confirmed by many bone biomechanical studies. For example, compression tests have consistently shown that PTH treatment of osteopenic OVX rats increases load to failure to a level greater than that of sham-operated control rats.[40,43,59,66,67] These positive results indicative of increased bone strength in PTH-treated OVX rats have been obtained from skeletal sites composed primarily of cancellous bone (lumbar vertebral body), cortical bone (femoral shaft), or a combination of the two (femoral neck). Mechanical strength of exclusively cancellous bone within the marrow cavity of the distal femur has also been shown to be increased by PTH treatment of OVX rats.[41] Therefore, PTH clearly improves the biomechanical competence of both cancellous and cortical bone in OVX rats. The observed increase in bone compressive strength correlates well with increments in bone mass and trabecular width.[41,43] Without question, PTH does not adversely affect bone quality but rather induces deposition of structurally sound lamellar bone that markedly improves the biomechanical competence of the estrogen-deplete skeleton of rats.

VI. CONCURRENT TREATMENT OF OVX RATS WITH PTH AND ANTIRESORPTIVE AGENTS

As detailed above, PTH is a powerful stimulator of bone formation that adds bone mass to the osteopenic skeleton. But perhaps the positive bone balance induced by treatment with PTH alone would be even greater if the hormone were administered in combination with an antiresorptive agent (estrogen, bisphosphonates, or calcitonin). If so, such concurrent treatments may allow PTH to be administered at a lower dose and still achieve the desired skeletal effect. Therefore, it is important to evaluate whether concurrent treatments with an inhibitor of bone resorption and a stimulator of bone formation would be more effective than single treatments to reverse osteopenia in OVX rats. It is also important to determine whether the bone anabolic effects of PTH would be maintained in a skeleton either concurrently or pretreated with an antiresorptive agent. This situation would be analogous to initiating PTH treatment in a postmenopausal woman on estrogen replacement therapy. Several recent studies in OVX rats have addressed these issues.

Concurrent treatments of osteopenic OVX rats with PTH and an antiresorptive agent (estrogen, the bisphosphonate risedronate, or calcitonin) were found to effectively restore lost cancellous bone and enhance bone strength to at least the level of sham-operated control rats.[25,31,40,43,59,66,67] However, these concurrent treatments were not more beneficial to the estrogen-deplete skeleton than treatment with PTH alone. Although the antiresorptive agents inhibited bone resorption, as expected, they also partially suppressed the stimulatory effect of PTH on bone formation. Consequently, the concurrent treatments did not have a greater positive cancellous bone balance in osteopenic OVX rats than treatment with PTH alone. These findings were similar in relatively young OVX rats treated during the early stages of estrogen depletion[31,59,66,67] and in aged OVX rats treated during the late stages of estrogen depletion.[25,40,43] In tibial shafts from these same animals, concurrent treatments with PTH and an antiresorptive agent did not have a greater, or lesser, anabolic effect on cortical bone mass than treatment with PTH alone.[58,60] However, it is important to note that the animals from these studies were treated with a moderate dose of PTH (80 μg/kg). With much lower doses of the hormone (2.5 to 40 μg/kg), Shen et al.[32,34] have reported that concurrent treatment with PTH + estrogen does have a greater positive effect on trabecular connectivity in osteopenic OVX rats than treatment with PTH alone. Therefore, the relative skeletal benefits of PTH monotherapy and cotherapy with an antiresorptive agent may be dependent on the dose of PTH.

Regardless of dose, it is noteworthy that all studies cited above support the concept that the bone anabolic effects of PTH in OVX rats are not blunted significantly by concurrent treatment with an antiresorptive agent. In addition, Shen et al.[44] have shown that extensive pretreatment of osteopenic OVX rats with estrogen does not block or diminish the bone anabolic effects of subsequent PTH treatment. These findings, which are consistent with those of a recent clinical trial,[68] suggest that PTH can still augment bone mass despite pretreatment or concurrent treatment with an antiresorptive agent.

VII. MAINTENANCE OF BONE AFTER WITHDRAWAL OF PTH TREATMENT

Gunness-Hey and Hock[69] first showed, in intact male rats, that new bone mass formed in response to PTH treatment is quickly lost after withdrawal of the hormone. This finding has since been confirmed in OVX rats.[24,28,49] Since it is not practical to treat osteoporotic patients indefinitely with an expensive, injectable peptide such as PTH, development of a therapeutic strategy to maintain the new bone induced by PTH treatment is essential. In this regard, antiresorptive agents seem to be a logical choice since bone resorption presumably increases soon after PTH withdrawal. This maintenance strategy was first tested by Jee and coworkers,[70] who used bisphosphonates to prevent bone loss in OVX rats after withdrawal of treatment with another anabolic agent, prostaglandin E_2. Similar positive results were obtained with bisphosphonates after discontinuation of PTH treatment,[28,49] with the added observation that cancellous bone continued to be maintained even after discontinuation of bisphosphonate treatment,[28] probably due to the long skeletal retention of the drug.[71] Not surprisingly, estrogen was also found to maintain the PTH-induced gains in bone mass, trabecular connectivity, and bone strength in OVX rats after withdrawal of the hormone.[44] As an alternative to maintenance therapy with drugs or hormones, exercise has been reported to be at least partially effective in this regard.[24] The results of these studies clearly indicate that the PTH-induced increment in cancellous bone in OVX rats is rapidly lost after withdrawal of the hormone, but that the bone gain can be preserved by subsequent treatment with an antiresorptive agent. These findings may have important implications for PTH therapy of osteoporotic patients.

VIII. POTENTIAL MEDIATORS OF THE SKELETAL EFFECTS OF PTH TREATMENT IN OVX RATS

Growth factors are considered to be potential mediators for the skeletal actions of PTH,[72] especially in view of evidence that ruled out such a role for prostaglandins.[8] Of the various growth factors, attention has focused primarily on IGF-I and TGF-β. Both are abundant in bone matrix and are liberated by osteoclastic activity to potentially affect the function of adjacent bone cells. Only *in vivo* evidence will be considered in this brief review. The reader is referred to Chapter 5 on PTH-induced osteogenic signaling for a more complete discussion of this topic.

Hock and Fonseca[73] first reported that the bone anabolic effects of PTH are dependent on growth hormone or IGF-I in intact rats. Another study in intact rats has shown that PTH treatment increases the bone concentration of both IGF-I and TGF-β.[74] However, these lines of evidence suggestive of a role of IGF-I in the skeletal effects of PTH were recently contradicted by Schmidt et al.[75] These investigators showed that growth hormone is not essential for PTH-mediated increases in either osteoblast number or bone matrix synthesis in intact rats. The most likely explanation for these conflicting results may be age differences in the experimental animals. In any case, *in situ* hybridization in the proximal tibia of OVX rats revealed that PTH enhanced IGF-I gene expression in cancellous osteoblasts.[27] This is the strongest evidence to date for a mediatory role for IGF-I in the bone anabolic effects of PTH specifically in OVX rats. Although the hormone induces a transient increase in IL-6 mRNA in cancellous bone cells of young intact rats,[76] the effect of PTH on gene expression of this and other growth factors in the skeleton of OVX rats has not yet been reported.

IX. SIDE EFFECTS OF PTH TREATMENT

PTH treatment has minimal side effects in intact and OVX rats. Even high doses of the hormone (400 to 1000 μg/kg) did not affect weight gain or serum calcium levels during an 8-week treatment period.[11] However, one should be aware that rats are much more resistant to the development of PTH-induced hypercalcemia than other mammals or birds.[77] Nevertheless, OVX rats treated for longer periods (15 weeks) with a much lower dose of PTH (80 μg/kg) may develop moderate hypercalcemia.[31] Other adverse effects such as marrow fibrosis or woven bone formation occur only in rats treated with the high doses of PTH referred to above.[11,23]

Long-term treatment of OVX rats with PTH may induce formation of excessive cancellous bone so that the metaphyseal marrow cavity of long bones becomes nearly totally occluded in some animals (Figure 3.3). This phenomenon has also been observed in the tibial shaft of OVX rats treated concurrently with PTH and estrogen (Figure 3.3), probably due to a PTH-

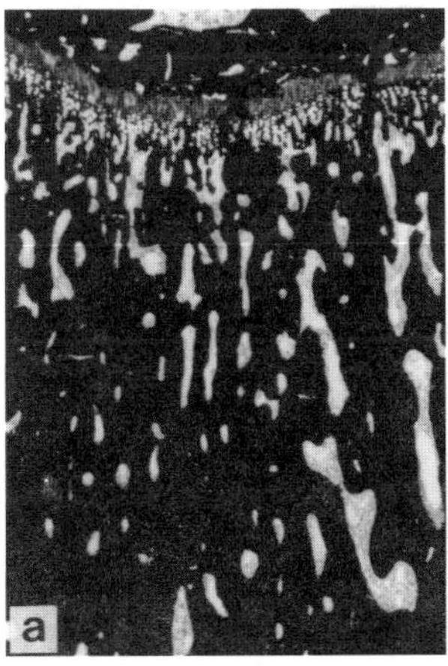

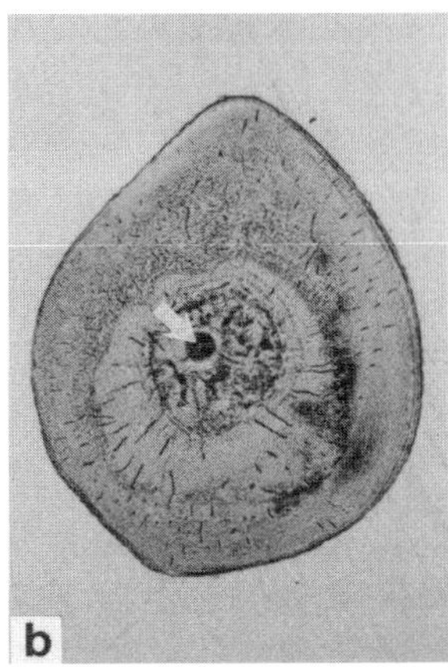

Figure 3.3
Longitudinal section of the proximal tibial metaphysis (a) from an OVX rat treated for 15 weeks with PTH alone. Note how the marrow cavity is nearly totally occluded with black-stained bone after long-term treatment with a moderate dose (80 μg/kg) of the hormone. In a cross section of the tibial diaphysis (b) from an OVX rat, the size of the marrow cavity (arrow) is markedly decreased by concurrent treatment with PTH and estrogen for 15 weeks. If this phenomenon is generalized throughout the skeleton, long-term treatment of rats with moderate to high doses of PTH may reduce the bone marrow area to such an extent as to diminish hematopoiesis.

induced stimulation of endocortical bone formation combined with an estrogenic suppression of endocortical bone resorption.[58] Although the skeletons of not all OVX rats respond to such a great extent to PTH, prolonged treatment with the hormone, either singly or in combination with antiresorptive agents, may produce abnormally dense bones in some animals with the potential for diminished hematopoiesis.

X. SUMMARY AND CONCLUSIONS

Unequivocal evidence supports the following statements regarding the skeletal effects of intermittent PTH treatment in OVX rats.

1. PTH augments both cancellous and cortical bone mass in OVX rats. The hormone is capable of preventing bone loss during the early stages of estrogen depletion. More importantly, PTH treatment completely restores lost bone mass in OVX rats with established osteopenia.
2. The PTH-induced increase in bone mass is due primarily to a powerful stimulation of bone formation. Both the numbers and activity of osteoblasts are increased markedly by PTH treatment. This anabolic effect has been consistently observed along cancellous bone surfaces of OVX rats as well as endocortical and, to a lesser extent, periosteal surfaces of cortical bone.

3. With the exception of very high doses, the new bone formed in response to PTH treatment is lamellar and biomechanically sound. The hormone clearly improves bone strength in both the axial and appendicular skeletons of OVX rats.
4. The ability of PTH to augment bone mass and strength in OVX rats is not dependent on age or stage of estrogen depletion at the beginning of treatment. However, the efficacy of PTH in restoring lost cancellous bone and trabecular connectivity may be compromised at a severely osteopenic skeletal site that lacks adequate numbers of bone spicules to serve as a template for new bone formation.
5. Concurrent treatment of PTH-treated OVX rats with an antiresorptive agent does not significantly blunt the anabolic response to PTH in either cancellous or cortical bone. On the other hand, such concurrent treatments are not more beneficial to the estrogen-deplete skeleton of rats than treatment with PTH alone, with the possible exception of OVX rats treated with low doses of PTH.
6. New cancellous bone formed in response to PTH treatment is lost after withdrawal of the hormone. However, this added bone can be maintained after PTH withdrawal by subsequent treatment with an antiresorptive agent such as estrogen or bisphosphonates.

The following skeletal effects of PTH in OVX rats are less well understood.

1. The response of bone resorption to intermittent PTH treatment is unclear because the hormone has been reported to increase, decrease, or have no effect on osteoclast variables in OVX rats. These inconsistent findings may be due in part to temporal variations in the effects of PTH on bone resorption. Results from long-term studies suggest that increased bone resorption may be a consequence of prolonged PTH treatment. Nevertheless, bone formation must exceed bone resorption in PTH-treated OVX rats to achieve the positive bone balance that obviously occurs in these animals.
2. The cell reserve that contributes to the increased osteoblast population in PTH-treated OVX rats is uncertain. The most likely candidates are osteoprogenitor cells in the bone marrow and bone lining cells. Both cell types have been reported to differentiate into osteoblasts soon after PTH treatment, but conflicting evidence makes their relative contributions to the osteoblast pool unclear.
3. The growth factor(s) that acts as a mediator for the bone anabolic effects of PTH in OVX rats has yet to be unequivocally identified. Available evidence strongly suggests that IGF-I is involved, but a cause-and-effect relationship has yet to be firmly established. The role of other growth factors in the skeletal effects of PTH in OVX rats has not been adequately investigated *in vivo*.

In conclusion, preclinical studies in OVX rats, an animal model for estrogen depletion, overwhelmingly support the potential of PTH as an osteoporosis therapy. The hormone stimulates bone formation and increases bone mass and strength substantially in the osteopenic skeleton of rats. Since agents with such a strong anabolic effect on bone are rare, the therapeutic potential of PTH is especially exciting. Unfortunately, clinical development of PTH is slowed by the need for frequent sc injections of the expensive peptide, which severely limits patient compliance with long-term therapy. The OVX rat model for postmenopausal bone loss will undoubtedly prove useful for testing new delivery systems for PTH and for determining the skeletal effects of smaller, more cost-effective PTH analogs. Positive results in such preclinical studies would contribute to the development and acceptance of PTH as an osteoporosis therapy.

REFERENCES

1. Parfitt, A. M., The actions of parathyroid hormone on bone: relation to bone remodeling and turnover, calcium homeostasis, and metabolic bone diseases, *Metabolism*, 25, 909, 1976.
2. Heaney, R. P., A unified concept of osteoporosis, *Am. J. Med.*, 29, 877, 1965.
3. Joborn, C., Ljunghall, S., Larsson, K., Lindh, E., Naessén, T., Wide, L., Åkerström, G., and Rastad, J., Skeletal responsiveness to parathyroid hormone in healthy females: relationship to menopause and oestrogen replacement, *Clin. Endocrinol.*, 34, 335, 1991.
4. Selye, H., On the stimulation of new bone-formation with parathyroid extract and irradiated ergosterol, *Endocrinology*, 16, 547, 1932.
5. Hefti, E., Trechsel, U., Bonjour, J. P., Fleisch, H., and Schenk, R., Increase of whole body calcium and skeletal mass in normal and osteoporotic adult rats treated with PTH, *Clin. Sci.*, 62, 389, 1982.
6. Tam, C. S., Heersche, J. N. M., Murray, T. M., and Parsons, J.A., Parathyroid hormone stimulates the bone apposition rate independently of its resorptive action: differential effects of intermittent and continuous administration, *Endocrinology*, 110, 506, 1982.
7. Gunness-Hey, M. and Hock, J. M., Increased trabecular bone mass in rats treated with human synthetic parathyroid hormone, *Metab. Bone Dis. Rel. Res.*, 5, 177, 1984.
8. Gera, I., Hock, J. M., Gunness-Hey, M., Fonseca, J., and Raisz, L. G., Indomethacin does not inhibit the anabolic effect of PTH on the long bones of rats, *Calcif. Tissue Int.*, 40, 206, 1987.
9. Mosekilde, Li., Søgaard, C. H., Danielsen, C. C., Torring, O., and Nilsson, M. H. L., The anabolic effects of human parathyroid hormone (hPTH) on rat vertebral body mass are also reflected in the quality of bone mass by biomechanical testing: A comparison study between hPTH (1-34) and hPTH (1-84), *Endocrinology*, 129, 421, 1991.
10. Mitlak, B. H., Williams, D. C., Bryant, H. U., Paul, D. C., and Neer, R. M., Intermittent administration of bovine PTH-(1-34) increases serum 1,25-dihydroxyvitamin D concentrations and spinal bone density in senile (23 month) rats, *J. Bone Min. Res.*, 7, 479, 1992.
11. Jerome, C. P., Anabolic effect of high doses of human parathyroid hormone (1-38) in mature intact female rats, *J. Bone Min. Res.*, 9, 933, 1994.
12. Ejersted, C., Andreassen, T. T., Hauge, E.-M., Melsen, F., and Oxlund, H., Parathyroid hormone (1-34) increases vertebral bone mass, compressive strength, and quality in old rats, *Bone*, 17, 507, 1995.
13. Kalu, D. N., The ovariectomized rat model of postmenopausal bone loss, *Bone Miner.*, 15, 176, 1991.

14. Wronski, T. J., and Yen, C.-F., The ovariectomized rat as an animal model for postmenopausal bone loss, *Cells and Materials* (Suppl. 1), 69, 1992.
15. Hock, J. M., Fonseca, J., Gunness-Hey, M., Kemp, B. E., and Martin, T. J., Comparison of the anabolic effects of synthetic parathyroid hormone-related protein (PTHrP) 1-34 and PTH 1-34 on bone in rats, *Endocrinology*, 125, 2022, 1989.
16. Leaffer, D., Sweeney, M., Kellerman, L. A., Avnur, Z., Krstenansky, J. L., Vickery, B. H., and Caulfield, J. P., Modulation of osteogenic cell ultrastructure by RS-23581, an analog of human parathyroid hormone (PTH)-related peptide-(1-34), and bovine PTH-(1-34), *Endocrinology*, 136, 3624, 1995.
17. Whitfield, J. F., Morley, P., Willick, G. E., Ross, V., Barbier, J.-R., Isaacs, R. J., and Ohannessian-Barry, L., Stimulation of the growth of femoral trabecular bone in ovariectomized rats by the novel parathyroid hormone fragment, hPTH-(1-31)NH2 (ostabolin), *Calcif. Tissue Int.*, 58, 81, 1996.
18. Lane, N. E., Kimmel, D. B., Nilsson, M. H. L., Cohen, F. E., Newton, S., Nissenson, R. A., and Strewler, G., Bone-selective analogs of human PTH(1-34) increase bone formation in an ovariectomized rat model, *J. Bone Miner. Res.*, 11, 614, 1996.
19. Hock, J. M., and Gera, I., Effects of continuous and intermittent administration and inhibition of resorption on the anabolic response of bone to parathyroid hormone, *J. Bone Miner. Res.*, 7, 65, 1992.
20. Podbesek, R., Edouard, C., Meunier, P. J., Parsons, J. A., Reeve, J., Stevenson, R. W., and Zanelli, J. M., Effects of two treatment regimens with synthetic human parathyroid hormone fragment on bone formation and the tissue balance of trabecular bone in greyhounds, *Endocrinology*, 112, 1000, 1982.
21. Hock, J. M., Gera, I., Fonseca, J., and Raisz, L. G., Human parathyroid hormone (1-34) increases bone mass in ovariectomized and orchidectomized rats, *Endocrinology*, 122, 2899, 1988.
22. Takahashi, H. E., Tanizawa, T., Hori, M., and Uzawa, T., Effect of intermittent administration of parathyroid hormone (1-34) on experimental osteopenia of rats induced by ovariectomy, *Cells and Materials* (Suppl. 1), 69, 1992.
23. Gasser, J. A., and Jerome, C. P., Parathyroid hormone: a cure for osteoporosis?, *Triangle*, 31, 111, 1992.
24. Yamamoto, N., Takahashi, H. E., Tanizawa, T., Fujimoto, R., Hara, T., and Tanaka, S., Maintenance of bone mass by physical exercise after discontinuation of intermittent hPTH (1-34) administration, *Bone Miner.*, 23, 333, 1993.
25. Qi, H., Li, M., and Wronski, T. J., A comparison of the anabolic effects of parathyroid hormone at skeletal sites with moderate and severe osteopenia in aged, ovariectomized rats, *J. Bone Min. Res.*, 10, 948, 1995.
26. Lane, N. E., Thompson, J. M., Strewler, G. J., and Kinney, J. H., Intermittent treatment with parathyroid hormone (hPTH 1-34) increased trabecular bone volume but not connectivity in osteopenic rats, *J. Bone Min. Res.*, 10, 1470, 1995.
27. Watson, P., Lazowski, D., Han, V., Fraher, L., Steer, B., and Hodsman, A., Parathyroid hormone restores bone mass and enhances osteoblast insulin-like growth factor I gene expression in ovariectomized rats, *Bone*, 16, 357, 1995.
28. Takano, Y., Tanizawa, T., Mashiba, T., Endo, N., Nishida, S., and Takahashi, H. E., Maintaining bone mass by bisphosphonate incadronate disodium (YM175) sequential treatment after discontinuation of intermittent human parathyroid hormone (1-34) administration in ovariectomized rats, *J. Bone Min. Res.*, 11, 169, 1996.
29. Liu, C-C., and Kalu, D. N., Human parathyroid hormone (1-34) prevents bone loss and augments bone formation in sexually mature ovariectomized rats, *J. Bone Min. Res.*, 5, 973, 1990.
30. Liu, C-C., Kalu, D. N., Salerno, E., Echon, R., Hollis, B. W., and Ray, M., Pre-existing bone loss associated with ovariectomy in rats is reversed by parathyroid hormone, *J. Bone Min. Res.*, 6, 1071, 1991.

31. Wronski, T. J., Yen, C.-F., Qi, H., and Dann, L. M., Parathyroid hormone is more effective than estrogen or bisphosphonates for restoration of lost bone mass in ovariectomized rats, *Endocrinology*, 132, 823, 1993.
32. Shen, V., Dempster, D. W., Birchman, R., Xu, R., and Lindsay, R., Loss of cancellous bone mass and connectivity in ovariectomized rats can be restored by combined treatment with parathyroid hormone and estradiol, *J. Clin. Invest.*, 91, 2479, 1993.
33. Kimmel, D. B., Bozzato, R. P., Kronis, K. A., Kwong, P., and Recker, R. R., The effect of recombinant human (1-84) or synthetic human (1-34) parathyroid hormone on the skeleton of adult osteopenic ovariectomized rats, *Endocrinology*, 132, 1577, 1993.
34. Shen, V., Dempster, D. W., Mellish, R. W. E., Birchman, R., Horbert, W., and Lindsay, R., Effects of combined and separate intermittent administration of low-dose human parathyroid hormone fragment (1-34) and 17β-estradiol on bone histomorphometry in ovariectomized rats with established osteopenia, *Calcif. Tissue Int.*, 50, 214, 1992.
35. Heaney, R. P., Recker, R. R., and Saville, P. D., Menopausal changes in bone remodeling, *J. Lab. Clin. Med.*, 92, 964, 1978.
36. Stepan, J. J., Pospichal, J., Presl, J., and Pacovsky, V., Bone loss and biochemical indices of bone remodeling in surgically induced postmenopausal women, *Bone*, 8, 279, 1987.
37. Hori, M., Uzawa, T., Morita, K., Noda, T., Takahashi, H., and Inoue, J., Effect of human parathyroid hormone (PTH (1-34)) on experimental osteopenia of rats induced by ovariectomy, *Bone Miner.*, 3, 193, 1987.
38. Kalu, D. N., Echon, R., and Hollis, B. W., Modulation of ovariectomy-related bone loss by parathyroid hormone in rats, *Mech. Ageing Dev.*, 56, 49, 1990.
39. Ibbotson, K. J., Orcutt, C. M., D'Souza, S. M., Paddock, C. L., Arthur, J. A., Jankowsky, M. L., and Boyce, R. W., Contrasting effects of parathyroid hormone and insulin-like growth factor I in an aged ovariectomized rat model of postmenopausal osteoporosis, *J. Bone Min. Res.*, 7, 425, 1992.
40. Mosekilde, Li., Danielsen, C. C., and Gasser, J., The effect on vertebral bone mass and strength of long term treatment with antiresorptive agents (estrogen and calcitonin), human parathyroid hormone-(1-38), and combination therapy, assessed in aged ovariectomized rats, *Endocrinology*, 134, 2126, 1994.
41. Meng, X. W., Liang, X. G., Birchman, R., Wu, D. D., Dempster, D. W., Lindsay, R., and Shen, V., Temporal expression of the anabolic action of PTH in cancellous bone of ovariectomized rats, *J. Bone Min. Res.*, 11, 421, 1996.
42. Mitlak, B. H., Burdette-Miller, P., Schoenfeld, D., and Neer, R. M., Sequential effects of chronic human PTH (1-84) treatment of estrogen-deficiency osteopenia in the rat, *J. Bone Min. Res.*, 11, 430, 1996.
43. Li, M., Mosekilde, Li., Søgaard, C. H., Thomsen, J. S., and Wronski, T. J., Parathyroid hormone monotherapy and cotherapy with antiresorptive agents restore vertebral bone mass and strength in aged ovariectomized rats, *Bone*, 16, 629, 1995.
44. Shen, V., Birchman, R., Xu, R., Otter, M., Wu, D. D., Lindsay, R., and Dempster, D. W., Effects of reciprocal treatment with estrogen and estrogen plus parathyroid hormone on bone structure and strength in ovariectomized rats, *J. Clin. Invest.*, 96, 2331, 1995.
45. Dobnig, H., and Turner, R. T., Evidence that intermittent treatment with parathyroid hormone increases bone formation in adult rats by activation of bone lining cells, *Endocrinology*, 136, 3632, 1995.
46. Hock, J. M., Hummert, J. R., Boyce, R., Fonseca, J., and Raisz, L. G., Resorption is not essential for the stimulation of bone growth by hPTH-(1-34) in rats in vivo, *J. Bone Min. Res.*, 4, 449, 1989.
47. Hodsman, A. B. and Steer, B. M., Early histomorphometric changes in response to parathyroid hormone therapy in osteoporosis: evidence for de novo bone formation on quiescent cancellous surfaces, *Bone*, 14, 523, 1993.

48. Nishida, S., Yamaguchi, A., Tanizawa, T., Endo, N., Mashiba, T., Suda, T., Yoshiki, S., and Takahashi, H. E., Increased bone formation by intermittent parathyroid hormone administration is due to the stimulation of proliferation and differentiation of osteoprogenitor cells in bone marrow, *Bone*, 15, 717, 1994.
49. Cheng, P.-T., Chan, C., and Müller, K., Cyclical treatment of osteopenic ovariectomized adult rats with PTH(1-34) and pamidronate, *J. Bone Min. Res.*, 10, 119, 1995.
50. Li, M., and Wronski, T. J., Response of femoral neck to estrogen depletion and parathyroid hormone in aged rats, *Bone*, 16, 551, 1995.
51. Zerwekh, J. E., Hagler, H. K., Sakhaee, K., Gottschalk, F., Peterson, R. D., and Pak, C. Y. C., Effect of slow-release sodium fluoride on cancellous bone histology and connectivity in osteoporosis, *Bone*, 15, 691, 1994.
52. Reeve, J., Williams, D., Hesp, R., Hulme, P., Klenerman, L., Zanelli, J. M., Darby, A. J., Tregear, G. W., and Parsons, J. A., Anabolic effect of low doses of fragment of human parathyroid hormone on the skeleton in postmenopausal osteoporosis, *Lancet*, 1, 1035, 1976.
53. Reeve, J., Bradbeer, J. N., Arlot, M., Davies, U. M., Green, J. R., Hampton, L., Edouard, C., Hesp, R., Hulme, P., Ashby, J. P., Zanelli, J. M., and Meunier, P. J., hPTH 1-34 treatment of osteoporosis with added hormone replacement therapy: Biochemical, kinetic, and histological responses, *Osteoporosis Int.*, 1, 162, 1991.
54. Hodsman, A. B., Fraher, L. J., Ostbye, T., Adachi, J. D., and Steer, B. M., An evaluation of several biochemical markers for bone formation and resorption in a protocol utilizing cyclical parathyroid hormone and calcitonin therapy for osteoporosis, *J. Clin. Invest.*, 91, 1138, 1993.
55. Hesp, R., Hulme, P., Williams, D., and Reeve, J., The relationship between changes in femoral bone density and calcium balance in patients with involutional osteoporosis treated with human PTH fragment 1-34, *Metab. Bone Dis. Rel. Res.*, 2, 331, 1981.
56. Neer, M., Slovik, D. M., Daly, M., Potts Jr., T., and Nussbaum, S. R., Treatment of postmenopausal osteoporosis with daily parathyroid hormone plus calcitriol, *Osteoporosis Int.*, Suppl. 1, S204, 1993.
57. Boyce, R. W., Paddock, C. L., Franks, A. F., Jankowsky, M. L., and Eriksen, E. F., Effects of intermittent hPTH(1-34) alone and in combination with $1,25(OH)_2D_3$ or risedronate on endosteal bone remodeling in canine cancellous and cortical bone, *J. Bone Min. Res.*, 11, 600, 1996.
58. Wronski, T. J. and Yen, C.-F., Anabolic effects of parathyroid hormone on cortical bone in ovariectomized rats, Bone, 15, 51, 1994.
59. Mosekilde, Li., Danielsen, C. C., Søgaard, C. H., McOsker, J. E., and Wronski, T. J., The anabolic effects of parathyroid hormone on cortical bone mass, dimensions and strength — assessed in a sexually mature, ovariectomized rat model, *Bone*, 16, 223, 1995.
60. Baumann, B. D. and Wronski, T. J., Response of cortical bone to antiresorptive agents and parathyroid hormone in aged ovariectomized rats, *Bone*, 16, 247, 1995.
61. Vigorita, V. J. and Suda, M. K., The microscopic morphology of fluoride-induced bone, *Clin. Orth. Rel. Res.*, 177, 274, 1983.
62. Lundy, M. W., Stauffer, M., Wergedal, J. E., Baylink, D. J., Featherstone, J. D. B., Hodgson, S. F., and Riggs, B. L., Histomorphometric analysis of iliac bone biopsies in placebo-treated versus fluoride-treated subjects, *Osteoporosis Int.*, 5, 115, 1995.
63. Søgaard, C. H., Mosekilde, Li., Richards, A., and Mosekilde, Le., Marked decrease in trabecular bone quality after five years of sodium fluoride therapy — assessed by biomechanical testing of iliac bone biopsies in osteoporotic patients, *Bone*, 15, 393, 1994.
64. Riggs, B. L., Hodgson, S. F., O'Fallon, W. M., Chao, E. Y. S., Wahner, H. W., Muhs, J. M., Cedel, S. L., and Melton, L. J., Effect of fluoride treatment on the fracture rate in postmenopausal women with osteoporosis, *N. Engl. J. Med.*, 322, 802, 1990.
65. Kleerekoper, M., and Balena, R., Fluorides and osteoporosis, *Ann. Rev. Nutr.*, 11, 309, 1991.

66. Søgaard, C. H., Wronski, T. J., McOsker, J. E., and Mosekilde, L., The positive effect of parathyroid hormone on femoral neck bone strength in ovariectomized rats is more pronounced than that of estrogen or bisphosphonates, *Endocrinology*, 134, 650, 1994.
67. Mosekilde, Li., Søgaard, C. H., McOsker, J. E., and Wronski, T. J., PTH has a more pronounced effect on vertebral bone mass and biomechanical competence than antiresorptive agents (estrogen and bisphosphonate) — assessed in sexually mature, ovariectomized rats, *Bone*, 15, 401, 1994.
68. Lindsay, R., Cosman, F., Nieves, J., Dempster, D. W., and Shen, V., A controlled clinical trial of the effects of 1-34 hPTH in estrogen treated osteoporosis, *J. Bone Min. Res.*, 8 (Suppl 1), S130, 1993.
69. Gunness-Hey, M. and Hock, J. M., Loss of the anabolic effect of parathyroid hormone on bone after discontinuation of hormone in rats, *Bone*, 10, 447, 1989.
70. Jee, W. S. S., Tang, L. Y., Ke, H. Z., Setterberg, R. B., and Kimmel, D. B., Maintaining restored bone with bisphosphonate in the ovariectomized rat skeleton: dynamic histomorphometry of changes in bone mass, *Bone*, 14, 493, 1993.
71. Lin, J. H., Bisphosphonates: a review of their pharmacokinetic properties, *Bone*, 18, 75, 1996.
72. Dempster, D. W., Cosman, F., Parisien, M., Shen, V., and Lindsay, R., Anabolic action of parathyroid hormone on bone, *Endocrine Rev.*, 14, 690, 1993.
73. Hock, J. M. and Fonseca, J., Anabolic effect of human synthetic parathyroid hormone-(1-34) depends on growth hormone, *Endocrinology*, 127, 1804, 1990.
74. Pfeilschifter, J., Laukhuf, F., Müller-Beckmann, B., Blum, W. F., Pfister, T., and Ziegler, R., Parathyroid hormone increases the concentration of insulin-like growth factor-I and transforming growth factor beta 1 in rat bone, *J. Clin. Invest.*, 96, 767, 1995.
75. Schmidt, I. U., Dobnig, H., and Turner, R. T., Intermittent parathyroid hormone treatment increases osteoblast number, steady state messenger ribonucleic acid levels for osteocalcin, and bone formation in tibial metaphysis of hypophysectomized female rats, *Endocrinology*, 136, 5127, 1995.
76. Onyia, J. E., Bidwell, J., Herring, J., Hulman, J., and Hock, J. M., In vivo, human parathyroid hormone fragment (hPTH 1-34) transiently stimulates immediate early response gene expression, but not proliferation, in trabecular bone cells of young rats, *Bone*, 17, 479, 1995.
77. Parsons, J. A., Reit, B., and Robinson, C. J., A bioassay for parathyroid hormone using chicks, *Endocrinology*, 92, 454, 1973.

Chapter **4**

Parathyroid Hormone: The Clinical Experience and Prospects

A. B. Hodsman, L. J. Fraher, and P. H. Watson

CONTENTS

0-8493-8556-3/98/$0.00+$.50

I. INTRODUCTION

Current concepts of therapy to reduce the fracture risk consequences of osteoporosis can be divided into antiresorptive and anabolic approaches. These are schematically shown in Figure 4.1. As bone mass falls with age, antiresorptive drugs (e.g., estrogen, calcitonin, and the bisphosphonates) have been shown to arrest bone loss and even increase bone mass. As will be discussed later, small gains in bone mass in patients with osteoporosis and established fractures translate into clinically important reductions in future fracture risk. By contrast, anabolic agents such as sodium fluoride and parathyroid hormone (PTH) have the potential to cause accelerated gains in bone mass over short periods (2 to 4 years), which might offer particular protection to patients with very low bone mass. Recent studies of PTH and several peptide analogs of PTH have provided evidence for a potent anabolic action on bone in both laboratory and clinical osteoporosis. This chapter focuses on the clinical information currently available and, when possible, contrasts this with the established efficacy of antiresorptive therapy.

It is just over 20 years ago that Reeve et al.[1,2] published the first clinical report describing the use of synthetic parathyroid hormone (hPTH-(1-34)) to treat four women with severe osteoporosis. The researchers reviewed circumstantial evidence in clinical hyperparathyroid states and animal experiments dating back to 1929 to support the hypothesis that under appropriate conditions, PTH might be a potent anabolic agent rather than the conventional assumption that it acts as a bone-resorbing agent. From the first study, and a subsequent larger clinical trial involving 21 subjects, Reeve et al.[3] concluded that daily injections of 500 "house units" of hPTH-(1-34) over 6 months resulted in histological and radiokinetic evidence for dramatic increases in bone turnover, histomorphometric evidence of structural trabecular growth, and a positive dietary calcium balance. Histologically, the new bone was of normal lamellar structure and mineralization.

Despite such promising findings, it has taken a further 20 years to bring the development of PTH as an anabolic treatment for osteoporosis into the commercial arena. In the interim, sporadic reports from five

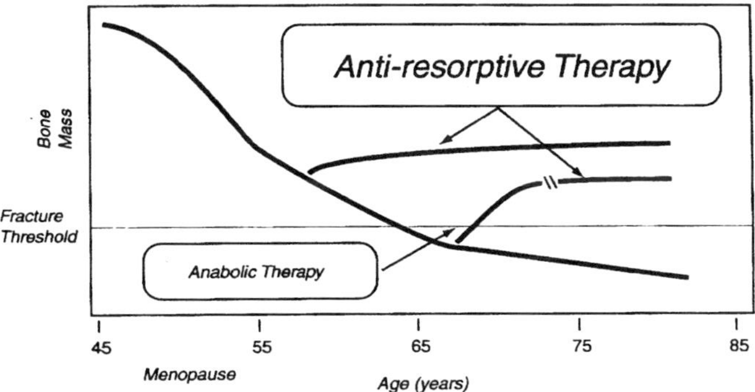

FIGURE 4.1
The relative efficacy of different strategies to maintain bone mass. Antiresorptive strategy: Various agents (i.e., estrogens, bisphosphonates, calcitonin) will arrest ongoing age-related and postmenopausal bone loss. Reductions in bone resorption and turnover are observed, and gains in skeletal bone mass may occur due to the reduced bone resorption and perhaps to a reversal of the remodeling deficit. Anabolic therapy: Agents such as PTH and sodium fluoride directly stimulate osteoblastic activity to increase bone mass, despite concurrent increases in bone turnover (i.e., there is an increase in both bone formation and resorption). The rapid increase in bone mass should accelerate the reduction in future fracture risk more effectively than the use of antiresorptive agents alone.

clinical centers have been published, involving small, largely uncontrolled clinical studies (Table 4.1). All conclude that PTH is an anabolic rather than a catabolic therapy in bone with as yet no demonstrable major adverse side effects. The absence of full-scale randomized controlled clinical trials exploring the full potential of PTH as an agent for the treatment of osteoporosis may seem surprising, but there are several reasons for this.

1. Large-scale synthesis of the hPTH-(1-34) amino-terminal fragment by the solid-state methods available in the 1970s and 1980s was very expensive, and this has resulted in very limited availability of the drug for clinical trials.
2. Commercialization of the natural sequence of human peptides presents significant risks because of current international patent laws. The pharmaceutical industry has now developed novel methods of peptide production and/or novel peptide analogs of hPTH which mimic the anabolic action of the native hormone. These conditions were not met until the 1980s.
3. The development of dual energy absorptiometry led to a rapid development in epidemiological aspects of osteoporosis, which initiated an understanding of the full societal impact of this condition, together with tools for risk management. Concurrently, the development of bisphosphonates for treatment of osteoporosis led not only to regulatory guidelines for licensing new therapeutic agents, but also to a new awareness that clinical reversal of osteoporosis was an achievable goal.

TABLE 4.1

Clinical Protocols used in PTH Studies

Author (year)	Age (yrs)	Gender ♀:♂	PTH Dose	Study Duration (Mon)	Concomitant Therapy	Controls	Main Outcome	Other Outcomes
Reeve[1] (1976)[1]	N/A	4:0	500 units	6	None	None	Histology	Diet Ca balance, markers
Reeve[2] (1976)[1]	N/A	4:0	500–2000 units	1–6	None	None	Diet Ca balance	
Reeve[3] (1980)[2]	61	16:5	500 units	6–24	None	None	Histology	^{47}Ca bone accretion, diet Ca balance, markers
Hesp[29] (1981)[2]	53–77	?	500 units	12	None	None	BMD	Diet Ca balance
Reeve[46] (1981)[2]	61	18:5	500 units	6	None	4 patients untreated	Ca balance	Histology ^{47}Ca accretion
Slovik[30] (1981)	50–70	5:1	450–750 units	1	None	None	Diet Ca balance	^{47}Ca-labeled bone accretion rate
Slovik[22] (1986)	50	0:8	400–500 units	12	Calcitriol	None	BMD	Diet Ca balance
Reeve[5] (1987)[2]	64	12:1	1000–1500 units, 7-day cycles	12	Calcitriol	None	BMD	^{47}Ca bone accretion, diet Ca balance, histology, anti-PTH-antibodies
Neer[48] (1987)	65	16:8	400–500 units either daily or in 6-week cycles	18–24	Calcitriol	7 ♀ on Ca or Calcitriol	BMD	Diet Ca balance
Hesch[6] (1989)	50	2:6	750 units, hPTH-(1-38), 70-day cycles	14	Calcitonin	5 ♀ on other treatments	BMD	Markers
Reeve[23] (1990)[2]	64	11:1	500 units	12	Estrogen or androgen	12 patients on fluoride	BMD	None

Hodsman[7] (1990)[3]	70	17:3	400 units PTH-(1-38), 14-day cycles	6	Calcitonin	None	Biochemistry	Markers
Reeve[35] (1991)[2]	64	11:1	500 units	12	Estrogen or androgen	None	Diet Ca balance	Histology, Markers, PTH antibodies
Hodsman[8] (1991)[3]	70	17:3	400 units PTH-(1-38), 14-day cycles	6	Calcitonin	None	BMD	Histology
Neer[25] (1991)	N/A	15:0	400–500 units	12–24	Calcitriol	15 women on Ca	BMD	None
Bradbeer[34] (1992)[2]	64	11:0	450–750	6–12	Estrogen or androgen	None	Histology	None
Hodsman[9] (1993)[4]	66	20:0	800 units, 28-day cycles	3	Calcitonin	None	Markers	Histology
Reeve[32] (1993)[2]	64	11:1	500 units	12	Estrogen or androgen	None	BMD	Diet Ca balance, histology
Finkelstein[4] (1994)	30	20:0	40 μg, daily	6	Calcium and naferelin	20 women on Ca and naferelin	BMD	Markers
Lindsay[24] (1995)	N/A	5:10	400 units daily	36	Estrogen	6 women on estrogen alone	BMD	Markers
Sone[65] (1995)	80	14:2	20 units daily	6	None	None	BMD	Phalangeal radiogrammetry
Hodsman[10] (1997)[4]	67	39:0	800 units, 28-day cycles	24	Calcitonin	None	BMD	Markers

Note: Superscript on author's name indicates published data from the same study cohort. Age: arithmetic means. Gender: numbers do not include controls who did not receive PTH.

4. Commercial development of PTH now includes completed preclinical trials. A large body of literature now exists and is summarized in other sections of this book. Properly designed, controlled clinical trials are currently in progress.

It is therefore timely to review the existing clinical experience of PTH to treat human osteoporosis. The focus of this chapter will be strictly clinical, since the experimental evidence is extensively reviewed elsewhere in this book.

II. CLINICAL PROTOCOLS

Table 4.1 summarizes the available clinical literature in which PTH has been given as a therapeutic agent either with the intention of treating patients with osteoporosis or exploring the biological mechanisms underlying its actions. Clearly these protocols are very heterogeneous. Although most researchers selected patients with osteoporosis, Finkelstein et al.[4] treated young hypoestrogenemic women treated with the gonadotrophin-releasing hormone antagonist, nafarelin, to determine whether PTH treatment could prevent bone loss under these conditions. Most subjects have been women with osteoporotic compression fractures in the spine, but men with osteoporosis have not been excluded. The duration of PTH treatment has varied from 1 to 36 months with an average of 11 months. Many protocols have incorporated concomitant antiresorptive therapy, but few have used clinically controlled therapeutic controls. Six of the 22 published studies employed a cyclical regimen in which PTH was given periodically rather than continuously.[5-10] The therapeutic peptide used has generally been hPTH-(1-34), but hPTH-(1-38) was used in three reports.[6-8]

A. Therapeutic Regimes

1. Daily or intermittent PTH therapy: dosing by daily subcutaneous injections
2. Cyclical PTH therapy: dosing by daily injections for defined temporal cycles (e.g., for 1 month at a time repeating four times per 12-month period)
3. Continuous PTH: given by continuous intravenous infusion, usually short-term over 12 to 48 hours

B. Doses

Throughout this chapter, doses of PTH are given in international units defined by bioassay. Earlier studies used less purified extracts of bovine parathyroid glands; later studies have used purified synthetic PTH peptides. Most authors have chosen to use doses of 500 IU PTH-peptide equivalent. It is difficult to obtain assay data regarding the purity and specific activity of commercially available PTH peptides. For the hPTH-(1-34) preparation used in our study,[8,10] 1 mg of hPTH-(1-34) had 13,530 units (U) of activity in an independent UMR 106 osteoblast adenylyl cyclase system.[11] Therefore 500 U are obtained with 37 μg, or approximately 8 nmoles, of pure peptide.

III. CLINICAL OUTCOMES

As can be seen from Table 4.1, the clinical outcomes of PTH therapy have varied because of the technology available at the time. In this section, clinical outcomes will be discussed in the order in which an ideal drug for the management of patients with osteoporosis might be evaluated.

A. Fractures Due To Osteoporosis

Since fractures are the principal consequences of osteoporosis, the current regulatory guidelines for the development of new treatments for osteoporosis require evidence that such treatments reduce the fracture incidence. The controversial studies of the use of sodium fluoride and bisphosphonates have not universally supported the assumption that increased bone mass (assessed by bone densitometry) reduces fracture risk.[12,13] Nor are there definitive studies that indicate whether increases in bone mass induced by PTH will translate into a reduced fracture risk. It is therefore of some comfort that new vertebral fractures occurring during a two-year study of cyclical hPTH-(1-34) injections given to osteoporotic women at high risk for such fractures were documented at less than 25 new fractures/100 patient years in the recent study of Hodsman et al.[10] No new appendicular fractures occurred during the trial.

B. Bone Mass

There are strong epidemiological associations between bone mass measurements at either central (lumbar spine) or appendicular sites (femoral neck, distal radius, os calcis) and the current or future risk for osteoporotic fractures.[14,15] Current estimates suggest a twofold increase in the risk of fracture for every 1.0 standard deviation (SD) below the average age- and sex-matched bone mineral density (BMD); this risk increases dramatically if there are pre-existing fragility fractures in an individual with a low BMD.[14,15] Figure 4.1 describes the strategic objectives of treatment for osteoporosis. It is apparent that low bone mass defines the risk for fragility fractures. For the purposes of this figure a fracture threshold has been indicated, but the gradient of risk is probably continuous, (as it

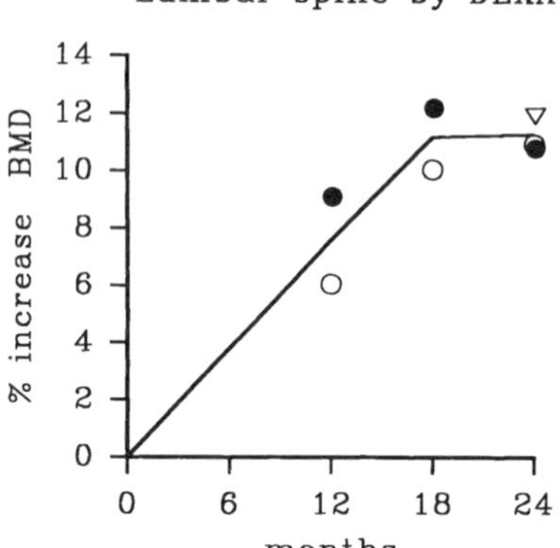

FIGURE 4.2
Changes in lumbar spine BMD measured by dual energy X-ray absorptiometry (DEXA) during the first two years of therapy with PTH. The plot shows the average change in BMD with time, and the individual points represent the data from individual publications: (●, Hodsman et al.[10]); (○, Lindsay et al.[24]); (▽, Neer et al.[25]).

is for many biological variables such as blood pressure and cholesterol in ischemic vascular disease). The most important role for an anabolic agent in bone would be the rapid induction of "new" bone formation in the skeleton to rapidly reduce the risk of fragility fractures. It is against this background that the role of PTH therapy is discussed.

In preliminary clinical studies, BMD measurements have been used as "surrogate" measures of reduced fracture risk, some justification for which exists in the published literature of antiresorptive agents such as estrogen[16] and bisphosphonates,[17-19] together with more recent literature of anabolic treatment of osteoporosis with fluoride preparations.[20,21]

Figure 4.2 shows changes in BMD measurements in reported studies in which responses to PTH treatments have been followed by dual energy absorptiometry of the lumbar spine. Other studies using quantitative computerized tomography (QCT) show even greater increments of 25 to 100% over baseline.[6,22,23] It is important to note in Figure 4.2 that the changes in lumbar spine BMD average 7.6% during the first year[10,24] and 11.3% by the end of the therapy.[10,24,25]

It is apparent that the increment in BMD levels off during the second year of therapy, and the question of developing "resistance" to PTH therapy over time has not been resolved clinically. The composite of data in Figure 4.2 is the result of different protocols using relatively small groups of subjects. Moreover, most studies using PTH therapy have been restricted to two years or less because of the limited availability of the peptide.

This compares with average increments during fluoride therapy of 9% in the first year and 14% by the end of the second year.[12,26,27] Increments in lumbar spine BMD during antiresorptive therapy average less than 6% after two years with bisphosphonates,[17-19] less than 3% with intranasal

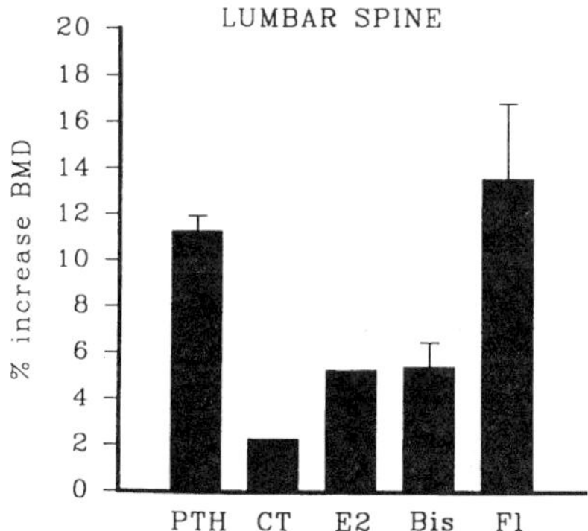

FIGURE 4.3
Average changes in lumbar spine BMD measurements in response to at least two years of treatment with anabolic agents including parathyroid hormone (PTH),[10,24,25,65] and sodium fluoride (Fl),[12,20,27,66] or antiresorptive agents, estrogen (E2),[16] calcitonin (CT),[28] bisphosphonates (Bis).[17-19,67]

calcitonin,[28] and less than 6% with estrogen after one year.[16] These comparative changes in lumbar spine BMD are illustrated in Figure 4.3.

Although the extended data on incremental lumbar spine BMD following PTH therapy are comparable to fluoride therapy, there are no comparative data on actual fracture incidence. Clearly this is an important gap in our clinical information.

Extended data on appendicular BMD changes during PTH treatment is limited. There is a widespread belief that PTH results in a decreased BMD at appendicular sites, mainly attributed to Neer et al.[25] who have reported a transient (but nonprogressive) reduction in distal radial BMD of 5.7% during the first year of PTH therapy. Hesp et al.[29] did not find an improved external calcium balance in patients with osteoporosis treated with daily injections of hPTH-(1-34) for 12 months, while Slovik et al.[30] came to a similar conclusion after short-term (one month) treatment. This has led to the hypothesis that anabolic agents used to treat osteoporosis may improve trabecular bone mass at the expense of diminishing cortical bone mass. Further evidence for this hypothesis has been supplied from the literature of fluoride therapy, in which patients who gained significant amounts of bone mass in the lumbar spine, lost significant bone mass at the distal radius site.[12,31] However, there are several other reports of no significant changes (either improved or decreased) in distal radius or femoral neck BMD over extended periods of PTH therapy.[4-6,10,22,23,32,33]

At the current time, the evidence suggests that PTH therapy rapidly improves spinal bone mass without convincing evidence for either a positive or deleterious effect on the appendicular skeleton. Further exploration of any effects of PTH on the appendicular skeleton or on any beneficial effects of the improved axial skeletal mass upon fracture rates requires that appropriate controlled clinical trials answer this question.

C. Histology

As described in earlier sections of this book, changes in bone histology can be detected in animal experiments very early on in the course of PTH therapy. Similar changes have been recorded in clinical studies.[9]

After only 28 days of hPTH-(1-34) injections, changes in both formation and resorption surfaces were increased 2 to 5 times those measured in a control panel of osteoporotic bone biopsies.[9] Similar findings were observed for bone formation rates and the activation frequency of bone remodeling. There was also no evidence for impaired mineralization as measured by mineral apposition rates, and trabecular architecture was apparently normal.[9] Reeve and co-workers have reported changes in bone histomorphometry after 6 to 12 months of daily PTH therapy.[3,5,32,34,35] Using each patient as an internal control, significant increases in trabecular area, trabecular width, and mean trabecular osteon wall thickness of between 5 and 25% over baseline measurements were documented.[34,35] Although the earlier study by Reeve et al. demonstrated increased trabecular osteoid surfaces (from 23.3% to 35.2%) and resorption surfaces (from 3.9% to 6.2%),[3] their later study demonstrated that, if anything, these same parameters tended to decrease with time.[32] Although little kinetic data (based on *in vivo* tetracycline labels) are available from Reeve and co-workers, the available evidence suggests that long-term PTH therapy (i.e., of more than 6 to 12 months' duration) favors a positive osteon remodeling balance and normal bone architecture, while the dramatic short-term histological evidence for increased bone turnover is not sustained over time.

D. Calcium Balance Studies

Before 1980, there were few ways to measure changes in bone mass in response to any agent. Bone biopsies yield important information, but the measured parameters are not precise (typical CV ± 20%).[36] Therefore, early studies relied on classical dietary calcium balance studies and radioisotopic techniques of assessing skeletal calcium accretion to determine the extent to which new therapies for osteoporosis improved skeletal "bone mass." The methodology of the reports discussed below is not easy to follow even for a reader trained in these techniques, but the cited references should help. Moreover, the reader should appreciate that the cited clinical protocols vary widely with respect to dose of PTH, duration of therapy, and concurrent medication (see Table 4.1). Given these limitations, the results are consistent enough to describe them in general terms (see Table 4.2).

In the initial report by Reeve et al.,[1] four patients treated with PTH (500 units/day), demonstrated an improved dietary calcium balance averaging 7.3 mmole/day. Net diet absorption of ^{47}Ca averaged 3.4

TABLE 4.2

Reported Calcium Kinetic Data in Patients with Osteoporosis Treated with Daily hPTH-(1-34) Injections for at Least One Year

Author (Year)	Diet Calcium Balance (mmol/day)	Diet Calcium Absorption (% Dose)	Skeletal Calcium Accretion (mmol/l/day)
Reeve (1976)[1]	+7.3	+3.4	+6.3
Reeve (1976)[5]	+1.4	+11.9	+0.1
Reeve (1980)[3]	No change	N/A	+7
Slovik (1986)[22]	+3	N/A	N/A
Reeve (1991)[35]	+1.7	+1.2	+3.4

All data are arithmetic means, as reported by the authors, with no clinically significant differences demonstrated across pre- and post-treatment intervals.

mmol/d. Measured accretion of ^{47}Ca by the skeleton averaged 6.3 mmole/day. These data seemed to confirm that the observed improvements in bone histology were indeed due to an anabolic effect of the injected hPTH-(1-34). A subsequent report on the short-term changes (less than one month) measured in the same subjects defined dose-dependent effects, with calcium balance improving with doses of 500 to 1000 U hPTH-(1-34)/day, but deteriorating at a dose of 1500 U/day.[2] In a small group of four patients treated with 450 to 750 U hPTH-(1-34) for one month by Slovik et al.,[30] a similar dose dependency was observed, with a positive dietary calcium balance (2.2 mmole/day) seen only at the lower doses of PTH.

In longer-term studies in which PTH was given for at least 12 months, the calcium kinetics appear to be reasonably consistent (Table 4.2), even though the treatment protocols with PTH are somewhat different. In summary, these calcium kinetic data demonstrate small trends toward positive dietary calcium balances during a variety of therapeutic PTH protocols. These techniques have not been as sensitive to changes in bone mass as dual energy absorptiometry, but they have provided the only evidence that prolonged PTH treatment does not consistently deplete total body calcium. However, two reports suggest that higher doses of PTH (>1000 units/day) may upset total body calcium balance.[2,30]

IV. SERUM BIOCHEMICAL CHANGES DURING PTH THERAPY

For the purposes of this section, only the expected physiological changes in the bone–calcium endocrine axis will be discussed. They form a background for the apparent safety of PTH therapy and provide a context against which to review other biochemical changes that are more directly related to the anabolic actions of PTH.

Changes in serum calcium are an important safety issue regarding the use of PTH to treat osteoporosis. Infusion of PTH over prolonged periods consistently and significantly increases the serum calcium concentration. In response to total infused doses of 400 to 800 U hPTH-(1-34), serum calcium increments of approximately 0.37 mM, have been reported during 12 to 24 hrs.[7,9,11,37] By contrast, single subcutaneous injections of 400 to 800 U produce a slow rise of about 0.10 mM in the serum calcium concentration which peaks at 4 to 8 hours.[9,38] With prolonged daily injections of comparable doses of PTH, the fasting serum calcium concentration at 24 hours after the injection is generally unchanged or only minimally increased over the baseline value, with the total serum calcium concentration remaining within the normal reference range.[3-5,7,9,22,30,35]

Not surprisingly, these rises in the serum calcium concentration to some degree suppress endogenous PTH release. Hodsman et al.[9] and Finkelstein et al.[4] reported an approximately 50% reduction in the level of endogenous immunoreactive PTH by 24 hours after exogenous PTH injection. Although the PTH level did not fall into the "hypoparathyroid" range, this trend to decreased endogenous PTH secretion may be important. Audran et al.[39] have reported one case of transient functional hypoparathyroidism after discontinuing prolonged daily PTH injections, probably due to the development of anti-PTH antibodies. Hesch and coworkers,[40,41] have speculated that altered endogenous pulsatile (minute-to-minute) PTH secretion may be associated either with the development of the osteoporotic condition or the anabolic actions ascribed to exogenous PTH therapy, but this hypothesis has not yet been confirmed. As expected, serum and urinary phosphate concentrations respond to PTH injections with there being either no change or a transient reduction in the serum phosphate concentration and a modestly increased phosphaturia.[1-3,5,22,30,35]

The conventional role for PTH action on the renal tubule is that of increased reabsorption of filtered calcium. This indeed occurs transiently over the first four hours after injection.[2] However, the balance of the published literature suggests a 15 to 70% increase in urinary calcium excretion.[1,3-5,9,22,30] This hypercalciuric effect has not been adequately explained. Coupled to only modest increments in absorbed dietary calcium, enhanced urinary calcium losses explain the minimally positive dietary calcium balance seen in PTH-treated patients.

Does PTH increase bone resorption? In fact it has been hypothesized that trabecular bone is made at the expense of cortical bone. This was first suggested by the decreasing bone mineral density at appendicular sites following fluoride therapy (see Section III.B). Apart from the decreased radial bone density reported by Neer et al.,[25] there is little evidence from BMD studies so far published that this occurs during PTH therapy.

Is the hypercalciuria due to increased fractional absorption of dietary calcium as a result of PTH-induced renal calcitriol synthesis? Hodsman and Fraher reported that increased circulating calcitriol levels after PTH therapy were probably physiologically significant,[7] although the dietary calcium balance studies do not support this (see Section III.D). While the reality may lie somewhere between these two explanations, it is clear that PTH induces mild hypercalciuria.

The response of the vitamin D metabolic pathway to prolonged PTH therapy is a contentious issue. At the heart of this is the possibility that older subjects with or without osteoporosis may have an impaired ability to increase renal calcitriol (1,25 $(OH)_2$ vitamin D_3) synthesis in response to circulating PTH. Hodsman and Fraher[7] and Lindsay et al.[38] have reported significantly increased circulating calcitriol levels following a subcutaneous injection of 400 U of hPTH-(1-34) into elderly women with osteoporosis. For example, calcitriol levels remained above baseline values after 14 days of PTH injections (400 U/day), and were associated with significantly increased fractional absorption of ^{45}Ca from the intestine.[7] The direct evidence in women with osteoporosis treated with daily PTH injections suggests that the renal 25-hydroxycholecalciferol-1α hydroxylase is stimulated by the exogenous PTH.

V. BIOCHEMICAL MARKERS OF BONE METABOLISM

It is beyond the scope of this review to discuss the development of biochemical markers of bone turnover in metabolic bone diseases. Their advantage for research purposes is principally to provide noninvasive indicators of the balance between bone resorption and bone turnover.[42-44] In this section, the discussion of biochemical markers of bone resorption will be restricted to urinary hydroxy-proline (OH-Pro) and the collagen crosslinking pyridinolines. The markers of bone formation will be total serum alkaline phosphatase and osteocalcin.

Because PTH is regarded as a potent bone-resorbing hormone that increases urinary calcium excretion, other markers of bone resorption are of great importance. Reeve et al.[3] reported a 26% increase in OH-Pro excretion by patients treated with daily PTH, but there was either no change or a 100% drop in urinary OH-Pro in a small group of 12 patients who were treated with estrogen or androgen as concurrent antiresorptive therapy.[5,35] When using a "high" dose of PTH (i.e., 800 U/day), Hodsman et al.[9] reported a 53% increase in urine OH-Pro after one month of treatment with no significant changes in urine pyridinoline excretion. Finkelstein et al.[4] reported increases of both OH Pro and pyridinoline excretion of approximately 125% in acutely hypoestrogenemic younger women after six months of PTH therapy.

It is not surprising that PTH increases collagen breakdown and the subsequent excretion of breakdown products because there is ample evidence for increased bone turnover with concurrent bone resorption during anabolic therapy. However, the results reported by Reeve et al.[5,35] are at the lowest, and those of Finkelstein et al.[4] at the highest, end of the spectrum. One common link between these two studies is the use of concurrent estrogen replacement in elderly osteoporotic women by Reeve et al. and the therapeutic induction of acute estrogen deficiency (as treatment for endometriosis with naferelin) by Finkelstein. This provides evidence for the potential benefits of combining antiresorptive agents with PTH therapy in an attempt to maximize gains in bone mass achieved by PTH alone.

Despite rather variable changes in markers of bone resorption, indices of bone formation have shown consistent increments. In response to exogenous PTH therapy, serum total alkaline phosphatase (tAP) levels increased from 15 to 104%,[1,3,4,6,7,9] and averaged 40%. In the three studies reporting changes in the serum osteocalcin (OC) concentration, both short-[7,9] and long-term[10] PTH treatment resulted in increments of 60 to 160%. Increases in tAP and/or OC have been seen only inconsistently during other anabolic treatments, specifically fluoride therapy,[12,45] whereas acute, abrupt, and sustained reductions in both resorption and formation markers are seen with antiresorptive therapy (i.e., estrogen replacement or alendronate[43,44]).

In summary, the reported measurements of biochemical markers for bone resorption and formation support the rapid onset of skeletal activation and bone turnover in response to PTH as reported histologically by Hodsman et al.[9] Increases in bone formation markers are consistent and of considerable magnitude, in keeping with direct osteoblastic stimulation and bone anabolism. Increases in bone resorption markers are less consistent, but appear to be less pronounced during concomitant therapy with estrogen.

VI. ANALYSIS OF CONCURRENT THERAPIES USED WITH PTH PROTOCOLS

During the past 20 years, PTH has been given, with or without nutritional calcium and vitamin D supplements,[1-3,29,46,47] with calcitriol,[22,25,48] with estrogen or androgen as a concurrent antiresorptive agent,[23,24,32,34,35] and in several cyclical protocols with or without antiresorptive agents.[5-10] The *concept* for the cyclical use of PTH should be distinguished from its direct anabolic effects on the skeleton. Since PTH also activates bone remodeling, cyclical protocols have attempted to exploit the ADFR hypothesis (*A*: activate remodeling; *D*: depress resorption in the activated bone modeling units; *F*: allow for a treatment-free period of bone formation; *R*: repeat the treatment cycle). In fact, none of the cyclical protocols can be considered a true ADFR protocol, and these should be regarded as hybrid anabolic protocols.

Despite the differences in these protocols, the overall results of therapy have been remarkably consistent with an increase in trabecular bone (as measured by BMD in lumbar spine or histomorphometrically in iliac crest) and little evidence for changes in bone mass in the appendicular skeleton. All reported studies had small samples of treated subjects and were thus unable to clearly define the interactions of concurrent therapies. Only the brief report by Neer et al.[25] used a true control group of patients treated with no other bone-active agents except nutritional calcium supplements. Nevertheless, some guarded conclusions can be made.

1. The earliest studies by Reeve and co-workers, using daily PTH injections without concurrent therapy, unequivocally found increased trabecular bone mass (histological outcome) and increased bone formation (^{47}Ca kinetics) with a slight trend toward a positive calcium balance (classical diet balance techniques). Given the poor precision of dietary calcium balance techniques, (CV ± 2.1 mmole/day,[2] the reported changes in calcium balance ranged from –3.7 to + 2.2 mmole/d.[5,30,35] Much larger samples would have been needed to find out whether PTH therapy by itself is beneficial or injurious to the skeleton as a whole. Current clinical trials will answer this question more economically by measuring total body bone mass by DEXA.
2. The studies by Neer and co-workers combined calcitriol with daily PTH injection.[22,25,30,48] This strategy was adopted because the earlier dietary calcium balance studies of Reeve and co-workers demonstrated minimal adaptations of dietary calcium absorption despite obvious histomorphometric restoration of trabecular bone and increased urinary Ca excretion. Slovik et al.[22] performed dietary calcium balance studies in 4 of 8 men with osteoporosis before and after at least 12 months of hPTH-(1-34) (400 to 500 U/day). Although net calcium absorption increased in all four subjects, overall calcium balance remained negative (–1.5 to –5.3 mmol/d) in three of them. Since exogenous PTH increases serum calcitriol levels[7,38] and is associated with increased fractional ^{45}Ca absorption, the need for additional calcitriol therapy remains unproven. The changes in lumbar BMD reported by Neer and co-workers are comparable to those in other studies (see Section III.B), but theirs is the one group to report significant losses of BMD at the radius in a controlled clinical trial (15 patients on calcium, 15 patients on PTH + calcitriol 0.25 μg/d, over 2 years).[25] The control group lost 1.7% and the experimental group lost 5.7% BMD — all in the first year of treatment. The greater and abrupt loss of appendicular bone mass in the experimental group might indicate a permanent loss of cortical bone, but an alternative explanation includes the possibility of a "transient" effect of increased intracortical modeling.
3. The concurrent use of antiresorptive agents, specifically estrogen, is attractive. If estrogen can selectively blunt the resorptive action of PTH on bone without deleterious inhibition of its anabolic effects, this combination would be ideal.

   The experimental literature is confusing. Cosman et al.[49] infused PTH over 20 hours (approximately 800 U to each of 17 estrogen-treated and 15 estrogen-deficient osteoporotic postmenopausal women). The estrogen-deficient women excreted significantly larger amounts of bone resorption markers (urinary OH-Pro and deoxypyridinoline), suggesting a protective effect of estrogen on resorption. However, in a similar experiment Tsai et al.[37] infused 400 U/day for three days into premenopausal women and postmenopausal women with or without osteoporosis. They found no differences in serum calcium or urinary OH-Pro excretion and concluded that estrogen did not have such a protective effect. Using an alternative approach of calcium deprivation to induce endogenous 2° hyperparathyroidism, the same group reached similar conclusions.[50] Marcus et al.[51] gave acute (20 minutes) infusions of graded doses of PTH to 15 postmenopausal women before and after starting estrogen replacement, and no differences were found in serum calcitriol increments or urinary cAMP excretion as a result of estrogen therapy. They concluded that the renal–endocrine axis was not affected by estrogen deficiency. The flaw in these arguments is the fact that clinical responses to PTH infusion favor bone catabolism, while intermittent injections favor anabolism.[9]

In the study by Reeve et al.,[35] daily PTH injections and concurrent estrogen therapy were combined in nine women. By comparison with historical controls (women treated with PTH alone),[3] calcium balance studies were significantly improved; cotreatment with estrogen actually led to a 12% decrease in urinary calcium,[35] rather than the 14% increase seen historically.[3] The three-year study by Lindsay's group comparing estrogen-treated patients with and without daily PTH injection is now completed and partially reported in abstract form.[52] To date there are no controlled factorial studies to test the estrogen effect independently of PTH. Therefore the protective effect of estrogen remains speculative. No clinical studies combining bisphosphonates with PTH have been reported to date, although encouraging (but conflicting) data are available in animal studies.

4. Cyclical therapy with PTH is of interest insofar as it might provide insights as to how the hormone might ultimately be given in the most economical fashion, but the literature to date adds little that is not already known about the actions of PTH. Hesch and Hodsman[6-10] have combined cyclical PTH-(1-34) or PTH-(1-38) with concomitant or sequential cycles of calcitonin and found little evidence that the antiresorptive action of calcitonin provides any additional clinical benefit. Short cycles of PTH (400 to 500 U/day) for less than 14 days provide little evidence of skeletal activation of bone turnover or anabolism,[5,7,8] although biochemical responses are detectable within this time frame. However, 28-day cycles of a high dose of PTH (800 U/day) appear to strongly activate bone turnover[9] and increase bone mass.[9,10] The reported changes in lumbar spine BMD, with small increments in femoral neck BMD with 28-day cycles of high-dose PTH may provide an alternative approach to harnessing the anabolic effects of PTH, but there are no controlled trials comparing cycles of PTH therapy with daily injections.

VII. PHARMACOKINETICS OF PTH ADMINISTRATION

Plasma pharmacokinetics after intravenous bolus administration of hPTH-(1-34) were reported in two studies,[53,54] and pharmacokinetics following a subcutaneous injection were described in three publications.[38,53,55] Changes in serum calcium, phosphorus, and 1,25-dihydroxyvitamin D_3, and in urinary calcium, cAMP, and phosphate after single subcutaneous injection were also reported in two of these studies.[38,55]

One of the earliest published studies[53] reported plasma pharmacokinetics after both intravenous and subcutaneous administration of 100 μg of hPTH-(1-34), as well as pharmacodynamics following the subcutaneous dose; both serum immunoreactivity and bioactivity were assessed in this study. Peak plasma immunoreactive PTH concentration was observed two minutes after intravenous administration to two healthy male volunteers, with a biexponential disappearance and a calculated "mean transit time" of 14 to 16 minutes. A small amount of immunoreactivity was still detected 75 minutes after injection. When measured by a cytochemical bioassay, the peak plasma bioactivity was observed four to six minutes after injection with a single-exponential disappearance half-life of 1.5 to 2.6 minutes and a calculated mean transit time of 5.8 to 8.6 minutes. Plasma bioactivity returned to baseline by 25 minutes in both subjects. In the same study, following subcutaneous administration of 100 μg synthetic human PTH-(1-34), the time to reach maximum plasma concentration (T_{max}) of both PTH immunoreactivity and bioactivity was 15 minutes. The bioactivity persisted for only 35 minutes after injection, but the immunoreactivity did not completely disappear from the plasma until 180 to 240 minutes after injection. In the second report of plasma pharmacokinetics following intravenous administration,[54] peak plasma immunoreactivity was observed two to three minutes after intravenous administration of 10.7 nmole (about 44 μg) of synthetic hPTH-(1-34) to five young male and five young female volunteers. The peptide demonstrated a biexponential disappearance with a terminal half-life of 10 minutes.

In a study of PTH pharmacokinetics in postmenopausal women, Lindsay et al.[38] administered 25 μg of hPTH-(1-34) subcutaneously to 11 estrogen-treated postmenopausal patients, and blood and urine samples were obtained over the next four hours. The principal pharmacokinetic and pharmacodynamic results are summarized in Table 4.3. The concentration of immunoreactive hPTH-(1-34) increased from 6.5 pM to a peak of 92.5 pM at 30 minutes, and disappeared with a mean half-life of 75 minutes. It was still above baseline at 240 minutes, but had returned to baseline in the two patients who were examined 24 hours after injection. The clearance rate was 0.79 l/min and, based on a regression analysis, appeared to decline with increasing age and years since menopause. No other age-related associations were observed. Serum total and ionized calcium, and

TABLE 4.3

Pharmacokinetics and Pharmacodynamics Following a 25-μg Subcutaneous Dose of Synthetic Human PTH(1-34)

Parameter	Baseline	Peak or Nadir	Time to Peak or Nadir (Minutes)	p-Value[a]
Urinary calcium (mmol/mmol creatinine)	0.16 ± 0.024	0.25 ± 0.044	120	NS
Urinary phosphorus (mmol/mmol creatinine)	0.50 ± 0.09	1.27 ± 0.10	>240	p <.003
Urinary cAMP (mmol/mmol creatinine)	757 ± 183	2395 ± 508	120	p <.04
Serum total calcium (mmol/L)	2.32 ± 0.03	2.40 ± 0.04	>240	p <.05[b]
Serum phosphorus (mmol/L)	1.09 ± 0.04	0.94 ± 0.03	120	p <.05
1,25-dihydroxyvitamin D_3 (calcitriol) (pmol/L)	106 ± 10	139 ± 11	>240	p <.05
Endogenous PTH-(1-84) pmol/L	3.31 ± 0.31	2.39 ± 0.29	>240	p <.04
hPTH-(1-34) immunoreactivity (pmol/L)	6.51 ± 0.79	92.5 ± 13	30	p <.002

Note: Abbreviations: NS = not significant; cAMP = cyclic adenosine 3′,5′-monophosphate.

[a] Compared to baseline, except where indicated.

[b] By trend analysis only.

Source: Data from Lindsay, R., Vieves, J., Henneman, E., Shen, V., and Cosman, F., Subcutaneous administration of the amino-terminal fragment of human parathyroid hormone-(1-34): kinetics and biochemical response to estrogenized osteoporotic patients, *J. Clin. Endocrinol. Metab.*, 77, 1535, 1993.

serum calcitriol concentration did not start rising until 90 to 120 minutes after injection, and had not yet peaked at the final 240-minute sample. Endogenous PTH-(1-84) began to decline within 15 minutes after injection of hPTH-(1-34) and remained significantly suppressed from 45 minutes after injection throughout the 240-minute sampling period. None of the changes in calcium, phosphorus, vitamin D, or endogenous PTH were clinically significant. As noted previously, the patients studied by Lindsay et al.[38] were all receiving estrogen (and usually progestin) replacement therapy. The extent to which estrogens and progestins affect the pharmacodynamic response to PTH is unknown.

Fraher et al.[55] reported very similar data in abstract form that compared the pharmacokinetics in 10 young volunteers and 9 elderly osteoporotic women, following the subcutaneous injection of 44 μg hPTH-(1-34). The profiles of serum immunoreactive hPTH-(1-34) following subcutaneous injection are clearly identical for young (mean age 25 yrs) and elderly (mean age 67 yrs) subjects. In this study, the time to peak serum PTH-(1-34) concentration was approximately 16 minutes, with a fractional clearance rate of approximately 2.0 l/minute. Maximal increments in serum calcium averaged 0.15 mmole/L and occurred at eight hours after injection (see Figure 4.4).

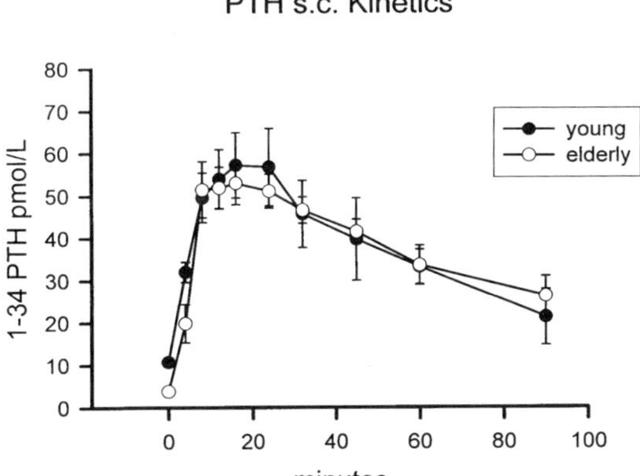

FIGURE 4.4
Serum concentrations of hPTH-(1-34) after subcutaneous injection of 800 IU PTH peptide in 10 young adults aged 25 ± 9 (S.D.) yrs., and 9 elderly women with osteoporosis, aged 67 ± 11 years. (Data from Fraher, L. J., Hodsman, A. B., Steer, B. M., and Freeman, A. A., Comparison of the pharmacokinetics of subcutaneous parathyroid hormone in healthy young and elderly osteoporotic subjects, [Abstract], *J. Bone Min. Res.*, 8, S253, 1993.)

A. Summary of Pharmacokinetics and Pharmacodynamics

Published literature on the pharmacokinetics and pharmacodynamics of hPTH-(1-34) indicates that single subcutaneous injections (25 to 100 μg) produced peak serum concentrations 10- to 14-fold higher than baseline endogenous PTH concentrations within approximately 15 to 30 minutes, and an apparent elimination half-life of about 75 minutes. Since administered PTH completely disappears from the circulation by 4 to 24 hours after injection, no accumulation is expected with repeated daily administration.

VIII. OTHER ANALOGS AND DELIVERY SYSTEMS

The principal analog used in the reported clinical literature was the presumed bioactive amino-terminal fragment of PTH, namely hPTH-(1-34). Several have used hPTH-(1-38) because it might be more potent than hPTH-(1-34),[6-8,40,56] but there is no compelling reason to accept this. The natural hPTH-(1-84) holohormone is currently under development for clinical trials and appears to be anabolically equipotent to PTH-(1-34). Other analogs include hPTH-(1-31)NH_2 which stimulates the adenylyl cyclase PTH, but, unlike the larger peptides, does not stimulate phospholipase-C and yet retains the anabolic properties of the larger PTH peptides in animal experiments.[57] Other PTH analogs have been published in abstract, appear to be potent bone anabolic agents in animal experiments,[58-60] but have not been fully evaluated at a clinical level.

While all PTH peptides are currently under clinical development using the subcutaneous injection route, alternative delivery systems include:

1. Automated injection or transcutaneous delivery
2. Intranasal delivery
3. Transpulmonary delivery of aerosolized peptide[61]

Alternative delivery systems are in the early stages of clinical evaluation. Intranasal delivery devices have been demonstrated for both PTH and calcitonin peptides, using lyophilized, microparticulate delivery systems.[61,62] Transpulmonary systems have been developed in which aerosol delivery to the bronchoalveolar tree leads to 30 to 40% bioavailability of PTH peptide compared with intravenous routes of administration, with profiles of peptide absorption which are very similar to those delivered by subcutaneous injection.[63] While noninjectable routes of PTH peptide delivery are still in the realm of experimental medicine, there is no reason to believe that this compliance barrier cannot be crossed in the near future. Meanwhile, clinical scientists must continue to answer the questions raised by the current body of clinical evidence supporting the use of PTH peptides as appropriate anabolic agents for the treatment of osteoporosis. In the short term, research using injectable PTH peptides has not been a significant barrier to patient compliance.

IX. IMMUNOLOGICAL RESPONSES TO EXOGENOUS PTH

Of the available reports in which antibody formation was deliberately sought, 8 of 75 patients apparently developed anti-hPTH-(1-34) antibodies in low titers.[1,5,6,10,35] Four patients discontinued hPTH-(1-34) therapy because of generalized urticarial reactions or local irritation at the injection site.[1,3] Although an 11% incidence of anti-PTH-(1-34) antibodies may seem high, it is likely that these early reports reflect impurities in the hPTH-(1-34) formulations that were used because hPTH-(1-34) is a naturally occurring peptide and should not be immunogenic. Whether the newer PTH analogs have this drawback awaits further clinical testing.

X. SIDE EFFECTS DURING PTH THERAPY

From Table 4.1, it can be seen that close to 140 patients with osteoporosis have been treated with PTH. Of these, no deaths have been reported. As discussed above, four patients probably experienced sufficiently severe immunological responses to hPTH-(1-34) to discontinue therapy. Eight patients may have demonstrated immunological reactions to an (impure) hPTH-(1-34) product, and/or local irritation at the injection site. Several patients developed mild nausea and arthralgia in one study.[4] Mild hypercalcemia and hypercalciuria have been observed, but neither appears to have had clinical consequences and no increased incidence of renal calculus formation has been reported to date. Hodsman et al.[10] have raised an issue about the long-term safety of PTH on renal function. In this report, 39 patients were treated with cyclical high-dose PTH (800 U/day for four 28-day cycles/year for two years). This patient group experienced a significant 10% increase in serum creatinine (albeit within the normal range of age-related serum creatinine). Thus, PTH-induced hypercalciuria might conceivably affect renal function.

XI. CONCLUSION

To date, the clinical experience with PTH as an anabolic agent in the treatment of osteoporosis is encouraging. The reported literature consistently reports improvements in trabecular bone mass without established evidence for detrimental effects on the appendicular skeleton or clinically important side effects. As such, PTH therapy holds the promise of being equal or superior to the alternative anabolic agent in bone, sodium fluoride. PTH therapy may be superior to current strategies using antiresorptive therapy, including bisphosphonates, estrogen replacement, or calcitonin. However, some important clinical issues remain to be defined.

1. The full safety profile of prolonged PTH therapy remains to be defined, but ongoing commercial clinical trials should establish this.
2. Does prolonged PTH therapy result in a net negative calcium balance to the detriment of the appendicular skeleton? Again, ongoing clinical trials employing total body bone mass measurements should address this question.
3. Will cyclical use of PTH prove to be as effective as continued daily dosing?
4. Despite impressive gains in bone mass during the period of PTH therapy, can this gain be maintained with less invasive treatment, i.e., the use of oral bisphosphonates? Preliminary data from the only study so far reported to employ such a strategy using 28-day cycles of clodronate (400 mg/d repeating every 3 months) suggests that this goal may not be as easy as it sounds.[64]
5. Is it necessary to add concomitant medication (i.e., calcitriol, estrogen, or bisphosphonates) to maximize the anabolic effects of PTH? While the published data employing such strategies are not convincing, factorially designed clinical trials have not been done.
6. Will analogs of PTH be better anabolic agents than hPTH-(1-34) or hPTH-(1-84)?

7. Will PTH-induced increments in BMD translate into reduced vertebral and apendicular fracture rates (the true indicators of the morbidity suffered by patients with osteoporosis)?

Clearly there is a large body of clinical work to occupy clinical scientists over the next five to ten years. Many of these questions should be resolved by then!

REFERENCES

1. Reeve, J., Hesp, R., Williams, D., Klenerman, L., Zanelli, J. M., Darby, A. J., Tregear, G. W., Parsons, J. A., and Hume, R., Anabolic effect of low doses of a fragment of human parathyroid hormone on the skeleton in postmenopausal osteoporosis. *Lancet*, 1, 1035, 1976.
2. Reeve, J., Tregear, G. W., and Parsons, J. A., Preliminary trial of low doses of human parathyroid hormone 1-34 peptide in treatment of osteoporosis, *Clin. Endocrinol.*, 21, 469, 1976.
3. Reeve, J., Meunier, P. J., Parsons, J. A., Bernat, M., Bijvoet, O. L. M., Courpron, P., Edouard, C., Lenerman, L., Neer, R. M., Renier, J. C., Slovik, D., Vismans, F. J. F. E., and Potts, J. T. J., Anabolic effect of human parathyroid hormone fragment on trabecular bone in involutional osteoporosis: a multicentre trial, *Br. Med. J.*, 1340, 1980.
4. Finkelstein, J. S., Klibanski, A., Schaefer, e. H., Hornstein, M. D., Schiff, I., and Neer, R. M., Parathyroid hormone for the prevention of bone loss induced by estrogen deficiency, *N. Engl. J. Med.*, 331, 1618, 1994.
5. Reeve, J. Arlot, M., Price, T. R., Edouard, C., Hesp, R., Hulme, P., Ashley, J. P., Zanelli, J. M., Green, J. R., Tellez, M., Katz, D., Spinks, T. J., and Meunier, P. J., Periodic courses of human 1-34 parathyroid peptide alternating with calcitriol paradoxically reduce bone remodelling in spinal osteoporosis: *Eur. J. Clin. Invest.*, 17, 421, 1987.
6. Hesch, R. D., Busch, U., Prokop, M., Delling, G., and Rittinghaus, E. F., Increase of vertebral density by combination therapy with pulsatile 1-38 hPTH and sequential addition of calcitonin nasal spray in osteoporotic patients, *Calif. Tissue Int.*, 44, 176, 1989.
7. Hodsman, A. B. and Fraher, L. J., Biochemical responses to sequential human parathyroid hormone (1-38) and calcitonin in osteoporotic patients, *Bone Miner.*, 9, 137, 1990.
8. Hodsman, A. B., Steer, B. M., Fraher, L. J., and Drost, D. J., Bone densitometric and histomorphometric responses to sequential human parathyroid hormone (1-38) and salmon calcitonin in osteoporotic patients, *Bone Miner.*, 14, 67, 1991.
9. Hodsman, A. B., Fraher, L. J., Ostbye, T., Adachi, J. D., and Steer, B. M., An evaluation of several biochemical markers for bone formation and resorption in a protocol utilizing cyclical parathyroid hormone and calcitonin therapy for osteoporosis, *J. Clin. Invest.*, 91, 1138, 1993.
10. Hodsman, A. B., Fraher, L. J., Watson, P. H., Ostbye, T., Stitt, L. W., Adachi, J. D., Taves, D. H., and Drost, D., A randomized controlled trial to compare the efficacy of cyclical parathyroid hormone versus cyclical parathyroid hormone and sequential calcitonin to improve bone mass in post-menopausal women with osteoporosis, *J. Clin. Endocrinol. Metab.*, 82, 620, 1997.
11. Fraher, L., Hodsman, A. B., Jonas, K., Saunders, D., Rose, C. I., Henderson, J. E., Hendy, G. N., and Goltzman, D. A., Comparison of the in vivo biochemical responses to exogenous parathyroid hormone (1-34) and parathyroid hormone-related peptide (1-34) in man, *J. Clin. Endocrinol. Metab.*, 75, 417, 1992.

12. Riggs, B. L., Hodgson, S. F., O'Fallon, W. M., Chao, E. Y. S., Wahner, H. W., Muhs, J. M., Cedel, S. L., and Melton, L. III, Effect of fluoride treatment on the fracture rate in postmenopausal women with osteoporosis, *N. Engl. J. Med.*, 322, 802, 1990.
13. Lindsay, R. and Cosman, F., Estrogen in prevention and treatment of osteoporosis, *Ann. NY Acad. Sci.*, 592, 326, 1990.
14. Cummings, S. R., Black, D. M., Nevitt, M. C., Browner, W., Cauley, J., Ensrud, K., Genant, H. K., Palermo, L., Scott, J., and Vogt, T. M., Bone density at various sites for prediction of hip fractures, *Lancet*, 341, 72, 1993.
15. Ross, P. D., Davis, J. W., Epstein, R. S., and Wasnich, R. D., Pre-existing fracture and bone mass predict vertebral fracture incidence in women, *Ann. Int. Med.*, 114, 919, 1991.
16. Lufkin, E. G., Wahner, H. W., O'Fallon, W. M., Hodgson, S. F., Kotowicz, M. A., Lane, A. W., Judd, H. L., Caplan, R. H., and Riggs, B. L., Treatment of postmenopausal osteoporosis with transdermal estrogen, *Ann. Int. Med.*, 117, 1, 1992.
17. Storm, T., Thamsborg, G., Steiniche, T., Genant, H. K., and Sorensen, O. H., Effect of intermittent cyclical etidronate therapy on bone mass and fracture rate in women with postmenopausal osteoporosis, *N. Engl. J. Med.*, 322, 1265, 1990.
18. Watts, N. B., Harris, S. T., Genant, H. K., Wasnich, R. D., Miller, P. D., Jackson, R. D., Licata, A. A., Ross, P., Woodson, G. C. III, Yanover, J. M., Mysiw, W. J., Kohse, L., Rao, M. B., Steiger, P., and Richmond, B., Intermittent cyclical etidronate treatment of postmenopausal osteoporosis, *N. Engl. J. Med.*, 323, 73, 1990.
19. Liberman, U. A., Weiss, S. R., Broll, J. Minne, H. W., Quan, H., Bell, N. H., Rodriguez-Portales, J., Downs, R. W., Dequiker, J., Favus, M., Seeman, E., Recker, R. R., Capizzi, T., Santora, A. C., and Lombardi, A., Effect of oral alendronate on bone mineral density and the incidence of fractures in postmenopausal osteoporosis, *N. Engl. J. Med.*, 333, 1437, 1995.
20. Pak, C. Y. C., Sakhaee, K., Adams-Huet, B., Piziak, V., Peterson, R. D., and Poindexter, J. R., Treatment of postmenopausal osteoporosis with slow-release sodium fluoride — Final report of a randomized control group, *Ann. Int. Med.*, 123, 401, 1995.
21. Riggs, B. L., O'Fallon, W. M., Lane, A., Hodgson, S. F., Wahner, H. W., Muhs, J., Chao, E., and Melton, L. J., Clinical trial of fluoride therapy in postmenopausal osteoporotic women: extended observations and additional analysis, *J. Bone Min. Res.*, 9, 265, 1994.
22. Slovik, D. M., Rosenthal, D. I., Doppelt, S., Potts, J. T. J., Daly, M. A., Campbell, J. A., and Neer, R. M., Restoration of spinal bone in osteoporotic men by treatment with human parathyroid hormone (1-34) and 1,25-dihydroxyvitamin D, *J. Bone Min. Res.*, 1, 377, 1986.
23. Reeve, J., Davies, U. M., Hesp, R., McNally, E., and Katz, D., Treatment of osteoporosis with human parathyroid peptide and observations on the effect of sodium fluoride, *Br. Med. J.*, 301, 314, 1990.
24. Lindsay, R., Cosman, F., Nieves, J., Dempster, D. W., and Shen, V. A., Controlled clinical trial of the effects of 1-34hPTH in estrogen treated osteoporotic women, *J. Bone Min. Res.*, 8, S130, 1995.
25. Neer, R., Slovik, D., Daly, M., Lo, C., Potts, J., and Nussbaum, S., Treatment of postmenopausal osteoporosis with daily parathyroid hormone plus calcitriol, in *Osteoporosis*. Christiansen, C. and Overgaard, K., Eds., Osteopress APS, Copenhagen, 1991.
26. Black, D. M., Bauer, D. C., and Lu, Y., Should BMD be measured at multiple sites to predict fractures in elderly women? *J. Bone Min. Res.*, 10, S140, 1995.
27. Sebert, J. L., Richard, P., Mennencier, I., Bisset, J. P., and Loeb, G., Monofluorophosphate increases lumbar bone density in osteopenic patients: A double-masked randomized study, *Osteoporosis Int.*, 5, 108, 1995.
28. Reginster, J. Y., Deroisy, R., Lecard, M. P., Sarlet, N., Zegels, B., Jupsin, I., De Longueville, M., and Franchimont, P., A double-blind, placebo-controlled, dose-finding trial of intermittent nasal salmon calcitonin for prevention of postmenopausal lumbar spine bone loss, *Am. J. Med.*, 98, 452, 1995.

29. Hesp, R., Hulme, P., Williams, D., and Reeve, J., The relationship between changes in femoral bone density and calcium balance in patients with involutional osteoporosis treated with human parathyroid hormone fragment (hPTH 1-34), *Metab. Bone Dis. Rel. Res.*, 2, 331, 1981.
30. Slovik, D. M., Neer, R. M., and Potts, J. T. J., Short-term effects of synthetic human parathyroid hormone-(1-34) administration on bone mineral metabolism in osteoporotic patients, *J. Clin. Invest.*, 68, 1261, 1981.
31. Hodsman, A. B. and Drost, D. J., The response of vertebral bone mineral density during the treatment of osteoporosis with sodium fluoride, *J. Clin. Endocrinol. Metab.*, 69, 1, 1989.
32. Reeve, J., Arlot, M. E., Bradbeer, J. N., Hesp, R., Mcally, E., Meunier, P. J., and Zanelli, J. M., Human parathyroid peptide treatment of vertebral osteoporosis, *Osteoporosis Int.*, 3, S199, 1993.
33. Lindsay, R., Cosman, F., Nieves, J., Dempster, D. W., and Shen, V. A., Controlled clinical trial of the effects of 1-34hPTH in estrogen treated osteoporotic women, [Abstract], *J. Bone Min. Res.*, 9, S130, 1993.
34. Bradbeer, J. N., Arlot, M. E., Meunier, P. J., and Reeve, J., Treatment of osteoporosis with parathyroid peptide (hPTH 1-34) and oestrogen: Increase in volumetric density of iliac cancellous bone may depend on reduced trabecular spacing as well as increased thickness of packets of newly formed bone, *Clin. Endocrinol.*, 37, 282, 1992.
35. Reeve, J., Bradbeer, J. N., Arlot, M., Davies, U. M., Green, J. R., Hampton, L., Edouard, C., Hesp, R., Hulme, P., Ashby, J. P., Zanelli, J. M., and Meunier, P. J., hPTH 1-34 treatment of osteoporosis with added hormone replacement therapy: biochemical, kinetic and histological responses, *Osteoporosis Int.*, 1, 162, 1991.
36. Chavassieux, P. M., Arlot, M. E., and Meunier, P. J., Intersample variation in bone histomorphometry: comparison between parameter values measured on two contiguous transilica bone biopsies, *Calcif. Tissue Int.*, 37, 345, 1985.
37. Tsai, K.-S., Ebeling, P. R., and Riggs, B. L., Bone responsiveness to parathyroid hormone in normal and osteoporotic postmenopausal women, *J. Clin. Endocrinol. Metab.*, 69, 1024, 1989.
38. Lindsay, R., Nieves, J., Henneman, E., Shen, V., and Cosman, F., Subcutaneous administration of the amino-terminal fragment of human parathyroid hormone-(1-34): kinetics and biochemical response to estrogenized osteoporotic patients, *J. Clin. Endocrinol. Metab.*, 77, 1535, 1993.
39. Audran, M., Basle, M. F., Defontaine, A., Jallet, P., Bidet, M. T., Ermias, A., Tanguy, G., Pouplard, A., Reeve, J., Zanelli, J., and Renier, J. C., Transient hypoparathyroidism induced by synthetic human parathyroid hormone-(1-34)-treatment, *J. Clin. Endocrinol. Metab.*, 64, 937, 1987.
40. Hesch, R. D., Busch, U., Prokop, M., Delling, G., Harms, H., and Rittinghaus, E. F., Increase in bone mass and turnover in low turnover osteoporosis by combined (1-38) hPTH and Calcitonin nasal spray, in *Calcitonin 88: New Therapeutic Perspectives; the Nasal Spray*, Mazzuoli, G. F., Ed., Sandos AG, Basel, 1989, 139.
41. Prank, K., Nowlan, S. J., Harms, H. M., Koppstech, M., Brabant, G., and Hesch, R., Time series prediction of plasma hormone concentration, *J. Clin. Invest.*, 95, 2910, 1995.
42. Delmas, P. D., Schlemmer, A., Gineyts, E., Riis, B., and Christiansen, C., Urinary excretion of pyridinoline crosslinks correlates with bone turnover measured on iliac crest biopsy in patients with vertebral osteoporosis, *J. Bone Min. Res.*, 6, 639, 1991.
43. Riis, B. J., Overgaard, K., and Christiansen, C., Biochemical markers of bone turnover to monitor the bone response to postmenopausal hormone replacement therapy, *Osteoporosis Int.*, 5, 276, 1995.
44. Garnero, P., Shih, W. J., Gineyts, E., Karpf, D. B., and Delmas, P. D., Comparison of new biochemical markers of bone turnover in late postmenopausal osteoporotic women in response to alendronate treatment, *J. Clin. Endocrinol. Metab.*, 79, 1693, 1994.

45. Hodsman, A. B. and Drost, D. J., The response of vertebral bone mineral density during the treatment of osteoporosis with sodium fluoride, *J. Clin. Endocrinol. Metab.*, 69, 932, 1989.
46. Reeve, J., Arlot, M., Bernat, M., Charhon, S., Edouard, C., Slovik, D., Vismans, F. J. F. E., and Meunier, P. J., Calcium-47 kinetic measurements of bone turnover compared to bone histomorphometry in osteoporosis: the influence of human parathyroid (hPTH 1-34) therapy, *Metab. Bone Dis. Rel. Res.*, 3, 23, 1981.
47. Reeve, J., Arlot, M., Bernat, M., Edouard, C., Hesp, R., Slovik, D., Vismans, F. J. F. E., and Meunier, P. J., Treatment of osteoporosis with human parathyroid fragment 1-34: a positive final tissue balance in trabecular bone, *Metab. Bone Dis. Rel. Res.*, 2, 355, 1980.
48. Neer, R. M., Slovik, D., Doppelt, S., Daly, M., Rosenthal, D., Lo, C., and Potts, J., The use of parathyroid hormone plus 1,25-dihydroxyvitamin D to increase trabecular bone in osteoporotic men and postmenopausal women, in *Osteoporosis 1987*, Christiansen, C., Johansen, J. S., and Riis, B. J., Eds., Osteopress Aps, Copenhagen, Denmark, 1987, 929.
49. Cosman, F., Shen, V., Xie, F., Seibel, M., Ratcliffe, A., and Lindsay, R., Estrogen protection against bone resorbing effects of parathyroid hormone infusion, *Ann. Intern. Med.*, 118, 337, 1993.
50. Ebeling, P. R., Jones, J. D., Burritt, M. F., Duerson, C. R., Lane, A. W., Hassager, C., Kumar, R., and Riggs, B. L., Skeletal responsiveness to endogenous parathyroid hormone in postmenopausal osteoporosis, *J. Clin. Endocrinol. Metab.*, 75, 1033, 1992.
51. Marcus, R., Villa, M. L., Cheema, M., Cheema, C., Newhall, K., and Holloway, L., Effects of conjugated estrogen on the calcitriol response to parathyroid hormone in postmenopausal women, *J. Clin. Endocrinol. Metab.*, 74, 413, 1992.
52. Lindsay, R., Cosman, F., Shen, V., Nieves, J., and Dempster, D. W., Bone mass increments induced by PTH treatment can be maintained by estrogen, [Abstract], *J. Bone Min. Res.*, 10, S200, 1995.
53. Kent, G. N., Loveridge, N., Reeve, J., and Zanelli, J. M., Pharmacokinetics of synthetic human parathyroid hormone 1-34 in man measured by cytochemical bioassay and radioimmunoassay, *Clin. Sci.*, 68, 171, 1985.
54. Fraher, L. J., Klein, K., Marier, R., Freeman, D., Hendy, G. N., Goltzman, D., and Hodsman, A. B., Comparison of the pharmacokinetics of parenteral parathyroid hormone (1-34) {PTH-(1-34)} and PTH-related peptide (1-34) in healthy young humans, *J. Clin. Endocrinol. Metab.*, 80, 60, 1995.
55. Fraher, L. J., Hodsman, A. B., Steer, B. M., and Freeman, A. A., Comparison of the pharmacokinetics of subcutaneous parathyroid hormone in healthy young and elderly osteoporotic subjects, [Abstract], *J. Bone Min. Res.*, 8, S253, 1993.
56. Hesch, R. D., Heck, J., and Auf'mkolk, B., First clinical observations with hPTH (1-38), a more potent human parathyroid hormone peptide, *Horm. Metab. Res.*, 16, 559, 1984.
57. Whitfield, J. F., Morley, P., Ross, V., Preston, E., Soska, M., Barbier, J.-R., Isaacs, R. J., Maclean, S., Ohannessian-Barry, L., and Willick, G. E., The hypotensive actions of osteogenic and non-osteogenic parathyroid hormone (PTH) fragments, *Calif. Tissue Int.*, 60, 302, 1997.
58. Yee, J. P., Monroe, S. E., and Thiene, K., The effects of RS-66271, a novel hPTHrP(1-34) analog, on serum and urinary markers of PTH-like activity in healthy postmenopausal women, *J. Bone Min. Res.*, 11, S254, 1996.
59. Yee, J. P., Friday, K. J., Monroe, S. E., Fine, G. D., and Thiene, K. A., Double-blind, controlled, crossover study on the effects of subcutaneous injections of RS-66271, a novel analog of hPTHrP(1-34), on blood pressure in postmenopausal women, *J. Bone Min. Res.*, 11, S454, 1996.
60. Henry, J. G., Mitnick, M. A., and Stewart, A. F., Subcutaneous administration of PTHrP(1-36) to humans: a dose-finding study, *J. Bone Min. Res.*, 11, S453, 1996.

61. Deftos, L. J., Nolan, J. J., Seely, B. L., Clopton, P. C., Cote, G. J., Witham, c. L., Florek, L. J., and Christenson, T. A., Intrapulmonary drug delivery of bone-active peptides: bioactivity of inhaled calcitonin approximates injected calcitonin, *J. Bone Min. Res.*, 11, S95, 1996.
62. Nomura, M., Okuno, T., Yanagawa, A., and Kono, T., Studies on intranasal absorption of new formulation of 1-34 PTH in healthy volunteers, *Osteoporosis Int.*, 6, 269, 1996.
63. Patton, J. S., Trinchero, P., and Platz, R. M., Bioavailability of pulmonary delivered peptides and proteins: α-interferon, calcitonins and parathyroid hormones, *J. Controlled Release*, 28, 79, 1994.
64. Hodsman, A. B., Fraher, L., and Adachi, J. A., Clinical trial of cyclical clodronate as maintenance therapy following withdrawal of parathyroid hormone, in the treatment of post-menopausal osteoporosis, *J. Bone Min. Res.*, 10, kS200, 1995.
65. Sone, T., Fukunaga, M., Ono, S., and Nishiyama, T. A., A small dose of human parathyroid hormone (1-34) increased bone mass in the lumbar vertebrae in patients with senile osteoporosis, *Min. Electrol. Metab.*, 21, 232, 1995.
66. Pak, C. Y. C., Sakhaee, K., Piziak, V., Peterson, R. D., Breslau, N. A., Boyd, P., Poindexter, J. R., Herzog, J., Heard-Sakhaee, A., Haynes, S., Adams-Huet, B., and Reisch, J. S., Slow-release sodium fluoride in the management of postmenopausal osteoporosis, *Ann. Int. Med.*, 120, 625, 1994.
67. Adami, S., Baroni, M. C., Broggini, M., Carratelli, L., Caruso, I., Gnessi, L., Laurenzi, M., Lombardi, A., Norbiato, G., and Ortolani, S., Treatment of postmenopausal osteoporosis with continuous daily oral alendronate in comparison with either placebo or intranasal salmon calcitonin, *Osteoporosis Int.*, 3, S21, 1993.

Chapter 5

Adenylyl Cyclase-Activating Anabolic Agents: Parathyroid Hormone and Prostaglandins E

James F. Whitfield, Paul Morley, R. M. Langille, and G. E. Willick

CONTENTS

0-8493-8556-3/98/$0.00+$.50

I. INTRODUCTION

Osteoporosis silently stalks 1 of 3 women after she reaches menopause.[1-3] This disease is said currently to afflict about 26 million people in Canada and the U.S. and 200 million worldwide. However, this number is challenged in Chapter 1 by Frost, who believes that true osteoporosis is much rarer and that most of these 26 million people really have a physiological osteopenia (i.e., they simply have less bone than their normal peers). Nevertheless, the number of elderly women (and men) with the osteopenia, bone pain, and the "spontaneous" fractures of true osteoporosis is growing as the populations of the two nations age. Indeed, both osteopenia and osteoporosis in both sexes will claim an increasingly large fraction of shrinking health budgets.[1]

Postmenopausal osteoporosis is a term coined by Albright et al.[4] to describe the reduced bone mass in women after menopause. It and the associated bone fragility are caused by an approximately 10-year acceleration of bone remodeling, bone loss, and a mounting burden of microdamage (see Chapter 1). Between the ages of 30 and 80 women lose about half their peak trabecular bone mass and one third of their peak cortical bone mass through normal continuous remodeling activity.[5-8] If a woman has not banked enough bone in her first 30 years, she may emerge from the menopausal burst of bone loss with a skeleton that cannot support her normal mechanical usage.[6] The strain at key points throughout her skeleton will exceed the microfracture threshold and microfractures will accumulate. The resulting fragility will cause her to start breaking and crushing hips, vertebrae, and wrists with once-normal movements and blows that were innocuous and unnoticed in the past. She may also get shorter and stoop into the "dowager's posture" as her vertebrae crush. And the older she is, the more likely she is to further weaken her bones by increasing immobility and ultimately succumb to the stresses of fracturing, prolonged hospitalization, and depression from a real or imagined inability to carry out her normal daily routine.

II. OSTEOPOROSIS

At first sight a bone is a rock-like thing — lifeless, changeless, but very unforgiving if broken, cracked, hit, punctured, or twisted. If it were, in fact, lifeless, the continuous loading surges would cause increasingly extensive matrix microdamage and failure which would lead ultimately to cracks and breaks. Actually bone is seething with activity, albeit in glacier-like slow motion. It is being continuously torn down, rebuilt, reshaped, and its matrix repaired and fresh cement lines laid down under the control of the mechanosensitive osteocytes of the strain-and microdamage-sensing *mechanostat mechanism* (see Frost's Chapter 1 for a detailed discussion). The osteocyte's mechanosensors are probably its integrin receptors which are "signal wires" that are induced by external Mg^{2+}, but particularly by the relatively high Mn^{2+} concentration (50 μM) in bone, to anchor the osteocyte to matrix proteins (e.g., fibrillar type-I collagen, fibronectin, laminin, osteopontin, osteonectin) and respond to deformation of the bone matrix and compression-induced pulses of fluid and electric (ion) currents surging through the extracellular space by generating signals which stimulate the production and secretion of products that mobilize the cells that will resorb or make bone depending on strain characteristics.[9-12] Bone must be repetitively loaded to maintain its normal mass. When the strain in a part of the skeleton drops below a certain threshold because of disuse, the mechanostat senses this and mobilizes and activates the cellular machinery needed to resorb the now excess, deloaded bone (by ceasing to make a resorption inhibitor?). Conversely, when the strain exceeds a certain threshold and the integrin signal wires are pulled hard enough, the mechanostat will order the production of new bone to reduce the added strain and drop the pulling to a subthreshold level. The result of the continuous remodeling, microdamage repair, and strain management in a normal adult is the complete replacement of the skeleton about every 8 to 10 years.

The continuous remodeling and microdamage repair in the adult skeleton are the jobs of the usually tightly coupled tandem efforts of bone-destroying osteoclasts and bone-building osteoblasts.[5,6,13-16] Provided skeletal size and turnover are normal, there are about 21 million of these remodeling teams at work on about 10% of the cortical bone and about 20% of trabecular bone at any moment, and these turn the mature skeleton over at a rate of about 10%/year.[5] These teams were recognized and called BMUs (Basic Multicellular Units) by Frost[15,16] or BRUs (Bone-Remodeling Units) by others.[5] Each BMU cycle consists of activation (A), resorption (R), and formation (F) phases. The ARF cycle starts with monocytes, the osteoclast precursors located in the blood or adjacent bone marrow which have been differentiated from early precursors by GM-CSF (granulocyte-macrophage colony-stimulating factor), M-CSF (macrophage colony-stimulating factor), and $1\alpha,(OH)_2$vitamin D_3. They fuse into large multinuclear osteoclasts adjacent to the resorption site and are then activated by a combination of factors such as IL-1, PGE_2, TGF-α, TNF-α, and TNF-β that are generated at the right spot by the strain-responsive, load- and microdamage-sensing osteocytes of the mechanostat.[6,17] This is followed by the assembly of a team of mature osteoclasts, syncytial microbeavers with 3 to 20 nuclei, who clamp with their sealing zones onto a patch of old, possibly microfractured, bone. Then they start digging Howship's lacunae in trabeculae, endosteum, or periosteum; or boring cutting cones through cortical bone with protons, phosphatases, and matrix-hydrolyzing proteases streaming from their densely ruffled microsuction cups, leaving a trail of Ca^{2+}, hydroxyproline, collagen crosslinkers, and crosslinked type-I collagen telopeptides as they go.[6,18] This releases and activates several osteogenic factors from the bone matrix which, together with the Ca^{2+}

released from the hydroxyapatite crystals, make up the coupling mechanism. Among these are TGF-βs, such as TGF-β3, a lot of which are stored in the matrix in a latent form in proteolysis-resistant fibrillar complexes with a specific binding protein belonging to the fibrillin family, LTBP (latent TGF-β-binding protein).[6,19-22] Another is the very important IGF-I (insulin-like growth factor-I) (see also Chapter 8 by Johansson and Rosen) which, when released from IGF-binding protein-5 (IGFBP-5) attached to hydroxyapatite crystals in the mineralized bone matrix, or released by cells that have been stimulated to make and secrete it by signals from surface polyvalent cation receptors activated by the released Ca^{2+}, can promote cell cycle transit of, and collagen production by, preosteoblasts.[23-29] Still others are BMPs (bone morphogenic proteins) members of the TGF-β superfamily.[30] All of these factors were dumped into the matrix by the osteoblasts of the previous BMU that had made the matrix.

When the osteoclast team has finished excavating and its members have moved on, broken up into mononuclear cells, or committed apoptotic suicide, the large amount of locally released, active TGF-βs stimulate preosteoblasts to proliferate, invade the intracortical cutting cone or trabecular trench, and then differentiate, while at the same time they prevent further osteoclast recruitment.[19,21] About 50 osteoblasts will be needed to replace the amount of bone resorbed by only one member of the osteoclast team in one day.[14] The invading preosteoblasts express their proliferation-driving genes (e.g., c-*myc*, c-*fos*, c-*jun*, and *H4* histone), and generate the successive transient surges of the different cyclin-dependent "cycle-engine" protein kinases that specifically drive the different cell cycle stages.[31,32] While proliferating, these cells first briefly express osteopontin and lay it down on osteoclast-clipped collagen fibers to produce a noncollagenous cement line; then they lay down a new collagen matrix, install integrin signal wires on their surfaces to attach themselves to the matrix, and make and secrete more TGF-βs to promote further matrix/osteoid production in a paracrine fashion.[19,33,34] When the matrix accumulation has exceeded a threshold level and the specific integrin signaling gets "loud" enough, the cells stop expressing cell-cycle genes and making cycle-engine parts. Now they shift into the postproliferative (postmitotic) mode in which they switch on genes whose products, such as alkaline phosphatase, prepare the new matrix/osteoid for the deposition of hydroxyapatite crystals.[33,34] At some stage the postproliferative cells make and secrete the angiogenic vascular endothelium-specific growth factor (VEGF)[35] and load the new matrix/osteoid with various factors such as IGF-I, TGF-βs, and the related BMPs.[19,30] When the matrix/osteoid signals to the cells that it is ready, they down-regulate their matrix-preparing genes and start expressing another set of genes whose products, such as the bone-specific osteocalcin and once again osteopontin, induce the ordered and limited deposition of hydroxyapatite crystals to make new mineralized bone.[33,34] (As will be discussed in Section III.C, it is at this stage that they also turn on the gene(s) for PTH receptors.[36-39]) Finally, having made new, adequately vascularized and mineralized bone with a factor-loaded matrix, they wind their bone-building activities down and change their matrix-binding focal adhesion apparatus to become strain-sensing osteocytes or lining cells,[9] or some, failing to establish a matrix-binding niche, may kill themselves by apoptosis to reduce the population to a minimal maintenance size.[34]

BMUs on endosteal and trabecular surfaces in contact with the bone marrow make less bone than they resorb. On the other hand, periosteal BMUs make more bone than they resorb.[5,6] Therefore, bone cortices get thinner and more porous, bone diameters increase, and the amount of trabecular bone declines (as indicated by an increasing marrow "star volume," which is inversely proportional to the mean number of intersections with trabeculae of straight lines radiating star-like from arbitrarily placed points in marrow spaces). The strength of trabecular bone also declines with age in mature skeletons.[5,6] However, it is the horizontal trabecular struts that are increasingly perforated, deloaded, and promptly resorbed by the mechanostat with age, while the mean thickness of the main load-bearing vertical plates and bars does not change significantly with age probably because of the load-sensing mechanostat.[5,6] The disappearance of horizontal trabecular struts with age results in a progressively rising ratio of the distance between supporting struts to load-bearing columns. When this ratio exceeds a critical value, elastic and bending forces rather than compression force become predominant, and the bone is weakened.[5,6]

When the estrogen level crashes at menopause, BMUs behave as if a spurious disuse signal has been given to the mechanostat (see Frost's Chapter 1) which drives a decade-long acceleration of bone loss resulting from a surge of cortical thinning and trabecular perforation and disintegration. According to the stochastic simulation of Thomsen et al.[40] the actual clinical data for postmenopausal trabecular remodeling are consistent with a doubling of the BMU activation frequency plus an imbalance between resorption and formation in favor of resorption, i.e., an increasing resorption deficit with each ARF cycle. The reasons for this response to estrogen withdrawal are unknown. They probably include surges of previously estrogen-suppressed osteoclast-recruiting and -stimulating cytokines, such as IL-1 and IL-6, as well as a reduction of the matrix stores of the recruitment-blocking TGF-βs, such as TGF-β3, which would combine to expand the pool of osteoclast precursors and enhance osteoclast recruitment but reduce preosteoblast invasion and osteoblast buildup at excavation sites.[6,7,19-22] Interestingly, it is 17-epiestriol, a 17β-estradiol breakdown product, that stimulates TGF-β3 production: it attaches to the estrogen nuclear receptor to form a complex which is attached by adaptor proteins to the TGF-β3 gene's raloxifene-responsive enhancing element which is accessible for activation in bone cells but not breast or kidney cells.[41] In view of the large number of osteoblasts needed to replace the bone removed by a single osteoclast,[14] such a reduction of preosteoblast invasion and osteoblast buildup would tip the balance of BMU activity into negative values. Because BMUs in contact with the bone marrow and its host of osteoclast-promoting factors, such as GM-CSF, M-CSF, IL-1, IL-6, IL-11, TNF-α, and TNF-β, normally make less bone than they resorb, the loss of trabecular bone in postmenopausal women and ovariectomized (OVX) rats is particularly marked.[5,6] The lower level of crosslinking of trabecular type-I collagen filaments[42] must also contribute to this special trabecular responsiveness. The osteoclasts of the increasing numbers of BMUs gnaw through, disconnect, and thereby deload trabecular struts, and the marrow star volume rises.[5,6] The osteoblasts cannot reattach severed struts, which, because they have been deloaded, are then declared redundant by the aroused mechanostatic mechanism and are promptly resorbed.[5,6] Thus, there is an irreversible loss of trabecular connectivity, and bones rich in trabecular bone, such as the vertebrae, must increasingly rely on their cortical shells for mechanical support. But there is also an increased porosity and thinning of cortical bone in osteoporotics which is due to a doubling of turnover and the normally negative balance between resorption and formation on the endosteal surfaces.[6] However, the acceleration of bone loss is only temporary, and an osteoporotic does not lose all of her bones! Eventually the mechanostatic mechanism awakens to the rising microdamage and mounting strain and decelerates deterioration by reducing turnover and reinforcing or stabilizing the load-bearing trabecular columns.

The bone loss in an osteoporotic woman can be prevented, reduced, or even stopped by calcitonin or the cheaper, orally or transdermally administrable, bisphosphonates, estrogens, and estrogen analogs such as droloxifene or raloxifene, the 17-epiestriol-mimicking stimulator of TGF-β3 expression in bone, but not in breast or uterus.[8,41,43,44] But none of these is a true anabolic agent that can directly stimulate bone formation and strengthen bones *after* substantial loss has occurred. Estrogens work mainly by reducing BMU activation although they do stimulate osteoblasts to produce osteogenic TGF-βs.[20] Calcitonin inhibits the recruitment of mononuclear osteoclast precursors and binds to, and activates, receptors whose signals inhibit resorption by mature osteoclasts.[18] Bisphosphonates inhibit both BMU activation and resorption[5,6] and promote osteoclast death by apoptosis.[45] By inhibiting bone turnover they give the osteoblasts of *existing BMUs* the opportunity to fill the holes (the resorption space) left by the osteoclasts. This results in a transient 5 to 10% increase in bone mass which plateaus and is then maintained or eventually lost.[5] However, prolonged treatment with potent antiresorptive agents could be dangerous, because microdamage may accumulate without the activation of new BMUs to remodel and repair it.[46,47]

But since women do not feel oncoming osteoporosis (hence the term *silent epidemic*), they don't seek help until they have lost enough bone to start fracturing and hurting. Therefore, we also need a restorative or therapeutic drug that can selectively and directly stimulate osteoblasts to make mechanically normal, or preferably supranormally strong, bone to strengthen remaining trabecular struts, enlarge and strengthen the load-bearing columns, and repair or override microdamage. This drug should also increase the amount of mechanically normal bone in the thinned, porous cortices, especially because the fractures in osteoporotic and elderly adults start in epiphyseal, intertrochanteric, and femoral neck cortices.[48] Just such a therapeutic drug was discovered 65 years ago at McGill University in Montreal, Canada.

III. PARATHYROID HORMONE (PTH)

A. PTH, Stimulator of Bone Growth

The first hint of the surprises and excitement to come appeared in 1929 in a report by Bauer et al.[49] of the results of experiments using cats and rats to test the idea that trabecular bone serves as both a reinforcing lattice and a readily available (because of its close contact with marrow and thus extensive access to the general circulation) source of Ca^{2+}. In one experiment they treated growing rats with Eli Lilly's bovine parathyroid extract (parathormone) and found something odd which was left unexplained.

> X-ray examination of the bone of animals which had received extract appears to be much denser and shorter than their control siblings, and on cross-section they showed many trabeculae. We are unable to explain these findings.
>
> Parathormone administration to growing rats results in a diminution of length of bone and an increase in the number of trabeculae.

But the story really began in Paris on Saturday, July 4, 1931, with the appearance of a paper by M. Péhu et al. in *La Presse Médicale*.[50] They reported the case of an 8-year-old boy, Pierre M., who was killed by the anemia resulting from the obliteration of his marrow spaces by the excessive bone growth of osteopetrosis. At autopsy they found that the boy had hypertrophic parathyroids and suggested that his excessive bone growth was the work of the PTH secreted by these glands.

> Or, dans notre cas, on a pu noter une hypertrophie nette, sinon très considérable, des parathyroïdes. Ces glandes se sont trouvées plus volumineuses que normalement, à cet âge. On peut donc penser que le trouble initial, le *primum movens* de l'affection, se trouve dans la glande parathyroïde.

This suggestion was surprising because PTH's job according to the medical textbooks, then and now, was, and still is, supposed to stimulate osteoclasts to tear bone down and release its Ca^{2+} when more Ca^{2+} is needed in the blood. Indeed, an apparent hypersensitivity of osteoporotics to PTH prompted the suggestion in 1994 that the hormone plays a crucial role in the development of osteoporosis,[6] and it has been suggested that a change in the PTH secretion pulsing pattern may be involved in osteoporosis.[51] In an even more recent review of bone biology, no mention is made of PTH's anabolic action: only its osteoclast-stimulating action is discussed.[14] But H. Selye, then at McGill University, did not dismiss this suggestion out of hand, because when he was at Johns Hopkins University he had carried out experiments on the stimulation of skin fibroblasts and induction of a scleroderma-like condition in rats by the Eli Lilly bovine parathyroid extract and found that the hormone preparation could also produce a condition resembling osteopetrosis.[52] He then carried out the pathfinding experiments at McGill that were designed to mimic the 8-year-old's hypertrophic parathyroid glands by giving young (e.g., 14-day-old) rapidly growing rats small daily doses (such as one injection of 5 units each day for 30 days) of the Eli Lilly bovine parathyroid extract.[53] He wrongly assumed that a once-daily injection would produce a prolonged elevation of circulating PTH like the boy's hypertrophic parathyroid glands. Actually he was producing brief pulses of circulating PTH, which is the secret to producing the striking response he got. These intermittently injected small doses of extract directly stirred up a swarm of osteoblasts that built massive amounts of cortical and trabecular bone without the expected preliminary appearance of osteoclasts. However, larger doses of the extract did evoke a preliminary osteoclast response, but this was followed by a massive recruitment of osteoblasts and bone formation. Selye concluded from these observations that the *"hitherto unexplained observations"* of Bauer et al.[49] of parathyroid extract-enhanced bone density were due to *"the second stage of hyperparathyroidism, the osteoblastic reaction."*[53]

This was confirmed a year later by Pugsley and Selye.[54] They reported that daily injections of 20 units of extract into older rats (probably male; they did not specify the sex), weighing 175 to 225 g, initially stimulated the appearance of numerous osteoclasts, spindle-shaped osteoblasts, and a rise in the serum and urine Ca^{2+} contents. However, the osteoclasts disappeared by days 9 to 12 when the serum and urine Ca^{2+} levels had returned to normal. Continuation of the hormone injections past day 14 resulted in greatly increased numbers of osteoblasts surrounding the trabeculae and the formation of *"huge amounts of bone tissue."*[54] Thus, the two key requirements for getting PTH to build rather than resorb bone, intermittence and low dosage, had been identified by 1933.

But, this massive bone growth could have been the work of some potently anabolic contaminant in the bovine extract rather than PTH, or calcitonin released in response to PTH-induced hypercalcemia. But even if it were due to PTH, it would have been useless because the extract had to be injected, it was expensive, and it lost its effectiveness with prolonged treatment. Moreover, osteoporosis was predominantly a workforce-irrelevant disease of elderly women which was not considered to be a major problem in the very different political climate and the far less menacing demographics of the earlier part of this century.

Thirty-eight years later, Kalu et al.[55] proved that it was indeed PTH that was responsible for the osteogenic activity of the Eli Lilly parathyroid extract by showing that pure parathyroid hormone stimulated bone growth in thyroparathyroidectomized (TPTX) rats. They also noted the clinically known association of metaphyseal sclerosis with hyperparathyroidism. The bone-building effectiveness of PTH in TPTX rats eliminated calcitonin as a possible mediator of PTH action. They concluded that calcitonin increases bone formation by inhibiting resorption, while PTH directly stimulates bone formation in growing animals. In the same year, Walker[56] convincingly confirmed the seminal suggestion of Péhu et al.[50] by showing that PTH caused osteopetrosis only in very young intact rats as well as in hypophysectomized or TPTX rats which definitively eliminated the possibility of calcitonin or growth hormone mediating PTH's powerful osteogenic action.

Between 1970 and now, an ever-increasing number of reports (see references 57 through 64 and other chapters of this book for complete reference lists) have confirmed the Péhu–Selye effect mainly with the synthetic and fully bioactive hPTH-(1-34) fragment which was first synthesized in 1974 by Tregear et al.[65] But reports by Neer et al.[66,67] cast doubt on the prospects of PTH being used to treat osteoporosis. They treated osteoporotic women with a combination of PTH (50 to 100 μg/day) and calcitriol (0.25 μg/day) for 1 to 2 years and found that while the combination increased the spinal mineral density by an impressive 32%, it *reduced* the cortical mineral density of the radius by a net 4%. Such a reduction of cortical bone would be serious, if not fatal, for PTH's future as an osteoporosis therapeutic because fractures in osteoporotics start in epiphyseal, intertrochanteric, and femoral neck *cortices*.[48] However, Hodsman et al. (see Chapter 4 for more details) rode to the rescue by showing that calcitriol was the confounder in this combined treatment and that hPTH-(1-34) or hPTH-(1-84) *alone* can stimulate both trabecular and cortical bone growth in osteoporotic patients. And, Sone et al.[68] found that a 26-week treatment of senile osteoporotics with hPTH-(1-34) significantly increased lumbar bone mineral density without affecting cortical bone mass or increasing markers of bone resorption. Still in primates, Jerome et al.[69] (using dual energy X-ray absorptiometry and quantitative computerized tomography) have reported that injecting hPTH-(1-34) (10 μg/kg of body weight; 3 days/week for 3 months) into 5- to 12-year-old cynomolgus monkeys (*Macaca fascicularis*) 10 months after OVX caused dramatic, 5 to 6%, increases in vertebral (LV2-4) trabecular bone and 15 to 28.8% increases in tibial trabecular bone without causing cortical bone loss. Thus, it is now certain that intermittent subcutaneous injections of PTH can greatly, apparently harmlessly, and without prior activation of osteoclasts, stimulate the formation of biomechanically normal or supranormal lamellar bone in trabeculae and cortical bone (with greater effectiveness in endosteum than periosteum) in osteopenic OVX rats as well as osteoporotic men and women.[57-64] It can stimulate the osteoblasts in the formation zones of bones of growing animals and humans strongly enough to produce osteopetrosis or near-osteopetrosis.[57-64] It can stimulate osteoblasts in the BMUs of the bones of mature animals and humans to reversibly transform local lining cells into osteoblasts and to prematurely invade, and start working on, excavated surfaces even before the osteoclasts have finished digging and thus produce new packets of trabecular bone with thickened walls. However, PTH cannot stimulate the formation of new trabeculae: It needs pre-existing trabeculae to serve as templates for the formation of new bone. Therefore, the hormone becomes less effective with increasing trabecular loss and increasingly fewer trabeculae to build up.

B. The Osteogenic Signal

How does PTH signal osteoblasts to start making bone? We must know this in order to make the ultimate PTH-based drug to treat osteopenia and osteoporosis.

We know that both the h(human)PTH-(1-84) holohormone and its hPTH-(1-34) fragment activate two membrane-associated signal enzymes, triggering a cascade of widely ramifying reactions. One of these enzymes is adenylyl cyclase, which makes cyclic AMP that in turn activates the cyclic AMP-dependent protein kinases that phosphorylate and activate or inhibit cyclic AMP-responsive gene transcription factors and many enzymes.[32,63,70-72] The other signaler is phospholipase-Cβ (PLC), which hydrolyzes membrane phosphatidylinositol-*bis*phosphate (PIP_2) into two products.[32] One of these is inositol-1,4,5 *tris*phosphate (IP_3), which directly triggers the emptying of internal Ca^{2+} stores that, in turn, induces influx of external Ca^{2+}.[32] This stimulates another host of nuclear and cytoplasmic reactions.[32] The other of these is diacylglycerol, which stimulates membrane-associated protein kinase-Cs (PKCs).[32,70-72] In fact, this stimulation of membrane-associated PKCs is an indirect, but reliable measure of PLC activation.

hPTH-(1-84) optimally stimulates PLC activity, as indicated by peak increases in membrane-associated PKC activity in ROS 17/2 rat osteosarcoma cells (which are neoplastic osteoblasts that have retained the ability to form bone nodules in the rat), at two widely separated picomolar and nanomolar concentrations, but it additionally stimulates adenylyl cyclase only at the latter nanomolar concentrations.[71] Exactly the same two-peak relation for PKCs stimulation and one-peak/plateau relation for adenylyl cyclase stimulation was obtained with the hPTH-(1-34).[71]

Jouishomme et al.[71,72] and then Gagnon et al.[73] suggested that the two-peak PKCs and one-peak/plateau adenylyl cyclase curves meant that ROS 17/2 cells display two kinds of PTH/PTHrP receptor. One of these would be a high-affinity receptor, which, when activated by PTH or PTHrP, only switches on one of the five members of the PLC-activating Gq protein family.[74] The other would be the recently isolated and cloned, lower affinity receptor, the so-called conventional PTH/PTHrP receptor, which, when activated by PTH or PTHrP, activates both a PLC-stimulating Gq protein and the adenylyl cyclase-stimulating Gs protein.[74] This lower-affinity receptor was the most readily isolated and therefore regarded as the one-and-only PTH receptor, probably because the osteoblasts and kidney cells from which it was isolated display many more of it than the high-affinity receptor. This suggestion of the existence of more than one kind of PTH receptor is now gaining strong support.[75] Indeed, differently spliced receptor types could be expected because of the receptor gene's complex intron-exon structure.[76] Orloff et al.[77] and Whitfield et al.[78] have found that keratinocytes express a PTH/PTHrP receptor, which, like the putative high-affinity receptor of ROS 17/2 osteoblasts, stimulates PLC but does not activate the cells' available adenylyl cyclase-stimulating Gs protein and is probably the product of a different gene. Rat cardiomyocytes and lymphocytes also display PTH/PTHrP receptors which stimulate PLC but not adenylyl cyclase despite the presence of functional Gs protein.[79] It also seems that there is even an adenylyl cyclase-activating receptor, PTH2, which is particularly abundant in brain and pancreas and is activated by PTH but not PTHrP.[80]

We then had to answer two questions. Were different regions of the PTH molecule involved in stimulating adenylyl cyclase and PLC? If so, could these regions be separated and stay functional so we could assess the abilities of the two signaling mechanisms to stimulate bone formation? We set about answering these questions by using several PTH fragments and determining their abilities to stimulate adenylyl cyclase and membrane-associated PKCs in ROS 17/2 osteoblasts.

We knew at the outset that the hormone needs its first two N-terminal amino acids, i.e., an intact N-terminus, to stimulate adenylyl cyclase and that its receptor-binding region is an α-helix within the 14-34 region.[81] As expected, removing the first two N-terminal amino acids to make hPTH-(3-34) eliminated the ability to stimulate adenylyl cyclase, but it did not affect the ability to stimulate PLC as indicated by an undiminished stimulation of membrane-associated PKCs activity.[71,72] This was a very important finding in 1992, because until then all models of PTH action were based on the wrong assumption that because fragments such as PTH-(3-34), PTH-(7-34), or PTH-(13-34) did not stimulate adenylyl cyclase they were functionally inert competitive inhibitors of the binding of the active PTH-(1-34) and PTH-(1-84) to the PTH receptor. In fact, the peptide chain could be shortened up to and including residue 28 without affecting the ability to stimulate membrane-associated PKCs activity.[72] The still potent PKCs-stimulating activity of PTH-(28-34) was later confirmed by Janulis et al.[82] using primary cultures of rat proximal kidney tubules. We then found that amino acids 33 and 34 could also be removed without affecting PLC/PKCs stimulation.[72] This left us with the PTH-(29-32) fragment which, tiny though it was, could still stimulate membrane-associated PKCs activity.[72] Further removal of amino acid-32 finally eliminated PLC/PKCs stimulation.[72] At this point we had a set of functionally well-defined tools with which to find out whether one or both signal mechanisms are needed to boot the osteogenic mechanism.

In the first experiments, we used a rapid, preventative protocol.[62] We ovariectomized sexually mature, still-growing 3-month-old rats and two weeks later started a six-week series of once-daily subcutaneous injections of 1 nmole of fragment/100 g of body weight, which did not affect the blood Ca^{2+} concentration. Every second week we removed femurs and measured the total dry weights and Ca^{2+} contents of the cortical and trabecular bone in their distal halves. As expected of young growing rats (the bones of old rats are much less responsive), ovariectomy triggered a large loss of trabecular bone (Figure 5.1). But it did not cause a loss of cortical bone. Cortical bone actually continued to increase (Figure 5.1). Daily injections of hPTH-(1-34) at the maximally effective dose of 1 nmole/100 g of body weight, starting two weeks after OVX, which was before the rapid loss of trabecular bone mass and Ca^{2+} content had started, *prevented* the loss of trabecular bone which, after a 2- to 4-week delay, resumed growing as rapidly as the trabecular bone in Sham-OVX control rats (Figure 5.1). After six weeks of daily injections, the trabecular bone had become very dense with thickened, "corticalizing" trabeculae and shrunken marrow spaces exactly like those in the PTH-treated animals of Selye[53] and Walker.[56] hPTH-(1-34) also doubled, or nearly doubled, the growth of cortical bone (Figure 5.1). But hPTH-(3-34) and hPTH-(13-34), which potently stimulated membrane-associated PKCs activity, but not adenylyl cyclase, did not stop, or even reduce, the OVX-induced trabecular bone loss or stimulate cortical bone growth (Figure 5.1). 1-Desamino hPTH-(1-34), with its adenylyl cyclase-stimulating ability greatly reduced by having a disabled N-terminus, also could not significantly reduce OVX-induced trabecular bone loss or stimulate cortical bone growth (Figure 5.2) despite being able to normally and strongly stimulate membrane-associated PKCs activity.[62]

This failure of potent PLC/PKCs stimulators to stimulate bone growth was unexpected. Sömjen et al.[83] had reported that PTH needed its PLC-activating 28-34 region, but not its first two N-terminal amino acids (i.e., its adenylyl cyclase-activating capability), to stimulate rat osteoblast proliferation. Thus, they found that fragments such as hPTH-(25-39) and PTH-(28-48), which we[71] had found to stimulate PKCs but not adenylyl cyclase, stimulated DNA synthesis in bone cells both *in vivo* and

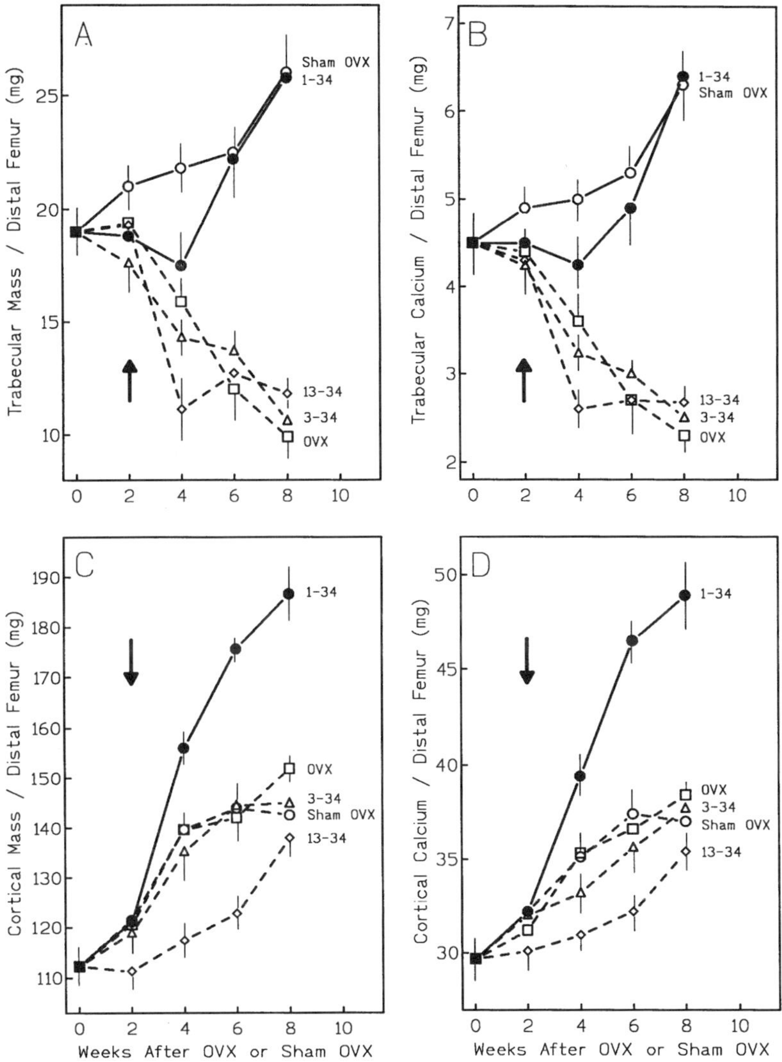

Figure 5.1
Effects of daily subcutaneous injections of different PTH fragments on the mass and calcium contents of trabecular (A and B) and cortical (C and D) bone in the distal halves of the femora of OVX rats. The PTH fragments were hPTH-(1-34), the fully bioactive fragment, which stimulated adenylyl cyclase and PKCs activity, and hPTH-(3-34) and PTH(13-34), which stimulated PKC but not adenylyl cyclase. Sham OVX rats were sham-operated and untreated. Experimental rats were ovariectomized at time 0, and the daily PTH injections began 2 weeks later, as indicated by the arrows. All fragments were injected at a dose of 1 nmole/100 g of body weight. (From Rixon, R. H., Whitfield, J. F., Gagnon, L., Isaacs, R. J., MacLean, S., Chakravarthy, B., Durkin, J. P., Neugebauer, W., Ross, V., Sung, W., and Willick, G. E., Parathyroid hormone fragments may stimulate bone growth in ovariectomized rats by activating adenylyl cyclase, *J. Bone Min. Res.*, 9, 1179, 1994. With permission.)

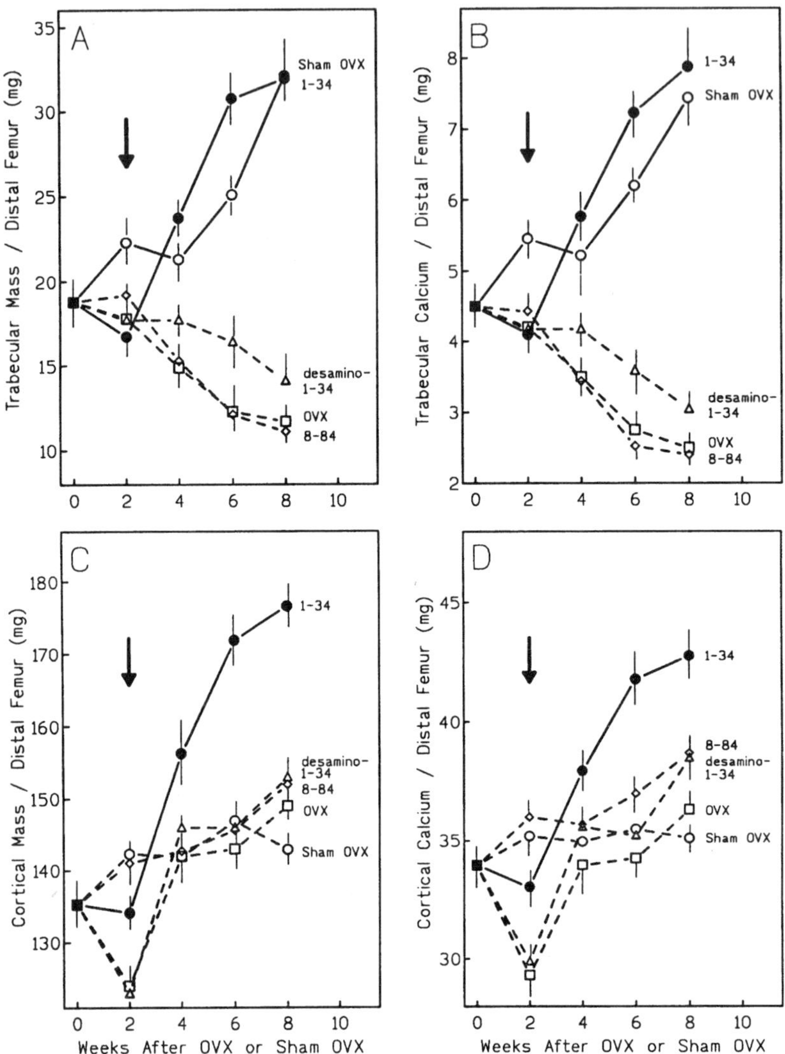

Figure 5.2
Effects of daily subcutaneous injections of different PTH fragments on the mass and calcium contents of trabecular (A and B) and cortical (C and D) bone in the distal halves of the femora of OVX rats. The PTH fragments were the standard, fully bioactive hPTH-(1-34), which stimulated adenylyl cyclase and PKC, 1-desamino-hPTH-(1-34), which stimulated PKC but had a much reduced ability to stimulate adenylyl cyclase, and rhPTH-(8-84), which stimulated PKC only. Sham OVX rats were sham-operated and untreated. Experimental rats were ovariectomized at time 0, and the daily PTH injections began 2 weeks later, as indicated by the arrows. All fragments were injected at a dose of 1 nmole/100 g of body weight. (From Rixon, R. H., Whitfield, J. F., Gagnon, L., Isaacs, R. J., MacLean, S., Chakravarthy, B., Durkin, J. P., Neugebauer, W., Ross, V., Sung, W., and Willick, G. E., Parathyroid hormone fragments may stimulate bone growth in ovariectomized rats by activating adenylyl cyclase, *J. Bone Min. Res.*, 9, 1179, 1994. With permission.)

in vitro.[83] Because of this we had predicted that potent PLC/PKCs-stimulating fragments such as hPTH-(13-34) would be novel and effective bone-building drugs for treating osteoporosis.[71] Therefore, we were relieved when our prediction was given a stay-of-execution by our finding that pieces of hPTH-(1-34) without their N-termini did not survive long enough in the blood to reach target cells in a functional state.[62] Thus, fragments such as hPTH-(3-34) and hPTH-(13-34) did not stimulate membrane-associated PKCs activity in spleen cells after intracardial injection in the rat. However, they strongly stimulated PKCs when added to freshly suspended spleen cells, while hPTH-(1-34) strongly stimulated spleen cell PKCs both in the rat after intracardiac injection and when added to freshly suspended cells. This failure of the two N-terminally truncated PKCs stimulators to stimulate target cells in the rat was probably due to their inactivation by the 230-kDa protein in rat blood plasma that Kukreja et al.[84] found to inactivate bPTH-(7-34) and PTHrP-(7-34), but not PTH-(1-34) or PTHrP-(1-34).

But our relief did not last long. Neither 1-desamino hPTH-(1-34), with its functionally disabled but still present N-terminus, nor the much larger PKCs-only stimulator, hPTH-(8-84), was inactivated by the 230-kDa plasma protein because it stimulated spleen cells' PKCs in the rat as strongly as hPTH-(1-34), but it did *not* stimulate bone growth.[62] We were then confirmed by Strein,[85] who reported that the PKCs-only stimulator PTH-(28-48) does not stimulate bone growth in the OVX rat despite its apparent ability to stimulate DNA synthesis in bone.[85] However, more recently, Sabatini et al.[86] have also cast doubt on the proliferogenic potencies of PLC/PKCs stimulators by showing that both the tiny PKCs-stimulating PTH-(28-34) and even PTH-(28-48) are at best only marginal stimulators of DNA synthesis in primary mouse calvarial cultures.

At this point we had to face the fact that it was adenylyl cyclase and its cyclic AMP product, and not PLC and its products, that drove the bone-building mechanism in our experiments. To prove this we needed a fragment that could stimulate adenylyl cyclase without stimulating PLC and the PKCs. But no one had ever made such a fragment because it would be necessary to disable the PLC/PKCs-activating domain by removing residues 32-34 and thus start biting into the 14-34 receptor-binding region. Nevertheless, we made an hPTH-(1-31) fragment ending with an NH_2 group rather than the normal COOH group (Figure 5.3). This fragment still had the PTH molecule's single large, amphiphilic α-helix which normally ends at Gln^{29} and whose hydrophobic face is the receptor-binding part of the molecule (see the legend of Figure 5.3 for more details). The C-terminal NH_2 group was put there to stabilize the receptor-binding α-helix because a C-terminal COOH group would have interacted unfavorably with the helix's macrodipole to destabilize it and thus reduce the fragment's receptor-binding affinity.[87] The C-terminal NH_2 group would also protect the peptide from peptidase attacks[88] and might be required for optimal binding if the receptor interacted with this part of the polypep-

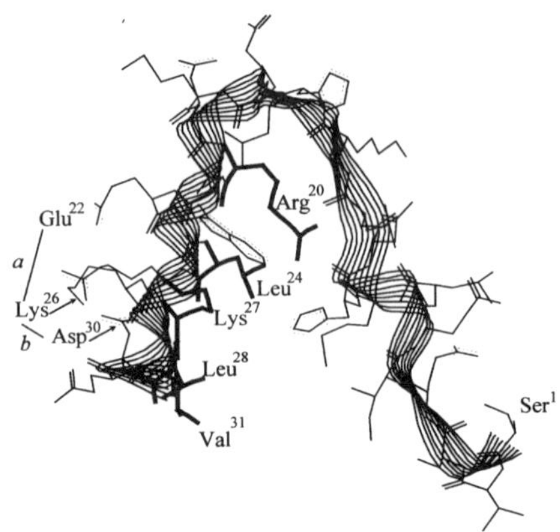

Figure 5.3
A model of hPTH-(1-31)NH_2 that has been adapted from the structure of hPTH-(1-37)NH_2 of Marx et al.,[138] with removal of residues 32-37. The features of this model are a well-defined stable α-helix extending between Ser[17] and Gln[29] and a less stable, small α-helix between Ile[5] and His[9]. Both are consistent with several circular dichroism and NMR studies of hPTH-(1-34) and hPTH-(1-37).[87,97,138-142] Part of the stable α-helix is amphiphilic (i.e., one face is predominantly hydrophobic while the other is hydrophilic), and it is the amino acids on the hydrophobic face (i.e., Arg[20], Leu[24], Leu[28], Lys[27], Val[31] indicated in **bold** letters) that have been shown to be critical for association with the receptor.[87,143-145] Also indicated are the lactam linkages between Glu[22] and Lys[26] and Lys[26] and Asp[30], either of which should conformationally restrict, and therefore stabilize, the receptor-binding α-helix and increase the fragment's resistance to proteolytic digestion.[146-149]

tide backbone. As we expected, the C-terminal truncated analog, hPTH-(1-31)NH_2, stimulated adenylyl cyclase as potently as hPTH-(1-34) and it did not stimulate membrane-associated PKCs activity.[62,87]

In our first experiment, using the rapid preventative protocol and what turned out to be a maximally effective dose of 1 nmole/100 g of body weight, we found that hPTH-(1-31)NH_2 stimulated femoral cortical bone growth as strongly as hPTH-(1-34), but it seemed to be a poor stimulator of trabecular bone growth.[62] This meant that either both adenylyl cyclase and PLC/PKCs stimulation were needed to stimulate trabecular bone growth, or there was such a massive increase in trabecular bone mass and hardness (i.e., "corticalization") that we could not remove all of it for weighing. In the next experiment we dug harder and found that there was indeed a massive stimulation of trabecular bone growth after six weeks of once-daily subcutaneous injections (i.e., 6 days/week, 36 total injections) starting two weeks after OVX.[64] During the first eight weeks after OVX, the amount of mainly nonlamellar or woven trabecular bone and trabecular Ca^{2+} in the distal femur dropped by 60 to 62%, but the mean trabecular thickness did not drop significantly because disconnected, hence deloaded, trabeculae were rapidly eliminated by the ever-vigilant mechanostat and thus did not stay around long enough to be measured (Figure 5.4). The hPTH-(1-31)NH_2 injections initially caused a

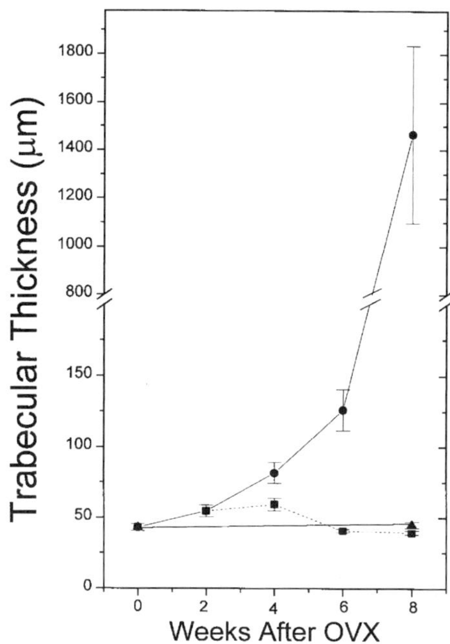

Figure 5.4
The ability of daily subcutaneous injections of hPTH-(1-31)NH_2, starting at 2 weeks after OVX, to increase the mean thickness of trabeculae in distal femoral bone. (▲) Distal femurs of sham OVX rats at 8 weeks after the operation. (■) Distal femurs from OVX rats injected daily with vehicle starting at 2 weeks and ending at 8 weeks. (●) Distal femurs from OVX rats injected daily with 1 nmole of PTH-(1-31)NH_2/100 g of body weight starting at 2 weeks and ending at 8 weeks. (From Whitfield, J. F., Morley, P., Willick, G. E., Ross, V., Barbier, J.-R., Isaacs, R., and Ohannessian-Barry, L., Stimulation of the growth of femoral trabecular bone in ovariectomized rats by the novel parathyroid hormone fragment, hPTH-(1-31)NH_2 (Ostabolin), *Calcif. Tissue Int.*, 58, 81, 1996. With permission.)

gradual, 4-to 5-week buildup to an apparently critical level, at which time it suddenly triggered a spurt of trabecular growth with a massive deposition of lamellae and an astonishing increase in the mean thickness of trabeculae. It seemed to be transforming into dense cortex-like lamellar bone while obliterating most of the marrow spaces (Figures 5.5 and 5.6). As we shall see in Section III.C, the trigger of this rapid bone growth could be the extensive conversion of quiescent bone-lining cells into active, PTH-responsive osteoblasts by paracrine factors such as IGF-I and TGF-βs diffusing from osteoblasts in BMUs and formation zones. It is important to note at this point that this extraordinarily osteogenic dose of hPTH-(1-31)NH_2 was still too low to affect the blood Ca^{2+} concentration or detectably damage kidneys. It should also be noted that Sabatini et al.[86] have found that hPTH-(1-31) stimulates DNA synthesis in primary cultures of mouse calvariae far more effectively than the PLC/PKCs-only stimulators, hPTH-(28-34) and hPTH-(28-48).

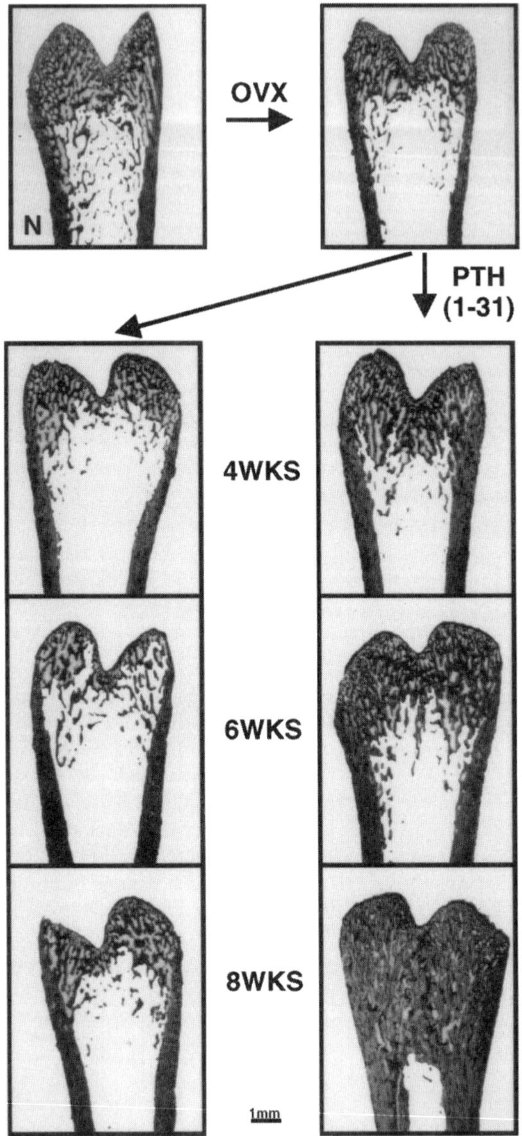

Figure 5.5
Representative samples from the distal femurs of animals in the experiment of Figure 5.4 showing the OVX-induced loss of trabecular bone and the increased trabecular thickness and overall trabecular bone density caused by daily injections of 1 nmole of hPTH-(1-31)NH_2/100 g body weight that began 2 weeks after OVX. The 10-μm sections were stained with Sanderson's rapid bone stain. (From Whitfield, J. F., Morley, P., Willick, G. E., Ross, V., Barbier, J.-R., Isaacs, R., and Ohannessian-Barry, L., Stimulation of the growth of femoral trabecular bone in ovariectomized rats by the novel parathyroid hormone fragment, hPTH-(1-31)NH_2 (Ostabolin), *Calcif. Tissue Int.*, 58, 81, 1996. With permission.)

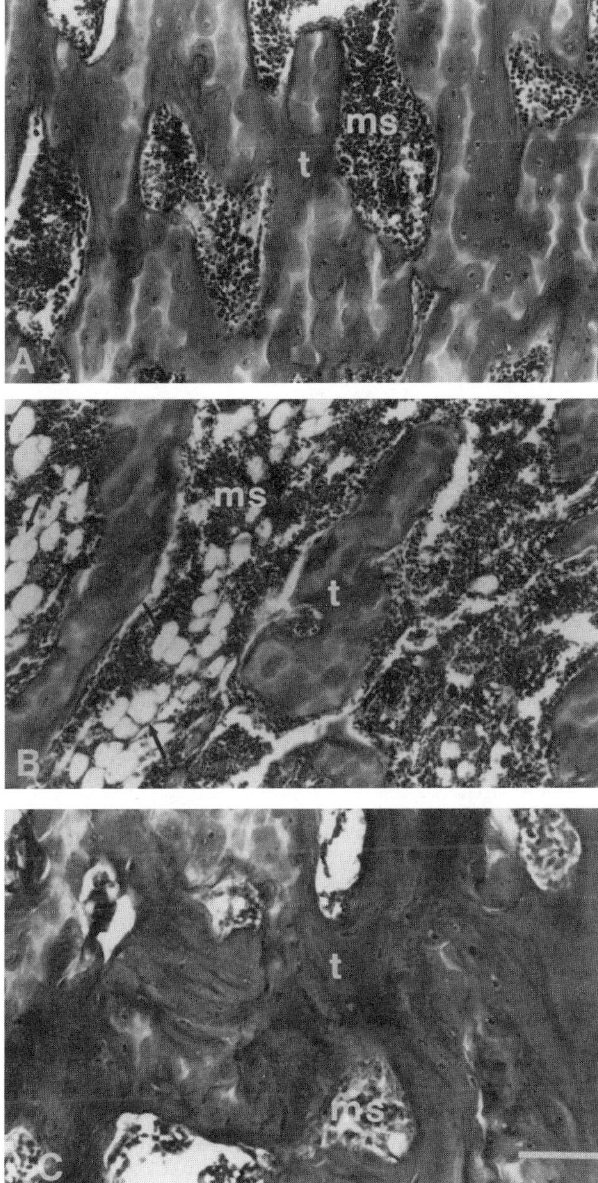

Figure 5.6
Compared with normal rat femoral metaphysis (A), ovariectomy over an 8-week period (B), depletes trabeculae (t) and increases the marrow space (ms), which display significant amounts of adipocytes (arrows). However, a 6-week treatment with 0.8 nmole/100 g of body weight of hPTH-(1-31)NH_2 started 2 weeks after OVX (C), dramatically builds up trabeculae while decreasing marrow space well below normal. H & E staining; bar = 0.2 mm.

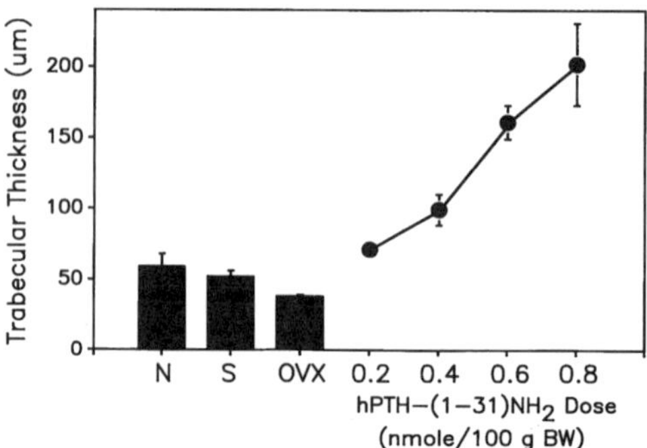

Figure 5.7
The dose-dependent ability of hPTH-(1-31)NH_2 to thicken trabeculae in the distal femur when subcutaneously injected daily between 9 and 15 weeks after OVX. The mean trabecular thickness in the distal femurs of sham-OVX and vehicle-treated (between 9 and 15 weeks) OVX rats at 15 weeks after the operations were not significantly different from each other or the values in the distal femurs from normal rats. However, daily injections of 0.4, 0.6, or 0.8 nmole, but not 0.2 nmole, of hPTH-(1-31)NH_2/100 g of body weight significantly ($P < 0.01$) increased trabecular thickness with respect to normal, sham OVX and OVX values. (From Whitfield, J. F., Morley, P., Willick, G. E., Ross, V., Barbier, J.-R., Isaacs, R., and Ohannessian-Barry, L., Stimulation of the growth of femoral trabecular bone in ovariectomized rats by the novel parathyroid hormone fragment, hPTH-(1-31)NH_2 (Ostabolin), *Calcif. Tissue Int.*, 58, 81, 1996. With permission.)

We then tested the bone-building potency of hPTH-(1-31)NH_2 using several doses (0.8, 0.6, 0.4, and 0.2 nmole/100 g of body weight) and a *regenerative* or treatment-assessing, rather than preventative, model.[64] In this experiment we did not use the excessively osteogenic 1 nmole/100 g of body weight. Again we started with ovariectomized 3-month-old rats, but we waited for nine weeks to let their mostly nonlamellar femoral trabecular bone be severely depleted before starting the six weeks of daily injections. By the end of the ninth week they had lost about 75% of their femoral trabecular bone mass. Figures 5.7 and 5.8 show the dose-dependent increases in the mean trabecular thicknesses caused by lamellar deposition that had been produced by the 36 injections of 4 different doses of the fragment. The fragment could also stimulate trabecular bone growth in much older rats. Thus, 36 injections of the mid-range dose of 0.6 nmole/100 g of body weight of hPTH-(1-31)NH_2 were able to significantly increase the mean trabecular thickness above the normal starting value in the predepleted (nine weeks after OVX) femoral trabecular bone of one-year-old rats, and they did so as effectively as hPTH-(1-84).[89]

The question then arose as to whether the much larger (139, 141, or 173 amino acids) hPTHrP (parathyroid hormone-related protein) is as osteogenic as hPTH. Indeed, in a tumor-bearing athymic rat model for PTHrP-produced humoral hypercalcemia of malignancy, the expression and growing production of PTHrP by the tumor cells produced an early twofold burst of bone formation before the switch-over to bone resorption

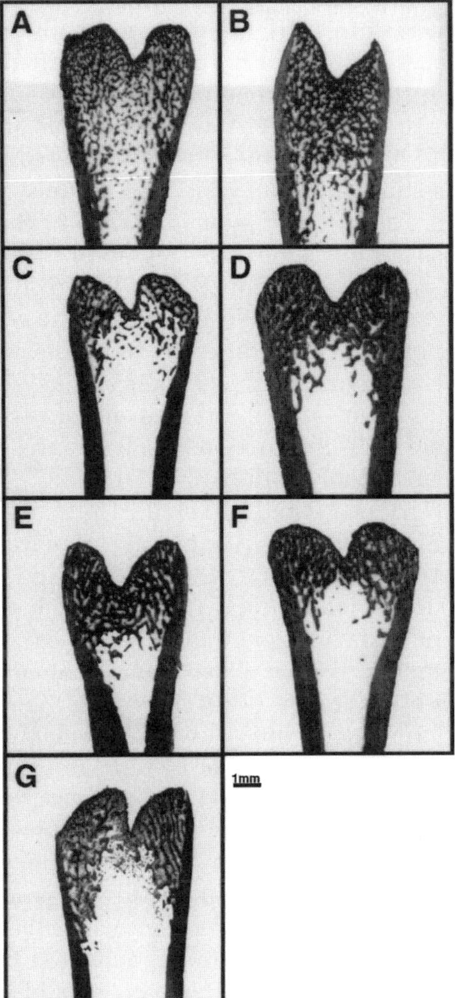

Figure 5.8
Representative examples of the reduction of femoral trabecular bone by 15 weeks after OVX and the ability of daily injections of various doses of hPTH-(1-31)NH_2 from 9 to 15 weeks to increase the density of the trabecular bone. (A) Normal demineralized distal femur. (B) Distal femur at 15 weeks after sham OVX. (C) Distal femur at 15 weeks after OVX. (D) Distal femur at 15 weeks after OVX and after daily injections of 0.8 nmole of hPTH-(1-31)NH_2/100 g of body weight from 9 to 15 weeks. (E) Distal femur at 15 weeks after OVX and after daily injections of 0.6 nmole of hPTH-(1-31)NH_2/100 g of body weight from 9 to 15 weeks. (F) Distal femur at 15 weeks after OVX and after daily injections of 0.4 nmole of hPTH-(1-31)NH_2/100 g of body weight from 9 to 15 weeks. (G) Distal femur at 15 weeks after OVX and after daily injections of 0.2 nmole of hPTH-(1-31)NH_2/100 g of body weight. The 10-μm sections of demineralized bone were stained with Sanderson's rapid bone stain. (From Whitfield, J. F., Morley, P., Willick, G. E., Ross, V., Barbier, J.-R., Isaacs, R., and Ohannessian-Barry, L., Stimulation of the growth of femoral trabecular bone in ovariectomized rats by the novel parathyroid hormone fragment, hPTH-(1-31)NH_2 (Ostabolin), *Calcif. Tissue Int.*, 58, 81, 1996. With permission.)

when the PTHrP production reached a critical threshold level.[90] Eight of the first 13 amino acids of PTHrP are the same as those of hPTH, but the amino acid sequences of the two hormones are different beyond amino acid 13.[73] However, their conformations in the receptor-binding region show some similarities[87] and N-terminal fragments such as hPTHrP-(1-34) and hPTH-(1-40) have the same affinity for the low-affinity, adenylyl cyclase-PLC/PKCs-stimulating and the high-affinity, PLC/PKCs-stimulating PTH receptors as hPTH fragments.[73] One of the two PLC/PKCs-activation domains is in the same 28-34 region of the PTHrP molecule as PTH's PLC/PKCs-activation domain.[73] But, PTHrP is far more complex than PTH and can be proteolytically processed into several potent autocrine/paracrine fragments with different receptors and different functions.[91] It has a nuclear translocation sequence in its 87-107 region which can promote proliferation and/or prevent apoptosis of target cells by promoting ribosomal RNA production,[92] as well as a second PLC/PKCs-activated domain next door in the 107-111 region.[73,91] It followed from these facts that hPTHrP-(1-34) and hPTH-(1-31)NH_2 should be as effective as the equivalent PTH fragments. Weir et al.[93] reported that hPTHrP-(1-74) was a more potent anabolic agent in male Sprague-Dawley rats than hPTH-(1-34), but Hock et al.[94] found that the much shorter hPTHrP-(1-34) was a less potent anabolic agent than hPTH-(1-34). The reason for this discrepancy is unknown. We have also found that 36 daily injections of 0.8 nmole/100 g of body weight of hPTHrP-(1-34) into rats, starting two weeks after OVX, stimulated bone growth less effectively than hPTH-(1-31)NH_2 as indicated by a much smaller increase in mean trabecular thickness, but the same dose of hPTHrP-(1-31)NH_2 was, unexpectedly, completely ineffective.[94a] While there are many possible reasons for the poor osteogenic performance of hPTHrP-(1-34) and the impotence of hPTHrP-(1-31)NH_2, there is one that merits future investigation — a significant role in the osteogenic response for the recently discovered PTH2 receptor that is coupled to adenylyl cyclase and is activated by PTH but *not* by PTHrP.[80] Therefore, could the lower effectiveness of hPTHrP-(1-34) be due to an activation of *both* PTH/PTHrP *and* the PTH2 receptors, to which PTHrP-(1-34) cannot bind, being needed to maximally stimulate bone growth? Another possibility, which could explain the observation of Weir et al.,[93] is that residues beyond amino acid-34 are needed for stability *in vivo,* and removing them reduces the fragment's survival in the blood. A possible explanation for the impotence of hPTHrP(1-31)NH_2 is that removing amino acids 32-34 further decreases its stability *in vivo* or disables its receptor-binding domain. The C-terminal α-helix of [Ala^{26}]-hPTHrP-(1-34)NH_2 has been reported to run from Phe^{21}/Phe^{22} to Ala^{34},[95] whereas that in hPTH extends from Leu^{15}/Ser^{17} to Gln^{29}.[96,97] Therefore, removing amino acids 32-34 would bite more deeply into hPTHrP's receptor-binding α-helix than hPTH's receptor-binding α-helix.

In conclusion, intermittent subcutaneous injections of PTH stimulate cortical and trabecular bone growth by causing a series of brief bursts of adenylyl cyclase activity and cyclic AMP synthesis, which trigger pulses of cyclic AMP-dependent protein kinase activity that stimulate a steady build-up of osteogenic products. The identification of adenylyl cyclase as the activator of the osteogenic mechanism is strongly supported by the potent osteogenic abilities of the adenylyl cyclase-stimulating prostaglandins to be discussed in Section IV. The osteogenic action of fluoride (see Lau et al.'s Chapter 9 for a detailed discussion of fluoride action) could in part be another example of bone-building by adenylyl cyclase and cyclic AMP, because fluoride has long been known to combine with traces of aluminum to form AlF_4^- complexes which bind beside the GDP in inactive $G_{s\alpha} \cdot$ GDP complexes where, by mimicking the γ-phosphoryl moiety of GTP, they form active adenylyl cyclase-stimulating $G_{s\alpha} \cdot$ GDP $\cdot$ AlF_4 complexes.[98]

C. A Plausible Osteogenic Mechanism

To find out how intermittent injections of an adenylyl cyclase-stimulating fragment, such as hPTH-(1-31)NH_2, and the pulses of cyclic AMP-dependent protein kinase activity it triggers stimulate bone formation we must first pinpoint the key target cells that display PTH receptors on their surfaces. Only certain members of the osteoblast lineage express and display PTH receptors. According to the latest information,[36-39] PTH receptors are transiently made and expressed in large numbers only by mature *postproliferative* osteoblasts on their way to becoming osteocytes or lining cells. At first sight this seems to conflict with the expression of PTH/PTHrP receptors by the proliferatively active, but still osteogenically competent, ROS 17/2 osteosarcoma cells that we used to test the abilities of PTH fragments to stimulate adenylyl cyclase and PLC. However, the osteocalcin gene, which is also normally expressed only by mature, postproliferative osteoblasts, is also dysregulated and constitutively expressed in proliferating ROS 17/2 cells.[34] In neoplastic cells such as ROS cells the nucleosome arrangements and the specific factor-mediated nuclear matrix attachments that grab promoters and twist them into their responsive configurations have been so radically changed that interactions of up-regulating transcription factors with the DNA of the promoters of replication-related genes (e.g., the genes encoding engine-kinases, replication enzymes, and histones) and differentiation-related genes (e.g., the genes encoding PTH receptors, alkaline phosphatase, osteocalcin, and osteopontin) become constitutive rather than restricted to the DNA-synthetic S phase of the cell cycle or to specific postproliferative maturation stages as in normal cells.[34] Normal osteoblasts start expressing PTH receptors (the number of which peaks at about 70,000/cell) along with the osteocalcin gene after the cell has shifted out of the proliferative mode and down-regulated the proliferation-driving AP-1(c-*fos*, c-*jun*) transcription factor complexes that were suppressing the osteocalcin gene,[34,36,37] and maybe the PTH receptor gene, in the mitotically active osteoblast precursors.

Where are these *first-response* cells? In the progressively modeling skeleton of a growing animal or human they will be clustered separately from osteoclasts in the bone-formation zones and in BMUs which are in the formation stage of the remodeling cycle. In the skeletons of mature animals and humans they will probably be found only in BMUs. However, Dobnig and Turner[99] and Leaffer et al.[100] appear to have found the *second-response* cells. Their key finding was that hPTH-(1-34) caused the accumulation of layers of plump osteoblasts on the surfaces of bones of 3- and 16-month-old female Sprague-Dawley rats without stimulating preosteoblast proliferation. Thus, despite the large increase in osteoblasts, the fraction of [^{3}H]-thymidine-labeled bone cells in the PTH-treated animals was not higher than in control animals, which could not have been the case if the new osteoblasts had come from proliferating preosteoblasts. Therefore, it appears that the PTH fragments in the studies of Dobnig and Turner[99] and Leaffer et al.,[100] as well as our hPTH-(1-31)NH_2, stimulated the rapid, reversible conversion of thin, osteogenically inactive, *lining cells* (lining cells in Figure 5.9 and the OC/L cells in Figure 5.10) into plump, active osteoblasts. This transformation of lining cells into osteoblasts was reversible, because the plump osteoblasts promptly reverted to thin lining cells when the fragment injections were stopped.

The bone-building scenario (Figure 5.10) starts with daily PTH injections briefly activating adenylyl cyclase-stimulating receptors on the surfaces of the first-response mature, postproliferative osteoblasts in BMUs as well as in the bone-formation zones if the individual is growing. The resulting, very brief, once-daily cyclic AMP surges stimulate a sustained expression of the cyclic AMP-responsive genes encoding IGF-I, IGFBP-5 (IGF-binding protein 5), TGF-βs, and VEGF (vascular endothelium growth factor) and a steady buildup of their products[23,24,62,64,101,102] (Figure 5.10). These products are autocrine/paracrine factors that stimulate the various matrix-making and other activities of the first-response osteoblasts and one of them, IGF-I, increases the cellular lifespan and thus increases the osteoblast population by inhibiting apoptotic suicide.[28] The TGF-βs would, in turn, stimulate the osteoblasts to produce the potently osteogenic BMP-2. They also trigger a self-propagating wave of reversible conversions of neighboring, thin lining cells with the condensed nuclei typical of relatively inactive cells into plump, probably PTH receptor-bearing, factor-secreting, matrix-making, second-response osteoblasts with active, large decondensed nuclei as they diffuse away from their natal BMUs and formation zones (if any) (Figures 5.9 and 5.10). The VEGF produced by the osteoblasts would stimulate the invasion of the new bone by the new blood vessels needed to feed it (Figure 5.10). However, the new bone is still vulnerable to the osteoporotic mechanism and would be

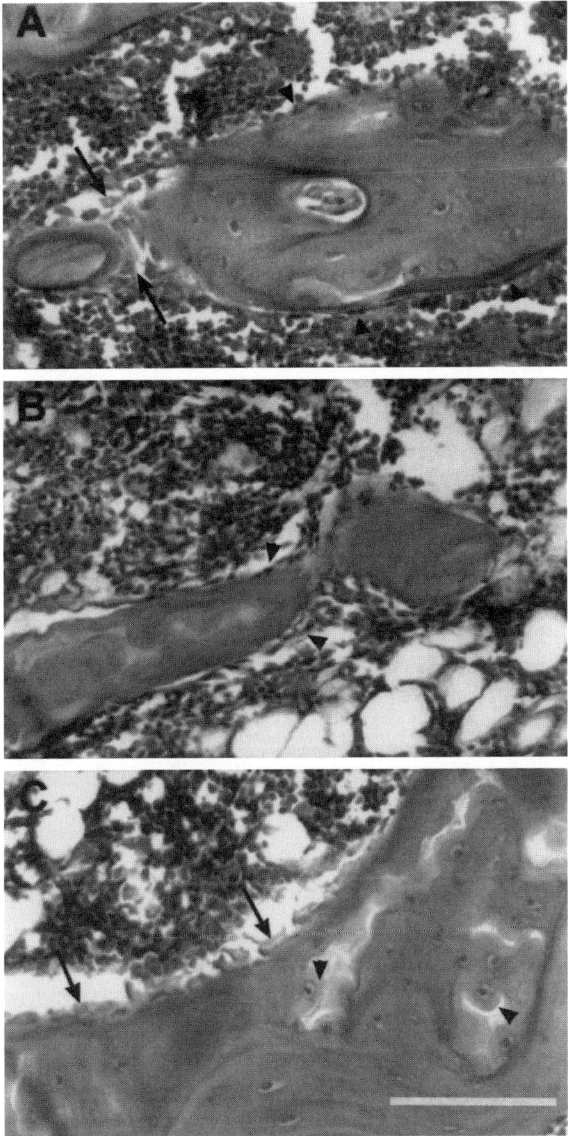

Figure 5.9
Under ordinary conditions (A), trabecular bone-lining cells are present in both a flattened (resting; arrowheads) and plump polygonal (active; arrows) forms. Eight weeks after OVX, (B) trabeculae are greatly reduced and most of the osteoblasts are present as flattened, resting cells (arrowheads). By contrast, trabeculae from OVX rats treated with daily injections of hPTH-(1-31)NH_2 (0.8 nmole/100 g of body weight) demonstrate a dramatic increase in active, plump polygonal osteoblasts lining the bone (arrows) as well as increased trabecular osteoblastic activity (arrowheads) probably associated with the conversion of osteoid and/or woven bone to lamellar bone. H & E staining; bar = 0.1 mm.

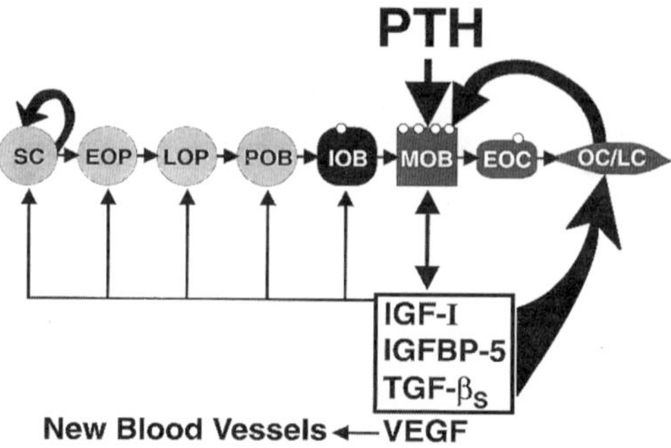

Figure 5.10
The PTH-triggered osteogenic mechanism. A once-daily pulse of an adenylyl cyclase-stimulating PTH fragment, such as hPTH-(1-34) or hPTH-(1-31)NH_2, activates the large number of receptors (O) that are selectively expressed by the mature, postproliferative osteoblasts (MOB) in a BMU or formation region. The resulting first cyclic AMP surge starts the expression of genes encoding IGF-I (insulin-like growth factor-I), IGFBP-5 (insulin-like growth factor-I binding protein-5), TGF-βs (tumor growth factor-βs) and possibly bone-morphogenic proteins of the TGF-β superfamily. Each subsequent cyclic AMP surge boosts the expression of these genes and thus drives the buildup of their products. These products are *autocrine* agents that stimulate matrix formation and other differentiated functions, but not proliferation, of the postproliferative producer osteoblasts. They are also *paracrine* agents that stimulate proliferation, matrix production, and other differentiation-related functions of local self-renewing stem cells (SCs), early and late proliferatively active osteoblast precursors (EOPs and LOPs), proliferatively active preosteoblasts (POBs), and early and mature osteocytes (EOCs and OCs). Most important, they start a local spreading wave of reversible transformation of thin lining cells (LCs) into mature, plump, and possibly PTH receptor-expressing osteoblasts. Another paracrine factor produced by the PTH-stimulated osteoblasts is VEGF (vascular endothelium growth factor), which stimulates the production of the blood vessels needed to supply the forming bone.

resorbed unless protected by an activation and/or resorption inhibitor according to the loss/restore/maintain (LRM) strategy of Jee et al.[103]

At this point we should try to explain why an intermittently injected dose of PTH stimulates bone growth while the same dose either does not affect bone or stimulates bone resorption when infused continuously. We should note at the outset that the results of preliminary experiments in our laboratory, like those of Tam et al.,[104] indicate that adenylyl cyclase stimulators such as hPTH-(1-84) and hPTH-(1-31)NH_2, stimulate bone resorption when continuously infused from subcutaneously inserted minipumps. But in our preliminary experiments, infusing an isomolar dose of a fragment such as hPTH-(28-48), which only stimulates PLC/PKCs, did not stimulate bone resorption. There are several possible reasons for these diametrically opposite responses to the intermittent versus continuous presence of adenylyl cyclase-stimulators. Unlike once-daily injections, a continuous infusion or closely spaced pulses of PTH would down-regulate the PTH receptors on mature osteoblasts.[74] Therefore, after an initial PTH-induced burst of activity and a transient surge of osteogenic and angiogenic factors, there would be no PTH receptors to provide the booster pulses of cyclic AMP needed to continue the buildup of these factors by the first-response osteoblasts that convert lining cells into amplifying second-response osteoblasts. The second possibility is that, while a brief cyclic AMP pulse triggers the production of osteogenic factors, a sustained elevation of cyclic AMP or closely spaced pulses of the cyclic nucleotide either inhibits the production of factors such as IGF-I or the subsequent cyclic AMP-independent osteogenic actions of these factors.[105] The result of this would be the inhibition of matrix production and acceleration of bone loss by impairing osteoblast action in BMUs and formation regions. A third possibility is that the osteoblasts need a continuous elevation, or at least closely spaced pulses, of cyclic AMP to build up and maintain a pool of more ephemeral resorption-related mRNA messages or their products such as GM-CSF, IL-1, or IL-6. These cytokines would override the actions of the anabolic factors by expanding the osteoclast population, giving the osteoclasts access to mineralized bone surfaces by stimulating the retraction of lining cells, and increasing the size and volume of the osteoclasts' bone-resorbing "suction cups."[14,106]

D. A Comparison of Anabolic Potencies

To compare the bone-building abilities of hPTH-(1-84), hPTH-(1-34), and hPTH-(1-31)NH_2 we ovariectomized 3-month-old rats and waited for nine weeks to let them lose about 75% of their trabecular bone before starting six weeks of once-daily subcutaneous injections (6 days/week for a total of 36 injections) of a submaximally effective, middle-range dose — 0.6 nmole/100 g of body weight. We focused on trabecular rather than cortical bone because the OVX-induced changes in trabecular bone are much larger, and hence trabecular responses to PTH can be measured more accurately. It turned out that hPTH-(1-84) and hPTH-(1-31)NH_2 were equally effective, but hPTH-(1-34) was more effective than the other two in increasing the mean trabecular thickness and total trabecular bone mass.[89,107]

Why was subcutaneously injected hPTH-(1-34) the most effective of the three osteogens at lower doses? It is not a significantly better stimulator of the ROS osteosarcoma cells' adenylyl cyclase.[87] Indeed, while the ability to stimulate ROS cells' adenylyl cyclase is the *sine qua non* of an osteogenic PTH fragment, it is not an absolute predictor of osteogenicity. Thus, hPTH-(1-30)NH_2, for example, does not stimulate bone growth despite being a potent stimulator of ROS cell adenylyl cyclase (albeit with a higher EC_{50} of 20 nM as opposed to hPTH-(1-34)'s 16 nM probably because Val^{31} removal destabilized the receptor-binding α-helix) and a potent producer of vascular smooth muscle relaxation and hypotension.[87,107] The osteogenic response also depends on several factors which combine to enable the arrival of enough active, adenylyl cyclase-stimulating hormone or hormone fragment at the PTH/PTHrP (and maybe PTH2) receptor-bearing mature osteoblasts.

An important factor governing the osteogenic response might be the kind of PTH/PTHrP receptor expressed by osteoblasts in the bone. This possibility is suggested by the observations of Dr. Peter Friedman of Dartmouth Medical School (personal communication) that hPTH-(1-30)NH_2, which stimulates adenylyl cyclase in ROS 17/2 cells but does not stimulate bone growth, cannot stimulate the adenylyl cyclase in primary proximal or distal convoluted rat kidney tubule cells that is strongly stimulated by hPTH-(1-31)NH_2. Thus, normal rat osteoblasts may express a kind of PTH receptor that, unlike those of neoplastic ROS 17/2 cells and the normal vascular smooth muscle cells to be discussed in the next paragraph are much less affected, or even unaffected, by hPTH-(1-30)NH_2.

One way to rapidly assess the movement of an osteogenic PTH fragment from the subcutaneous injection site into the circulation is based on PTH's well-known potent hypotensive action, which is due to the cyclic AMP-mediated relaxation of vascular smooth muscle cells.[107-110] The reduction of tail artery pressure in the ovary-intact rat following a single subcutaneous injection of the three osteogenic PTHs (e.g., at a dose of 0.8 nmole/100 g of body weight) paralleled their abilities to stimulate bone formation.[107] Indeed, hPTH-(1-34) was at least twice as effective as hPTH-(1-84) and hPTH-(1-31)NH_2.[107] However, shortening the PTH molecule C-terminally from 84 to 31 residues decreased by nine times the length of time required for the tail artery pressure to reach its minimum.[107] In other words, hPTH-(1-31)NH_2 got into the circulation from the injection site much faster than hPTH-(1-34), but less of it got to the target cells. However, that lesser amount was still potently osteogenic. Thus, it appears that hPTH-(1-34) has the optimal combination of penetrability and stability for optimal hypotensive and osteogenic responses. Clearly, if both the *in vivo* survival and receptor affinity of the rapidly penetrating hPTH-(1-31)NH_2 could be increased and its affinity for its receptor enhanced we would have a very potent osteogen. These ends could be achieved in two ways. First, intrahelix peptidase target sites could be blocked and the α-helix clamped in place and stabilized by forming a cyclizing lactam linkage between Glu^{22} and Lys^{26}. Second, the affinity for the receptor could be increased by enhancing the hydrophobicity of the helix's receptor-associating hydrophobic face by replacing the normal, hydrophilic Lys^{27} with the hydrophobic Leu^{27} (Figure 5.3). Indeed, the cyclized ([Leu^{27}]cyclo(Glu^{22}-Lys^{26})-hPTH-(1-31)NH_2 is a much more potent osteogen than linear hPTH-(1-31)NH_2, as indicated by a greater ability to stimulate the growth and corticalization of trabecular bone (Figures 5.11 and 5.12).[110a]

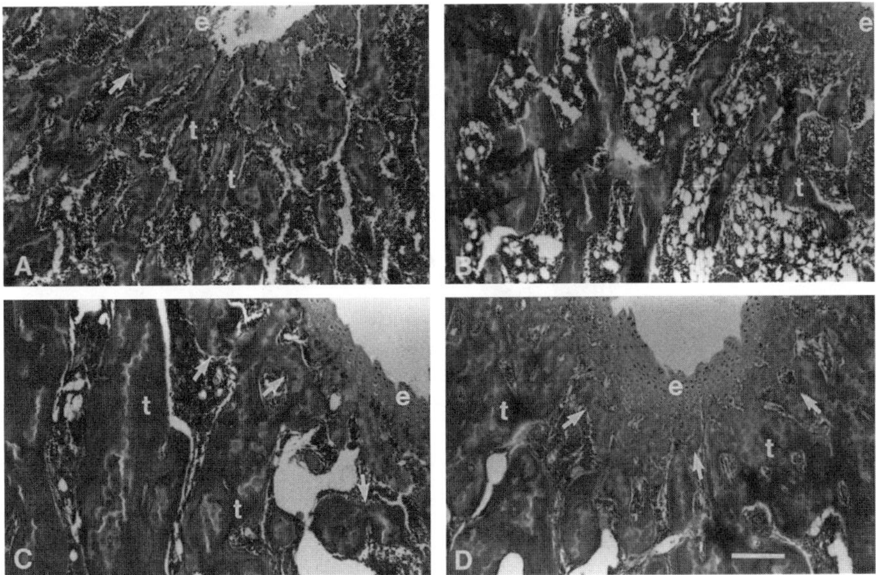

Figure 5.11
Comparison of the effectiveness of cyclized PTH fragments with hPTH-(1-31)NH_2 for building bone after OVX. Normal distal femoral metaphysis of the rat (A) displays a regular array of longitudinal trabeculae (t) radiating away from the epiphyseal plate (e) with abundant cross-bracing (arrows) between trabeculae. OVX over an 8-week period (B) results in a reduction of trabeculae, especially the cross-bracing units. By contrast, rats treated daily with subcutaneous injection of 0.8 nmole/100 g of body weight of hPTH-(1-31)NH_2 (C) or cyclized ([Leu^{27}]cyclo(Glu^{22}-Lys^{26})-hPTH-(1-31)NH_2 (D), show dramatic increases in longitudinal and cross-bracing trabeculae. Decrease in marrow space and thickening of the trabeculae is especially prominent after treatment with the cyclized hPTH (D). e-remnants of epiphyseal plate after removal of epiphysis prior to fixation is evident in all views. H & E staining; bar = 0.1 mm.

IV. PROSTAGLANDINS

The conclusion that it is adenylyl cyclase that boots bone formation is supported by a large body of evidence that the adenylyl cyclase-stimulating PGE_1 and PGE_2, but not the PLC/PKCs-stimulating prostaglandins are osteogenic and angiogenic.[111-114] Like PTH, the adenylyl cyclase-stimulating PGEs can stimulate either bone resorption or formation depending on the size of the dose and the dosing schedule. As expected of a cyclic AMP-driven mechanism, intermittence and low dosage are again the requirements for a PGE-triggered osteogenic response.

The first indication of the osteogenic potency of the prostaglandins came from an unusual source, a side effect of using PGE_1-induced cyclic AMP surges to relax the ductus arteriosus in children with cyanotic congenital heart disease.[115] This treatment eventually caused a massive periosteal hyperostosis which has since been confirmed by other groups such

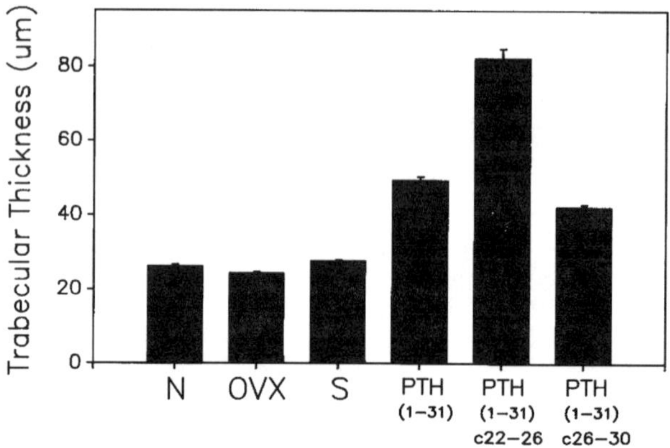

Figure 5.12
Comparison of the abilities of two lactam derivatives of hPTH-(1-31)NH_2 to stimulate bone growth as indicated by differences in the mean trabecular thickness in the distal femur. Young (3-month-old) Sprague-Dawley rats were OVX'd and injected subcutaneously once a day (6 days/week) with 0.6 nmole of fragment/100 g of body weight between 2 and 8 weeks after the operation. At the end of the 8th week, the mean trabecular thicknesses were determined. The 22-26 lactam, ([Leu^{27}]cyclo(Glu^{22}-Lys^{26})-hPTH-(1-31)NH_2, was significantly ($P < 0.01$) more effective than either the 26-30 lactam, ([Leu^{27}]cyclo(Lys^{26}-Asp^{30})-hPTH-(1-31)NH_2 or hPTH-(1-31)NH_2.[110a]

as Drvaric et al.[116] Since then, the anabolic action of the adenylyl cyclase-stimulating prostaglandins has been observed in many different models. Prostaglandin accumulation has been reported to be associated with proliferating periosteal bone in avian osteopetrosis.[117] Limb burning in rats causes a 250% increase in PGE_2 production, periosteal proliferation, and a 50% increase in bone cross-sectional area.[118] Feeding a diet rich in arachidonic acid, the precursor of prostaglandins, increases prostaglandin production and vertebral bone density in rats.[119] Oral or subcutaneously injected PGE_2 prevents the severe bone loss in male rats that is triggered by castration.[120] But most important for this discussion, daily subcutaneous injections of PGE_2 (e.g., at a dose of 6 mg/kg of body weight) prevents or reverses the severe bone loss in OVX'd rats and that the new bone, like PTH-induced new bone, can be maintained by an antiresorptive such as the bisphosphonate risedronate.[103,121-123] In fact, it has even been claimed that PGE_2 stimulates the formation of new trabeculae in OVX-rats.[123]

PGEs stimulate bone remodeling with an imbalance in favor of formation.[123] They are potent mitogens which stimulate DNA synthesis by cultured avian and rat calvarial cells.[124-126] But the duration of exposure (hence, as with PTH, the importance of intermittent dosing) is critical. A brief, 5-min, but not a 45-min, exposure to PGE_2 (or the adenylyl cyclase-stimulating forskolin, dibutyryl cyclic AMP, or the cyclic AMP-elevating cyclic nucleotide phosphodiesterase inhibitor isobutylmethylxanthine) stimulates the proliferation of chick osteoblast-like cells.[126] As would be expected from an adenylyl cyclase stimulator, PGE_2 also stimulates osteoblasts to make growth factors such as IGF-I, VEGF, and more PGEs.[35,127]

Similar though they are, the anabolic actions of the adenylyl cyclase-stimulating PGEs are different with respect to their target cells. As pointed out in Section III.C, only postproliferative mature osteoblasts in formation zones and BMUs express PTH receptors. Therefore, PTH can start osteogenesis and expand the osteoblast population by osteoblastic conversion of lining cells only by stimulating these postproliferative cells to produce, make and secrete paracrine growth factors, among which are IGF-I and the PGEs, some of which can reversibly transform quiescent lining cells into osteoblasts (Figure 5.10).[99,100] However, unlike IGF-I, PGEs do not play a significant role in PTH's osteogenic action, because this action is unaffected by blocking PGE synthesis with indomethacin.[128] By contrast, PGEs are promiscuous agents with a broad selection of targets in bone and other tissues. They can directly stimulate all members of the preosteoblast/osteoblast/osteocyte/lining cell lineage, as well as indirectly by stimulating their targets to express various cyclic AMP-responsive genes such as the gene encoding IGF-I.

Perhaps the most important role of the PGEs is their probable mediation of mechanostat action.[111,129,130] When the strain exceeds a certain threshold, the mechanostat activates a mechanism that changes local bone mass and shape to drop the strain below the threshold. Mechanically stressing osteoblasts/osteocytes in culture or bone stimulates PLA_2 by pulling "integrin wires," which in turn stimulate PGE production and thus cyclic AMP synthesis, which triggers changes in gene expression that lead ultimately to the initiation of DNA synthesis.[111,129] The first of these changes are increased *c-fos* gene expression and decreased alkaline phosphatase, osteocalcin, and osteopontin gene expression followed by increased IGF-I and TGF-β gene expression.[111,130] It is also possible that autocrine/paracrine PTHrP, depending on the length of the processed and secreted fragment(s) (see Section III.B), might also be involved in the mechanostat, because its expression in other organs is stimulated by mechanical stress,[131,132] and, providing that it has an intact N-terminus (to stimulate adenylyl cyclase) and the C-terminal regions responsible for PLC stimulation and cytosolic Ca^{2+} elevation,[73,91] it can stimulate PGE_2 production and secretion by osteoblasts.[133]

Finally, while the adenylyl cyclase-stimulating PGEs are potent bone-builders, they are not as tissue specific as PTH and have many unpleasant side effects.[112] Like IGF-I, they cannot selectively stimulate bone growth as the PTHs do and therefore might enhance the proliferation of carcinogenically initiated cells of, for example, breast, colon, and prostate in older patients. Clearly it would be unreasonable to use a PGE when we can more safely and selectively use the at least equally potent hPTH-(1-34) or hPTH-(1-31)NH_2 to stimulate bone growth.

V. PROSPECTS

Where do we go from here? We have developed the very potent anabolic hPTH-(1-31)NH_2, which, by stimulating only adenylyl cyclase, can avoid any potential side effects of the multitude of Ca^{2+}- and PKCs-mediated reactions that are also triggered by hPTH-(1-84) and hPTH-(1-34). But we have not addressed what many believe to be the most serious barrier to patients' acceptance of PTH — the need for subcutaneous injections (albeit painlessly through ultrafine 30-gauge syringe needles) for one or two years before switching over to oral resorption inhibitors to maintain the new bone. However, while oral delivery is clearly essential for long-term preventative treatment with an antiresorptive drug, it is far less important for an anabolic drug, because a woman normally does not realize that she is in trouble (osteoporosis is the "silent epidemic") until she starts breaking bones, that is, until she has an established severe osteopenia/osteoporosis and is therefore acutely aware of her need for, and is prepared to accept, a bone-builder such as PTH regardless of whether or not it is injectable. Also, Hodsman (see Chapter 4) has found that an effective treatment with PTH needs only 28-day cycles interrupted by 3-month rest periods.

To overcome this possibly unimportant barrier we should make smaller peptides that can be structurally modified or suitably packaged (e.g., in liposomes) for oral or intratracheal delivery. We have taken the first step toward this goal by learning to make even smaller, still potent, adenylyl cyclase-stimulating fragments such as hPTH-(1-30)NH_2, hPTH-(1-29)NH_2, and hPTH-(1-28)NH_2 by using the C-terminal-amide-group strategy.[87] But so far these fragments do not stimulate bone formation[64] probably because they take too long to enter the circulation from the injection site and they and their truncated receptor-binding α-helices are too unstable after entering the circulation to reach the waiting osteoblasts in a configurationally receptor-ready state. A possible way of configurationally constraining, and thus stabilizing, the receptor-binding α-helices and further increasing the protease resistance, of these smaller fragments is to cyclize them with the intramolecular lactam linkage that increases the anabolic effectiveness of hPTH-(1-31)NH_2. Of course, the smaller the fragment, the easier it will be to determine the minimal PTH/PTHrP receptor-binding adenylyl cyclase-stimulating molecular configuration needed to make the much-desired oral nonpeptide mimic.

While waiting for this ultimate oral therapeutic peptide mimic, we can use intermittent subcutaneous injections of a fragment such as hPTH-(1-31)NH_2 or one of its cyclized derivatives to stimulate bone growth in osteoporotic patients and then preserve this new bone with one of the rapidly growing family of potent bisphosphonates. In the world of drugs, smaller and simpler is better, so it seems to us that it would be prudent to use a fragment, such as hPTH-(1-31)NH_2, which approaches the ideal because it does its osteogenic job by stimulating adenylyl cyclase without the unnecessary clutter of PLC-induced reactions that are triggered by its larger relatives such as hPTH-(1-34), hPTH-(1-38), and hPTH-(1-84). The potential uses for such a small, signally simple fragment extend beyond osteoporosis therapy, especially if it can be given in some way other than by injection. It should promote fracture healing, reverse the bone loss resulting from immobilization for various reasons,[134-136] and be a type of "chemical gravity" to hold back an aroused mechanostat and restore bone lost during prolonged space missions.

Finally we must herald the emergence of a new gene-therapy technology for putting PTH-producing fibroblasts into fracture sites.[137] In the first demonstration of this technology, a collagen matrix was prepared and incubated with a DNA plasmid containing the gene for prepro-PTH-(1-34). When this gene-activated matrix was implanted into a break in rat femoral diaphyses, the fibroblasts in the fracture's granulation repair tissue picked up the DNA and became microbioreactors that locally produced PTH-(1-34) that stimulated fracture healing. Adding a second plasmid containing the gene for bone morphogenic protein-4 further enhanced the fracture repair. Clearly the door has been opened for repairing fractures with combinations of PTH and other anabolic agents that could not be safely used if injected systemically.

ACKNOWLEDGMENTS

We must acknowledge the immense contributions of Jean-René Barbier, Sasha Bidwell, Balu Chakravarthy, Rick Isaacs, Sue Maclean, Witold Neugebauer, Ray Rixon, Virginia Ross, and Mark Soska to our quest for an understanding of how PTH stimulates bone growth and for better bone-building bits of this remarkable hormone.

REFERENCES

1. Hughes, M. D., Biochemical markers for osteoporosis: Update on emerging diagnostic opportunities, *Spectrum*, 77, 1, 1995.
2. Russell, R., *Bone Diseases and Osteoporosis*, IBC Technical Services, London, 1994.
3. Stini, W. A., What does an epidemic of hip fractures tell us about human evolution? *South African J. Sci.*, 91, 455, 1995.
4. Albright, F., Bloomberg, E., and Smith, P. H., Postmenopausal osteoporosis, *Trans. Assoc. Am. Phys.*, 55, 298, 1940.
5. Eriksen, E. F., Axelrod, D. W., and Melsen, F., *Bone Histomorphometry*, Raven Press, New York, 1994.
6. Eriksen, E. F., Langdahl, B., and Klassen, M., The cellular basis of osteoporosis, *Spine:State of the Arts Revs.*, 8, 23, 1994.
7. Kalu, D. N., Evolution of the pathogenesis of bone loss, *Bone*, 17 (Suppl.), 135S, 1995.

8. Riggs, B. L. and Melton, L. J., Eds., *Osteoporosis*, 2nd Ed, Lippincott-Raven, Philadelphia, 1995.
9. Aarden, E. M., Nijweide, P. J., van der Plas, A., Alblas, M. J., Mackie, E. J., Horton, M. A., and Helfrich, M. H., Adhesive properties of isolated chick osteocytes in vitro, *Bone*, 18, 305, 1996.
10. Sanchez-Mateos, P., Cabanas, C., and Sanchez-Madrid, F., Regulation of integrin function, Seminars in Cancer Biology, 7, 99, 1996.
11. Sinha, R. K. and Tuan, R. S., Regulation of human osteoblast integrin expression by orthopedic implant materials, *Bone*, 18, 451, 1996.
12. Meredith, J. E., Winitz, S., Lewis, J. M., Hess, S., Ren, X.-D., Renshaw, M. W., and Schwartz, M. A., The regulation of growth and intracellular signaling by integrins, *Endocr. Rev.*, 17, 207, 1996.
13. Buckwalter, J. A., Glimcher, M. J., Cooper, R. R., and Recker, R., Bone biology, I, *J. Bone Jt. Surg.*, 77-A, 1256, 1995.
14. Buckwalter, J. A., Glimcher, M. J., Cooper, R. R., and Recker, R., Bone biology II, *J. Bone Jt. Surg.*, 77-A, 1276, 1995.
15. Frost, H. M., Tetracycline-based histological analysis of bone remodeling, *Calcif. Tissue Int.*, 3, 211, 1969.
16. Frost, H. M., *Intermediate Organization of the Skeleton*, Vol. 1, CRC Press, San Diego, 1986.
17. Yoneda, T., Cytokines in bone: Local translators in cell-to-cell communication, in *Cellular and Molecular Biology of Bone*, Noda, M., Ed., Academic Press, San Diego, 1993, Chap. 12.
18. Baron, R., Ravesloot, J.-H., Neff, L., Chakrabarty, M., Chatterjee, D., Lomrie, A., and Horne, W., Cellular and molecular biology of the osteoclast, in *Cellular and Molecular Biology of Bone*, Noda, M., Ed., Academic Press, San Diego, 1993, chap. 14.
19. Mundy, G. R., Ibbotson, K. G., and D'Souza, S. M., Tumor products and the hypercalcemia of malignancy, *J. Clin. Invest.*, 3, 211, 1985.
20. Linkhart, T. A., Mohan, S., and Baylink, D. J., Growth factors for bone growth and repair: IGF, TGFβ and BMP, *Bone*, 19 (Suppl.), 1S, 1996.
21. Riancho, R. and Mundy, G. R., The role of cytokines and growth factors as mediators of the effects of systemic hormones at the bone local level, *Crit. Rev. Eukaryot. Gene Express.*, 5, 193, 1995.
22. Kim, S.-J. and Ballock, R. T., Cellular and molecular biology of transforming growth factor β, in *Cellular and Molecular Biology of Bone*, Noda, M., Ed., Academic Press, San Diego, 1993, chap. 3.
23. Canalis, E., Insulin-like growth factors and their role in osteoporosis, *Calcif. Tissue Int.*, 58, 133, 1996.
24. Canalis, E., Pash, J., and Varghese, S., Skeletal growth factors, *Crit. Rev. Eukaryot. Gene Express.*, 3, 155, 1992.
25. Quarles, L. D., Hartle, J. E., Middleton, J. P., Zhang, J., Arthur, J. M., and Raymond, J. R., Aluminum-induced DNA synthesis in osteoblasts: Mediation by a G-protein couples cation sensing mechanism, *J. Cell. Biochem.*, 56, 66, 1994.
26. Rosen, C. J. and Donahue, L. R., Insulin like growth factors: Potential therapeutic options for osteoporosis, *Trends Endocrinol. Metab.*, 6, 235, 1995.
27. Rosen, C., Donahue, L. R., and Hunter, S. J., Insulin-like growth factors and bone: the osteoporotic connection, *Proc. Soc. Exp. Biol. Med.*, 206, 83, 1994.
28. Rubin, R. and Baserga, R., Biology of disease: Insulin-like growth factor-I receptor, *Lab. Invest.*, 73, 311, 1995.
29. Sugimoto, T., Kanatani, M., Kana, J., Kobayashi, T., Yamaguchi, T., Fukase, M., and Chihara, K., IGF-I mediates the stimulatory effect of high calcium concentration on osteoblastic cell proliferation, *Am. J. Physiol.*, 266, E709, 1994.
30. Mundy, G. R., Local control of bone formation by osteoblasts, *Clin. Orthop.*, 313, 19, 1995.

31. MacLachlan, T. K., Sang, N., and Giordano, A., Cyclins, cyclin-dependent kinases and Cdk inhibitors: Implications in cell cycle control and cancers, *Crit. Rev. Eukaryot. Gene Express.*, 5, 127, 1995.
32. Whitfield, J. F., *Calcium in Cell Cycles and Cancer*, CRC Press, Boca Raton, 1995.
33. Stein, G. S. and Lian, J. B., Molecular mechanisms mediating developmental and hormone-regulated expression of genes in osteoblasts: An integrated relationship of cell growth and differentiation, in *Cellular and Molecular Biology of Bone*, Noda, M., Ed., Academic Press, San Diego, 1993, chap. 2.
34. Stein, G. S., Lian, J. B., Stein, J. L., Van Wijnen, J., and Montecino, M., Transcriptional control of osteoblast growth and differentiation, *Physiol. Rev.* 76, 593, 1996.
35. Harada, S., Nagy, J. A., Sullivan, K. A., Thomas, K. A., Endo, N., Rodan, G. A., and Rodan, S. B., Induction of vascular endothelial growth factor expression by prostaglandin E_2 and E_1 in osteoblasts, *J. Clin. Invest.*, 93, 2490, 1994.
36. Aubin, J. E., Liu, F., Malaval, L., and Gupta, A. K., Osteoblast and chondroblast differentiation, *Bone*, 17, 77S, 1995.
37. Bos, M. P., van der Meer, J. M., Feyen, J. H. M., and Hermann-Erlee, M. P. M., Expression of the parathyroid hormone receptor and correlation with other osteblastic parameters in fetal rat osteoblasts, *Calcif. Tissue Int.*, 58, 95, 1996.
38. McCauley, L. K., Koh, A. H., Beecher, C. A., Cui, Y., Decker, J. D., and Franceschi, R. T., Effects of differentiation and transforming growth factor beta 1 on PTH/PTHrP receptor mRNA levels in MC3T3-E1 cells. *J. Bone Min. Res.*, 10, 1243, 1995.
39. Fermor, B. and Skerry, T. M., PTH/PTHrP receptor expression on osteoblasts and osteocytes but not resorbing bone surfaces in growing rats, *J. Bone Min. Res.*, 10, 1935, 1995.
40. Thomsen, J. S., Mosekilde, L., Boyce, R. W., and Mosekilde, E., Stochastic simulation of vertebral trabecular bone remodeling, *Bone*, 15, 655, 1994.
41. Yang, N. N., Venugopalan, M., Hardikan, S., and Glasebrook, A., Identification of an estrogen response element activated by metabolites of 17β-estradiol and raloxifene, *Science*, 273, 1222, 1996.
42. Suarez, K. N., Romanello, M., Bettica, P., and Mors, L., Collagen type I of rat cortical and trabecular bone differs in the extent of posttranslational modifications, *Calcif. Tissue Int.*, 58, 65, 1996.
43. Marcus, R., Ed., *Osteoporosis*, Blackwell Scientific Publications, Oxford, 1994.
44. Reginster, J.-Y., *Ostéporose Postménopausique*, Masson, Paris, 1993.
45. Hughes, D. E., Wright, K. R., Uy, H. L., Sasaki, A., Yoneda, T., Roodman, G. D., Mundy, G. R., and Boyce, B. F., Bisphosphonates promote apoptosis in murine osteoclasts in vitro and in vivo, *J. Bone Min. Res.*, 10, 1478, 1995.
46. Adami, S. and Zamberlan, N., adverse effects of bisphosphonates, *Drug Safety*, 14, 158, 1996.
47. Kleerekoper, M., Fluoride and the skeleton, *Crit. Rev. Clin. Lab. Sci.*, 33, 139, 1996.
48. Ferretti, J. L., Frost, H. M., Gasser, J. A., High, W. B., Jee, W. S. S., Jerome, C., Mosekilde, L., and Thompson, D. D., Perspectives on osteoporosis research: Its focus and some insights from a new paradigm, *Calcif. Tissue Int.*, 57, 399, 1995.
49. Bauer, W., Aub, J. C., and Albright, F., Studies of calcium and phosphorus metabolism, V. A study of the bone trabeculae as a readily available reserve supply of calcium, *J. Exp. Med.*, 49, 145, 1929.
50. Péhu, M., Policard, A., and Dufort, A., L'Ostéoporose ou maladie des os marmoréens, *La Presse Médicale*, 53, 999, 1931.
51. Prank, K., Nowlan, S. J., Harms, H. M., Kloppstech, M., Brabant, G., Hesch, R.-D., and Sejnowski, T. J., Time series prediction of plasma hormone concentration. Evidence for differences in predictability of parathyroid hormone secretion between osteoporotic patients and normal controls, *J. Clin. Invest.*, 95, 2910, 1995.
52. Selye, H., A condition simulating human scleroderma in rats injected with parathyroid hormone, *J. Am. Med. Assoc.*, 99, 108, 1932.

53. Selye, H., On the stimulation new bone-formation with parathyroid extract and irradiated ergosterol, *Endocrinology*, 16, 547, 1932.
54. Pugsley, L. T. and Selye, H., The histological changes in the bone responsible for the action of parathyroid hormone on the calcium metabolism of the rat, *J. Physiol.*, 79, 8, 1993.
55. Kalu, D. N., Doyle, F. H., Pennock, J., and Foster, G. V., Parathyroid hormone and experimental osteosclerosis, *Lancet* i, 1363, 1970.
56. Walker, D. G., The induction of osteopetrotic changes in hypophysectomized and thyroparathyroidectomized, and intact rats of various ages, *Endocrinology*, 89, 1389, 1971.
57. Boivin, G., Meunier, P. J., and Reeve, J., Treatments that are anabolic for osteoblasts, *Spine: State of the Art Revs.*, 8, 225, 1994.
58. Dempster, D. W., Cosman, F., Parisien, M., Shen, V., and Lindsay, R., Anabolic actions of parathyroid hormone on bone, *Endocrine Revs.*, 14, 690, 1993.
59. Gasser, J. A., Clinical and experimental results with PTH in the treatment of postmenopausal osteoporosis, in *Bone Diseases and Osteoporosis*, Russell, R. G., Chairman, IBC Technical Services Limited, London, 1994, article 15.
60. Gasser, J. A., Parathyroid hormone: a cure for osteoporosis? *Triangle*, 31, 111, 1992.
61. Reeve, J., PTH: A future role in the management of osteoporosis? *J. Bone Min. Res.*, 11, 440, 1996.
62. Rixon, R. H., Whitfield, J. F., Gagnon, L., Isaacs, R. J., MacLean, S., Chakravarthy, B., Durkin, J. P., Neugebauer, W., Ross, V., Sung, W., and Willick, G. E., Parathyroid hormone fragments may stimulate bone growth in ovariectomized rats by activating adenylyl cyclase, *J. Bone Min. Res.*, 9, 1179, 1994.
63. Whitfield, J. F. and Morley, P., Small bone-building fragments of parathyroid hormone: new therapeutic agents for osteoporosis, *Trends Pharmacol. Sci.*, 16, 382, 1995.
64. Whitfield, J. F., Morley, P., Willick, G. E., Ross, V., Barbier, J.-R., Isaacs, R., and Ohannessian-Barry, L., Stimulation of the growth of femoral trabecular bone in ovariectomized rats by the novel parathyroid hormone fragment, hPTH-(1-31)NH_2 (Ostabolin), *Calcif. Tissue Int.*, 58, 81, 1996.
65. Tregear, G. W., van Rietschofen, J., Greene, E., Niall, H. D., Keutman, H. T., Parsons, J. A., O'Riordan, J. L. H., and Potts, J. T. J., Solid phase synthesis of the biologically active N-terminal 1-34 peptide of human parathyroid hormone, *Hoppe-Seyler's Z. Physiol. Chem.*, 355 (S), 415, 1974.
66. Neer, R., Slovik, D., Daly, M., Lo, C., and Nussbaum, S. R., Treatment of postmenopausal osteoporosis with daily parathyroid hormone plus calcitriol, in *Osteoporosis*, Christiansen, C., and Overgaard, K., Eds., Osteopress, ApS, Copenhagen, 1990, Vol. 3, p. 1314.
67. Neer, R., Slovik, D. M., Daly, M., Potts, J. T., and Nussbaum, S. R., Treatment of postmenopausal osteoporosis with daily parathyroid hormone plus calcitriol, *Osteop. Int.* (Suppl.1), S204, 1993.
68. Sone, T., Fukunaga, M., Ono, S., and Nishiyama, T., A small dose of human parathyroid hormone (1-34) increased bone mass in the lumbar vertebrae in patients with senile osteoporosis, *Miner. Electrolyte Metab.*, 21, 232, 1995.
69. Jerome, C. P., Johnson, C. S., and Lees, C. J., Effect of treatment with human parathyroid hormone 1-34 peptide in ovariectomized cynomolgus monkeys (*Macaca fascicularis*), *Bone*, 17 (Suppl. 4), 415S, 1995.
70. Abou-Samra, A.-B., Jüppner, H., Westerberg, D., Potts, J. T., and Segre, G. V., Parathyroid hormone causes translocation of protein-kinase-C from cytosol to membranes in rat osteosarcoma cells, *Endocrinology*, 124, 1107, 1992.
71. Jouishomme, H., Whitfield, J. F., Chakravarthy, B., Durkin, J. P., Gagnon, L., Isaacs, R. J., MacLean, S., Neugebauer, W., Willick, G., and Rixon, R. H., The protein kinase-C activation domain of the parathyroid hormone, *Endocrinology*, 130, 53, 1992.

72. Jouishomme, H., Whitfield, J. F., Gagnon, L., MacLean, S., Isaacs, R., Chakravarthy, B., Durkin, J. P., Neugebauer, W., Willick, G., and Rixon, R. H., Further definition of the protein kinase C-activating domain of the parathyroid hormone, *J. Bone Min. Res.*, 9, 943, 1994.
73. Gagnon, L., Jouishomme, H., Whitfield, J. F., Durkin, J. P., MacLean, S., Neugebauer, W., Willick, G., Rixon, R. H., and Chakravarthy, B., Protein kinase C-activating domains of parathyroid hormone-related protein, *J. Bone Min. Res.*, 8, 497, 1993.
74. Brown, E. M., Segre, G. V., and Goldring, S. R., Serpentine receptors for parathyroid hormone, calcitonin and extracellular calcium ions, *Bailliere's Clinical Endocrinology and Metabolism*, 10, 123, 1996.
75. Seitz, P. K., Nickols, G. A., McPherson, M. B., and Cooper, C. W., Radioiodinated parathyroid hormone-(1-34) binds to its receptor on rat osteosarcoma cells in a manner consistent with two classes of binding sites. *J. Bone Min. Res.*, 5, 353, 1990.
76. Jüppner, H., Molecular cloning and characterization of a parathyroid hormone/parathyroid hormone-related peptide receptor: a member of an ancient family of G protein-coupled receptors, *Curr. Opin. Nephrol. Hypertens.*, 3, 371, 1994.
77. Orloff, J. J., Katz, Y., Urena, P., Schipani, E., Vasavada, R. C., Philbrick, W. M., Behal, A., Abou-Samra, A.-B., Segre, G. V., and Jüppner, H., Further evidence for a novel receptor for amino-terminal parathyroid hormone-related protein on keratinocytes and squamous carcinoma cell lines, *Endocrinology*, 136, 3016, 1995.
78. Whitfield, J. F., Chakravarthy, B. R., Durkin, J. P., Isaacs, R. J., Jouishomme, H., Sikorska, M., Williams, R. E., and Rixon, R. H., Parathyroid hormone stimulates protein kinase C but not adenylate cyclase in mouse epidermal keratinocytes, *J. Cell. Physiol.*, 150, 299, 1992.
79. Schlüter, K.-D., Weber, M., and Piper, H. M., Parathyroid hormone induces protein kinase C but not adenylate cyclase in adult cardiomyocytes and regulates cyclic AMP levels via protein kinase C-dependent phosphodiesterase activity, *Biochem. J.*, 310, 439, 1995.
80. Behar, V., Pines, M., Nakamoto, C., Greenberg, Z., Bisello, A., Stueckle, S. M., Bessalle, R., Usdin, T. B., Chorev, M., Rosenblatt, M., and Suva, L. J., The human PTH2 receptor: Binding and signal transduction properties of the stably expressed recombinant receptor, *Endocrinology*, 137, 2748, 1996.
81. Caulfield, M. P., McKee, R. L., Goldman, M. E., Duong, L. T., Fisher, J. E., Gay, C. T., DeHaven, P. A., Levy, J. J., Roubini, E., Nutt, R. F., Chorev, M., and Rosenblatt, M., Parathyroid hormone-related protein (PTHrP): studies with synthetic peptides indicate that parathyroid hormone and PTHrP interact with the same receptor. *Endocrinology*, 127, 83, 1990.
82. Janulis, M., Wong, M.-S., and Favus, M. J., Structure-function requirements of parathyroid hormone for stimulation of $1,25(OH)_2D_3$ production by rat renal proximal tubules, *Endocrinology*, 133, 713, 1993.
83. Sömjen, D., Schlüter, K.-D., Wingender, E., Mayer, H., and Kaye, A. M., Stimulation of cell proliferation in skeletal tissues of the rat by defined parathyroid hormone fragments, *Biochem. J.*, 277, 863, 1991.
84. Kukreja, S. C., D'Anza, J. J., Wimbiscus, S. A., Fisher, J. E., McKee, R. L., Caulfield, M. P., and Rosenblatt, M., Inactivation by plasma may be responsible for lack of efficacy of parathyroid antagonists in hypercalcemia of malignancy, *Endocrinology*, 134, 2184, 1994.
85. Strein, K., Are animal studies with bisphosphonates and PTH fragments predictive for the clinical situation? in *Bone Diseases and Osteoporosis*, Russell, R. G., Chairman, IBC Technical Services Limited, London, 1994, article 12.
86. Sabatini, M., Lesur, C., Pacherie, M., Pastoureau, P., Kucharczyk N., Fauchère, J.-L., and Bonnet, J., Effects of parathyroid hormone and agonists of the adenylate cyclase and protein kinase C pathways on bone cell proliferation, *Bone*, 18, 59, 1996.

87. Neugebauer, W., Barbier, J.-R., Sung, W. L., Whitfield, J. F., and Willick, G. E., Solution structure and adenylyl cyclase stimulating activities of C-terminal truncated human parathyroid hormone analogues, *Biochemistry*, 34, 8835, 1995.
88. Leslie, F. M. and Goldstein, V., Degradation of dynorphin-(1-13) by membrane-bound rat brain enzymes, *Neuropeptides*, 2, 185, 1982.
89. Whitfield, J. F., Morley, P., Willick, G. E., Ross, V., Maclean, S., Barbier, J.-R., Isaacs, R. J., and Ohannessian-Barry, L., Comparison of the ability of recombinant human parathyroid hormone, rhPTH-(1-84), and hPTH-(1-31)NH_2 to stimulate femoral trabecular bone growth in ovariectomized rats, *Calcif. Tissue. Int.*, 60, 26, 1997.
90. Yamato, H., Nagai, Y., Inoue, D., Ohnishi, Y., Ueyama, Y., Ohno, H., Matsumoto, T., Ogata, E., and Ikeda, K., In vivo evidence for progressive activation of parathyroid hormone-related peptide gene expression with tumor growth and stimulation of osteoblastic bone formation at an early stage of humoral hypercalcemia of malignancy, *J. Bone Min. Res.*, 10, 36, 1995.
91. Whitfield, J. F., Isaacs, R. J., Jouishomme, H., Maclean, S., Chakravarthy, B. R., Morley, P., Barisoni, D., Regalia, E., and Armato, U., C-Terminal fragment of parathyroid hormone-related protein, PTHrP-(107-111), stimulates membrane-associated protein kinase C activity and modulates the proliferation of human and murine keratinocytes, *J. Cell. Physiol.*, 166, 1, 1996.
92. Henderson, J. E., Amizuka, N., Warshawsky, H., Biasotto, D., Lanske, B. H. K., Goltzman, D., and Karaplis, A. C., Nuclear localization of parathyroid hormone-related peptide enhances survival of chondrocytes under conditions that promote apoptotic cell death, *Mol. Cell. Biol.*, 15, 4064, 1995.
93. Weir, E. C., Terwilliger, G., Sartori, L., and Insogna, K. L., Synthetic parathyroid hormone-like protein (1-74) is anabolic for bone *in vivo*, *Calcif. Tissue Int.*, 51, 30, 1992.
94. Hock, J. M., Fonseca, J., Gunness-Hey, M., Kemp, B. E., and Martin, T. J., Comparison of the anabolic effects of synthetic parathyroid hormone-related protein (PTHrP)1-34 or PTH-(1-34) on bone in rats, *Endocrinology*, 125, 2022, 1989.
94a. Whitfield, J. F., Morley, P., Willick, G. E., Ross, V., Langille, R., MacLean, S., Barbier, J.-R., Isaacs, R. J., and Ohannessian-Barry, L., Comparison of the abilities of human parathyroid hormone (hPTH)-(1-31)NH_2 and human parathyroid hormone-related protein (hPTHrP)-(1-31)NH_2 to stimulate femoral trabecular bone growth in ovariectomized rats, *Calcif. Tissue Int.*, in press, 1997.
95. Barden, J. A. and Kemp, B. E., Stabilized NMR structure of the hypercalcemia of malignancy peptide PTHrP[Ala-26](1-34)amide, *Biochem. Biophys. Acta*, 1208, 256, 1994.
96. Wray, V., Federau, T., Gronwald, W., Mayer, H., Schomburg, D., Tegge, W., and Wingender, E., The structure of human parathyroid hormone from a study of fragments in solution using H-1 NMR spectroscopy and its biological implications, *Biochemistry*, 33, 1684, 1994.
97. Neugebauer, W., Surewicz, W. K., Gordon, H. L., Somorjai, R. L., Sung, W., and Willick, G. E., Structural elements of human parathyroid hormone and their possible relation to biological activities, *Biochemistry*, 31, 2056, 1992.
98. Gilman, A. G., G-proteins and regulation of adenylyl cyclase, *Biosci. Reports*, 15, 65, 1995.
99. Dobnig, H. and Turner, R. T., Evidence that intermittent treatment with parathyroid hormone increases bone formation in adult rats by activation of bone lining cells, *Endocrinology*, 136, 3632, 1995.
100. Leaffer, D., Sweeney, M., Kellerman, L. A., Avnur, Z., Krstenansky, J. L., Vickery, B. H., and Caulfield, J. P., Modulation of osteogenic cell ultrastructure by RS23581, an analogue of human parathyroid hormone (PTH)-related peptide-(1-34), and bovine PTH-(1-34), *Endocrinology*, 136, 3624, 1995.

101. McCarthy, T. L., Thomas, M. J., Centrella, M., and Rotwein, P., Regulation of insulin-like growth factor I transcription by cyclic adenosine 3′,5′-monophosphate (cAMP) in fetal rat bone cells through an element within exon 1: protein kinase A-dependent control without a consensus cAMP response element, *Endocrinology*, 136, 3901, 1995.
102. Pfeilschifter, J., Laukhuf, F., Muller-Beckmann, B., Blum, W. F., Pfister, T., and Ziegler, R., Parathyroid hormone increases the concentration of insulin-like growth factor-I and transforming growth factor beta 1 in rat bone, *J. Clin. Invest.*, 96, 767, 1995.
103. Jee, W. S. S., Ma, Y. F., and Chow, S. Y., Maintenance therapy for added bone mass or how to keep the profit after the withdrawal of therapy of osteopenia, *Bone*, 17 (Suppl.), 309S, 1995.
104. Tam, C. S., Heersche, J. N. M., Marray, T. M., and Parsons, J. A., Parathyroid hormone stimulates the bone apposition rate independently of its resorptive action: Differential effects of intermittent and continuous administration, *Endocrinology*, 110, 506, 1982.
105. Canalis, E., Centrella, M., Burch, W., and McCarthy, T., Insulin-like growth factor 1 mediates selective anabolic effects of parathyroid hormone in bone cultures, *J. Clin. Invest.*, 83, 60, 1989.
106. Takahashi, T., Wada, T., Mori, M., Kokai, Y., and Ishii, S., Overexpression of the granulocyte colony-stimulating factor gene leads to osteoporosis in mice, *Lab. Invest.*, 74, 827, 1996.
107. Whitfield, J. F., Morley, P., Ross, V., Preston, E., Soska, M., Barbier, J.-R., Isaacs, R. J., MacLean, S., Ohannessian-Barry, L., and Willick, G. E., The hypotensive actions of osteogenic and non-osteogenic parathyroid hormone (PTH) fragments, *Calcif. Tissue Int.*, 60, 302, 1997.
108. Mok, L. L. S., Nickols, G. A., Thompson, J. C., and Cooper, C. W., Parathyroid hormone as a smooth muscle relaxant, *Endocrine Revs.*, 10, 420, 1989.
109. Nickols, G. A., Actions of parathyroid hormone in the cardiovascular system, *Blood Vessels*, 24, 120, 1987.
110. Pang, P. K., Hong, B. S., Yen, L., and Yang, M. C., Parathyroid hormone: A specific potent vasodilator, *Contrib. Nephrol.*, 41, 137, 1984.
110a. Whitfield, J. F., Morley, P., Willick, G. E., Langille, R., Ross, V., MacLean, S., and Barbier, J.-R., Cyclization by a specific lactam increases the ability of human parathyroid hormone (hPTH)-(1-31)NH_2 to stimulate bone growth in ovariectomized rats, *J. Bone Min. Res.*, 12, in press, 1997.
111. Bergman, P. and Schoutens, A., Prostaglandins and bone, *Bone*, 16, 488, 1995.
112. Norrdin, R. W., Jee, W. S. S., and High, W. B., The role of prostaglandins in bone in vivo, *Prost. Leuk. Essential Fatty Acids*, 41, 139, 1990.
113. Raisz, L. G. and Martin, T. J., Prostaglandins in bone and mineral metabolism, in *Bone and Mineral Research*, Peck, A. W., Ed., Elsevier Science Publishers, Amsterdam, 1983, Annual 2, chap. 6.
114. Raisz, L. G., Pilbeam, C. C., and Fall, P. M., Prostaglandins: Mechanisms of action and regulation of production in bone, *Osteop. Int.*, Suppl. 1, S136, 1993.
115. Ueda, K., Saito, A., Nakano, H., Aoshima, M., Yokota, M., Muraoka, R., and Iwaya, T., Cortical hyperostosis following long-term administration of prostaglandin E1 in infants with cyanotic congenital heart disease, *J. Pediatrics*, 97, 834, 1980.
116. Drvaric, D. M., Parks, W. J., Wyly, J. B., Dooley, K. J., Plauth, W. H., and Schmitt, E. W., Prostaglandin-induced hyperostosis, *Clin. Orthoped. Rel. Res.*, 246, 3000, 1989.
117. Norrdin, R. W., Powers, B. E., and Smith, R. E., Prostaglandin production in periosteal cells cultured from proliferating bone lesions in avian osteopetroses, *J. Bone Min. Res.*, 2 (Suppl.), S139, 1986.
118. Ho, S. S. W., Stern, P. J., Bruno, L. P., Wyrick, J. D., Waymack, J. P., and Alexander, J. W., Pharmacological inhibition of prostaglandin E_2 in bone and its effect on pathological new bone formation in a rat burn model, *Thirty-Fourth Ann. Meeting, Orthopedic Research Soc.*, Atlanta, GA, Feb. 1–4, 1989, p. 536.

119. Bartels, T., Hein, W., Taube, C., Runge, H., and Mest, H. J., Correlations between endogenous prostaglandin E formation in the bone and spongiosa density, *Biomed. Biochim. Acta*, 47, S278, 1988.
120. Li, M., Jee, W. S., Ke, H. Z., Tang, L. Y., Ma, Y. F., Liang, X. G., and Setterberg, R. B., Prostaglandin E_2 administration prevents bone loss induced by orchidectomy in rats, *J. Bone Min. Res.*, 10, 66, 1995.
121. Ma, Y., Chen, Y. Y., Jee, W. S. S., Ke, H. Z., and Ijiri, K., Co-treatment of PGE_2 and risedronate is better than PGE_2 alone in the long-term treatment of ovariectomized-induced osteopenic rats, *Bone*, 17 (Suppl.), 267S, 1995.
122. Ma, Y. F., Ke, H. Z., and Jee, W. S. S., Prostaglandin E_2 adds bone to a cancellous bone site with a closed growth plate and low bone turnover in ovariectomized rats, *Bone*, 17, 137, 1994.
123. Mori, S., Jee, W. S. S., and Li, X. J., Production of new trabecular bone in ovariectomized rats by prostaglandin E_2, *Calcif. Tissue Int.*, 50, 80, 1992.
124. Chyun, Y. S. and Raisz, L. G., Stimulation of bone formation by prostaglandin E_2, *Prostaglandins*, 27, 97, 1984.
125. Feyen, J. H. M., Di Bon, A., van der Plas, A., Löwik, C. W. G. M., and Nijweide, P. J., Effects of exogenous prostanoids on the proliferation of osteoblast-like cells in vitro, *Prostaglandins*, 30, 827, 1985.
126. Scutt, A., Duvos, C., Lauber, J., and Mayer, H., Time-dependent effects of parathyroid hormone and prostaglandin E_2 on DNA synthesis by periosteal cells from embryonic chick calvaria, *Calcif. Tissue Int.*, 55, 208, 1994.
127. McCarthy, T. L., Centrella, M., Raisz, L. G., and Canalis, E., Prostaglandin E_2 stimulates insulin-like growth factor I synthesis in osteoblast-enriched cultures from fetal rat bone, *Endocrinology*, 128, 2895, 1991.
128. Gera, T., Hock, J. M., Gunness-Hey, M., Fonesca, J., and Raisz, L. G., Indomethacin does not inhibit the anabolic effect of parathyroid hormone on the long bones of rats, *Calcif. Tissue Int.*, 40, 206, 1987.
129. Burger, E. H. and Veldhuijzen, J. P., Influence of mechanical factors on bone formation, resorption and growth *in vitro*, in *Bone: A Treatise*, Hall, K., Ed., CRC Press, Boca Raton, 1993, Chap. 2.
130. Raab-Cullen, D. M., Thiede, M. A., Petersen, D. N., Kimmel, D. B., and Recker, R. R., Mechanical loading stimulates rapid changes in periosteal gene expression, *Calcif. Tissue Int.*, 55, 473, 1994.
131. Daifotis, A. G., Weir, E. C., Dreyer, B. E., and Broadus, A. E., Stretch-induced parathyroid hormone-related peptide gene expression in the rat uterus, *J. Biol. Chem.*, 267, 23455, 1992.
132. Pirola, C. J., Wang, H. M., Strgacich, M. I., Kaymar, A., Cercek, B., Forrester, J. S., Clemens, T. L., and Fagin, J. A., Mechanical stimuli induce vascular parathyroid hormone-related protein gene expression *in vivo* and *in vitro*, *Endocrinology*, 134, 2230, 1994.
133. Mitnick, M., Isales, C., Poliwal, I., and Insogna, K., Parathyroid hormone-related protein stimulates prostaglandin E_2 release from human osteoblast-like cells: modulating effect of peptide length, *J. Bone Min. Res.*, 7, 887, 1992.
134. Ma, Y. F., Ferreti, J. L., Capozza, R. F., Cointry, G., Alippi, R., Zanchetta, J., and Jee, W. S. S., Effect of on/off anabolic PTH and remodeling inhibitors on metaphyseal bone of immobilized rat femurs. Tomographical (pQCT) description and correlation with histomorphometric changes in tibial cancellous bone, *Bone*, 17 (Suppl.), 321S, 1995.
135. Ma, Y. F., Jee, W. S. S., Ke, H. Z., Lin, B. Y., Liang, Y. G., Yamamoto, N., Human parathyroid hormone-(1-38) restores cancellous bone to the immobilized, osteopenic proximal-tibial metaphysis in rats, *J. Bone Min. Res.*, 10, 496, 1995.
136. Yuan, Z. Z., Jee, W. S. S., Ma, Y. F., Wei, W., and Ijiri, K., Parathyroid hormone therapy accelerates recovery from immobilization-induced osteopenia, *Bone*, 17 (Suppl.), 219S, 1995.

137. Fang, J. A., Zhu, Y.-Y., Smiley, E., Bonadio, J., Rouleau, J. P., Goldstein, S. A., McCauley, L. K., Davidson, B. L., and Roessler, B. J., Stimulation of new bone formation by direct transfer of osteogenic plasmid genes, *Proc. Natl. Acad. Sci. USA*, 93, 5753, 1996.
138. Marx, U. C., Austermann, S., Bayer, P., Aderman, K., Ejchart, A., Sticht, H., Walter, S., Schmid, F.-X., Jaenicke, R., and Forssmann, W.-G., Rösch structure of human parathyroid hormone 1-37 in solution, *J. Biol. Chem.*, 270, 15194, 1995.
139. Barden, J. A. and Cuthbertson, R. M., Stabilized NMR structure of human parathyroid hormone (1-34), *Eur. J. Biochem.*, 215, 315, 1993.
140. Klaus, W., Dieckmann, T., Wray, V., Schomberg, D., Wingender, E., and Mayer, H., Investigation of the solution structure of the human parathyroid hormone fragment (1-34) by H-1 NMR spectroscopy, distance geometry, and molecular dynamics calculations, *Biochemistry*, 30, 6936, 1991.
141. Smith, L. M., Jentoft, J., and Zull, J. E., Proton NMR studies of the biologically active 1-34 fragment of bovine parathyroid hormone: Examination of a structural model, *Arch. Biochem. Biophys.*, 253, 81, 1987.
142. Strickland, L. A., Bozzato, R. P., and Kronis, K. A., Structure of human parathyroid hormone (1-34) in the presence of solvents and micelles, *Biochemistry*, 32, 6050, 1993.
143. Barbier, J.-R., Neugebauer, W., Morley, P., Ross, V., Whitfield, J. F., and Willick, G., Bioactivities and secondary structures of constrained analogues of human parathyroid hormone: Cyclic lactams of the receptor binding region, *J. Med. Chem.*, 40, 1373, 1997.
144. Gardella, T. J., Wilson, A. K., Keutmann, H. T., Oberstein, R., Potts, J. T., Kronenberg, H. M., and Nussbaum, S. R., Analysis of parathyroid hormone's principal receptor-binding region by site-directed mutagenesis and analog design, *Endocrinology*, 132, 2024, 1993.
145. Surewicz, W. K., Neugebauer, W., Gagnon, L., Maclean, S., Whitfield, J. F., and Willick, G. E., Structure-function relationships in human parathyroid hormone: The essential role of amphiphilic α-helix, in *Peptides: Chemistry, Structure, and Biology 1993*, Smith, J. and Hodges, R., Eds., ESCOM, 1993, p. 556.
146. Bossus, M., Gras-Masse, H., Précheur, B., Craescu, G., and Tartar, A., Resistance to enzymatic degradation of conformationally constrained antigenic peptides, in *Innovation and Perspectives in Solid Phase Synthesis*, Epton, R., Ed., Mayflower Worldwide, Birmingham, U.K., 1994, 457.
147. Lung, F.-D., Collins, N., Stropova, D., Davis, P., Yamamura, H. I., Porreca, F., and Hruby, V. J., Design, synthesis, and biological activities of cyclic lactam peptide analogues of dynorphin A (1-11)-NH_2, *J. Med. Chem.*, 39, 1136, 1996.
148. Marqusee, S. and Baldwin, R. L., Helix stabilization by Glu^-...Lys^+ salt bridges in salt bridges in short peptides of *de novo* design, *Proc. Natl. Acad. Sci. USA*, 84, 8898, 1987.
149. Szewczuk, Z., Gibbs, B. F., Yue, S. Y., Purisima, E. O., and Konishi, Y., Conformationally restricted thrombin inhibitors resistant to proteolytic digestion, *Biochemistry*, 31, 9132, 1992.

Chapter 6

Bone Formation May be Uncoupled from Resorption, as Demonstrated by a New Class of hPTHrP (1-34) Analogs in Both Rapid and Slow Turnover Models of Osteopenia

Brian H. Vickery, Zafrira Avnur, Georgia I. McRae, Ruth Waters, Esther Hill, and John L. Krstenansky

CONTENTS

0-8493-8556-3/98/$0.00+$.50

I. INTRODUCTION

The association between parathyroid hormone, PTH, (as glandular extracts) and anabolic activity in bone has an extensive history, being first noted, although without comment, in 1929 by Fuller Albright.[1] The connection was more formally made three years later by Selye.[2] There was desultory interest in the phenomenon[3,4] until the 1980s and the demonstration that the desired activity resides in the N-terminal 34 amino acid sequence of the 84 amino acid hormone.[5,6] The availability of synthetic PTH-(1-34) enabled clinical trials for treatment of osteopenia,[7-10] and this in turn sparked a resurgence in animal experimentation.[11-13] Overlapping this time, an intriguing story of a ubiquitously expressed PTH-related peptide (PTHrP) family has emerged.[14] Although the alternatively spliced, full-size, expressed hormone family ranges from 139–173 amino acids, it now appears that, again, the N-terminal 34 amino acid sequence is a high-affinity agonist at one of the identified PTH receptors (PTH-1R)[15,16] and possesses all the bone activity of PTH-(1-34).[6,17,18] Clinical pharmacology studies are now being reported with fragments of PTHrP; PTHrP-(1-34) seems less potent than PTH-(1-34), perhaps because of increased metabolic lability.[19] However, hPTHrP-(1-36), which may be the endogenously secreted sequence, is reported to be equipotent to PTH-(1-34).[20]

Major increases in cancellous bone have been reported in response to PTH-(1-34) administration to osteopenic individuals.[21] However, with the exception of a handful of animal studies,[22,23] compact bone assessed either regionally or as total body bone mineral density (BMD) does not increase and may even decline.[24] This profile recalls the situation in the clinical condition of hyperparathyroidism, in which cancellous bone is well maintained but compact bone is resorbed, with accompanying hypercalcemia.[25] Animal studies have demonstrated overwhelming bone formation on all trabecular surfaces with PTH,[26] but others have shown cortical porosity and tunneling,[27] consistent with compartmentalization of anabolic and catabolic effects.

In light of the well-documented resorptive effects of PTH (and PTHrP) on bone *in vitro*,[28,29] researchers have questioned whether it is possible to separate anabolic and catabolic effects of PTH-like molecules. Indeed, some have suggested that PTH induces a high turnover state in which increase in resorption is the trigger for increased anabolic activity. Certainly, infusion of PTH causes rampant resorption with intolerable hypercalcemia.[30-32]

However, we have recently synthesized a new class of peptides, analogs of hPTHrP-(1-34), which when tested *in vivo* cause an extremely rapid, high-magnitude gain in bone in both trabecular and cortical compartments and whole body BMD.[33,34] The contrast from results obtained with PTH, as well as PTHrP, suggested that these new analogs are selectively anabolic. This chapter will summarize the experimental evidence recently obtained which further supports that conclusion.

TABLE 6.1

Sequences of hPTH(1-34), hPTHrP(1-34), and Analogs With Selected *In Vitro* Data

Name	Sequence[a]	Receptor Binding (IC_{50} nM)	cAMP (EC_{250} nM)
hPTH(1-34)	SVSEIQLMHN LGKHLNSMER VEWLRKKLQD VHNF	5.0	1.6
hPTHrP(1-34)	AVSEHQLLHD KGKSIQDLRR RFFLHHLIAE IHTA	1.3	0.3
RS-66271	AVSEHQLLHD KGKSIQDLRR RELLEKLLEK LHTA#	18	2.0
RS-23581	AVSEHQLLHD KGKSIQDLRR RELLEKLLEK LHT-Hsl	29	4.1

[a] Peptide sequences are given using the standard one-letter code, with the exception of the C-terminal residue of RS-23581 which is homoserine lactone, Hsl. The "#" symbol represents a C-terminal amide modification.

II. DESIGN OF MODEL α-HELICAL PEPTIDE (MAP) ANALOGS

Structure-activity relationship (SAR) studies on PTH-(1-34) have indicated that both N-terminal and C-terminal regions are important for binding, while the N-terminal residues are critical to agonist activity via cAMP.[17] The limited SAR that has been published on PTHrP-(1-34) suggests similar roles for its corresponding structural regions. The PTH/PTHrP receptor binding for the two peptides is equivalent, even though homology in the C-terminal half of the peptides is limited to residues 20, 24, and 32 (Table 6.1). It had been noted that the C-terminal region of PTH-(1-34) was amphipathic when placed in an α-helical conformation.[35] A number of reports of the solution conformation of PTH-(1-34), as determined by NMR spectroscopy, gave evidence for an α-helical structure in the C-terminal region.[36-40] In contrast, the solution conformation of PTHrP did not give evidence for α-helix in its C-terminal region, but did suggest a folded conformation.[41] Comparison of the C-terminal regions of PTH-(1-34) and PTHrP-(1-34) indicated that both could be amphipathic α-helices. This led us to the hypothesis that C-terminal regions of these two peptides were structurally homologous (both amphipathic α-helices), despite the lack of homology in terms of matching amino acid residues at corresponding positions in the peptide.

There are several approaches that can be taken to examining the nature and importance of an α-helical region in a molecule.

Maximal residue modification: This approach tests the importance of the overall structure for receptor interaction vs. the importance of individual residues. Operationally, in this method one changes the residues in the original sequence with residues that preserve (or enhance) the structure while preserving as few of the original amino acids as possible. This is the method pioneered by E.T. Kaiser and applied to several peptides (e.g., endorphin, glucagon, NPY).[42] We did not use this approach because nature had done this experiment for us. The lack of homology between the C-terminal regions of PTH-(1-34) and PTHrP-(1-34) and their comparable importance for receptor binding gave the original evidence for a structural role for this region.

Minimal residue modification: This approach seeks to enhance the structural stability of the region of interest by making minimal changes in the residues of the region. This type of modification has been used successfully with several peptides, such as glucagon.[43] Surewicz et al.[44] reported an enhancement of both α-helical content and cAMP potency by making such small changes in PTH-(1-34). The effects of these changes on *in vivo* activity was not reported.

Covalent structural stabilization: This approach makes use of covalent linkages to lock the molecule into the desired conformation. Such an approach has been successfully performed in α-helical peptides using linkages, such as amides [45] or D-Cys^{i}, Cys^{i+3} disulfides.[46] Neugebauer et al. [47] used amide linkages to demonstrate the effectiveness of stabilizing α-helical structure in PTH-(20-34) analogs for enhancing their PKC stimulatory activity.

Optimized structural replacement: This was an approach we developed for our PTH/PTHrP optimization program. The idea is to replace a structural region of the target molecule with a highly structurally optimized sequence that is not necessarily homologous to the original sequence. This approach makes use of "model" sequences that have been independently developed to exhibit high levels of a given structure (ideally, with the shortest sequence).

We tested the importance of a general amphipathic α-helical structure in the C-terminal 22-31 region of PTHrP-(1-34), by substituting a nonhomologous, model amphipathic α-helical peptide (MAP) sequence[48] in hPTHrP-(1-34), to give a series of $[MAP_{1-10}]^{22-31}$ hPTHrP-(1-34) analogs (Figure 6.1). The MAP sequence was chosen because it is a simple linear sequence composed entirely of natural amino acids that exhibits high levels of α-helical structure in aqueous solution at room temperature with only decapeptide lengths. By comparison, other reported model α-helical

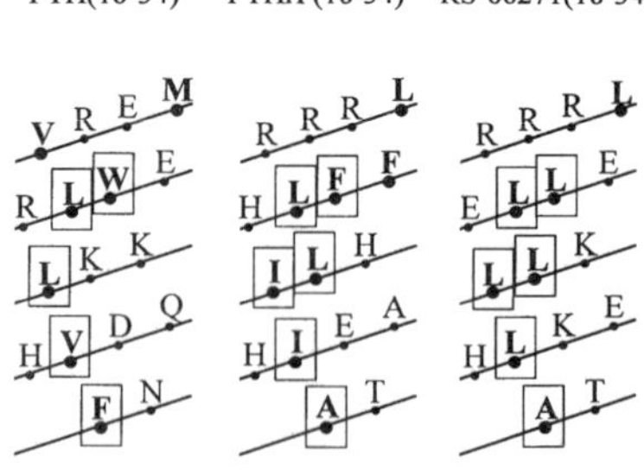

Figure 6.1
Helical net diagrams of PTH-(18-34), PTHrP-(18-34), and RS-66271-(18-34). Lipophilic residues representing the hydrophobic face of the C-terminal amphipathic α-helix of the peptides are enclosed in boxes. Note: A, Ala; D, Asp; E, Glu; F, Phe; H, His; I, Ileu; K, Lys; L, Leu; Q, Gln; R, Arg; T, Thr; V, Val; W, Tryp.

sequences [49-51] require longer peptide lengths and reduced temperatures to exhibit similar levels of α-helical content as the MAP peptide.

Substitution of the 22-31 region of hPTHrP-(1-34) with the model amphipathic α-helical peptide Glu-Leu-Leu-Glu-Lys-Leu-Leu-Glu-Lys-Leu (MAP_{1-10}) results in analogs having increased α-helical content as evidenced by the CD spectrum.[52] The introduction of the MAP sequence reduced receptor affinity and the corresponding second messenger potencies (cAMP and IP). Although the MAP analogs still retain nM affinity, their differences from the parent compound are significant (Table 6.1).

III. *IN VIVO* EFFECTS OF THE MAP ANALOGS

A. Studies in Rats

The anabolic activities of RS-66271 and hPTHrP-(1-34) were evaluated in rats, ovariectomized (OVX) at three months old, and dosed starting three weeks after OVX.[53,54] Daily subcutaneous injection for three weeks of hPTHrP-(1-34) at 80 µg/kg/day partially reversed estrogen depletion-induced loss in trabecular bone calcium content, but was ineffective in the cortex (Figure 6.2). bPTH-(1-34) dose-relatedly restored trabecular bone mass but again was ineffective at the cortex. In contrast, RS-66271 dose-relatedly reversed loss at both sites and, in this very short period of time at 80 µg/kg/day, returned both trabecular and cortical bone calcium to the level of sham-operated controls. Studies with the related analog, RS-23581, confirmed (by pQCT) changes in BMD at both trabecular and cortical sites (Figure 6.3). Histomorphometric analysis showed significantly elevated bone formation rates over vehicle-treated OVX in both trabecular and cortical tibial bone following treatment with RS-66271. We then hypothesized that the rapidity and magnitude of the bone accretion

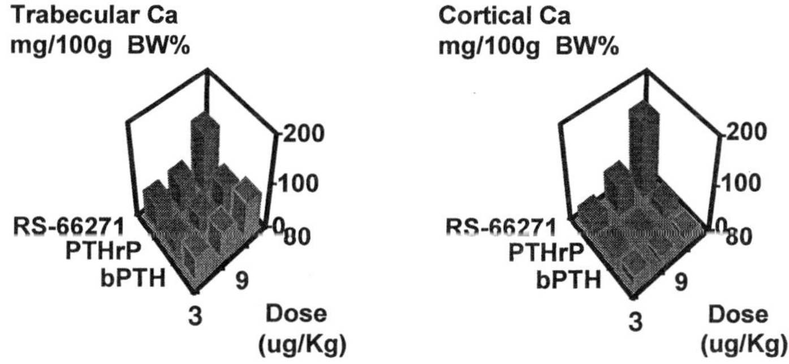

Figure 6.2
Trabecular vs. cortical Ca content in ovariectomized rats treated with bPTH, PTHrP, RS-66271.

SHAM
pQCT
Trabecular: 288.3 mg/cm³
Cortical: 916.1 mg/cm³
DEXA
0.2436 gm/cm²
OVX
pQCT
Trabecular: 163.6 mg/cm³
Cortical: 955.2 mg/cm³
DEXA
0.1218 gm/cm²

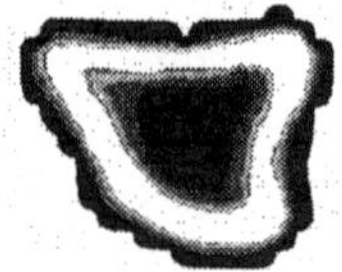

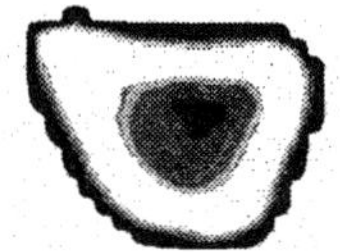

Figure 6.3
pQCT (peripheral quantitative computerized tomography) and DEXA (dual energy X-radiation absorptiometry) of proximal tibias of sham-operated rats, OVXed rats, and RS-23581-treated OVXed rats.

gained with RS-66271, particularly at cortical sites, reflected a kinetic difference in the rate of bone formation relative to the natural congeners, and that this could reflect a dissociation between formation and resorption, normally highly coupled.

More detailed studies were performed with the closely related MAP analog, RS-23581, again injected sc daily, in much older animals with established, stable osteopenia. These animals, which were OVX at eight months of age and not treated until a further four months had elapsed, had a significant, large-magnitude osteopenia which was stable throughout the duration of the study. In this model, we were able to confirm the restorative activity of the MAP peptide at both trabecular and cortical sites by DEXA, including a demonstration of increase in total body BMD.[54] Analysis of biochemical indices of formation (serum osteocalcin) and resorption (urinary pyridinoline, PYD) showed the former to be temporally and dose-relatedly correlated with the increases in bone density (Figure 6.4). In contrast, increases in resorptive markers, when they occurred, were associated only with times at which bone density, as well as biomechanical parameters, exceeded normal values for the treated animals, suggesting a response to mechanical factors[55] rather than to a direct

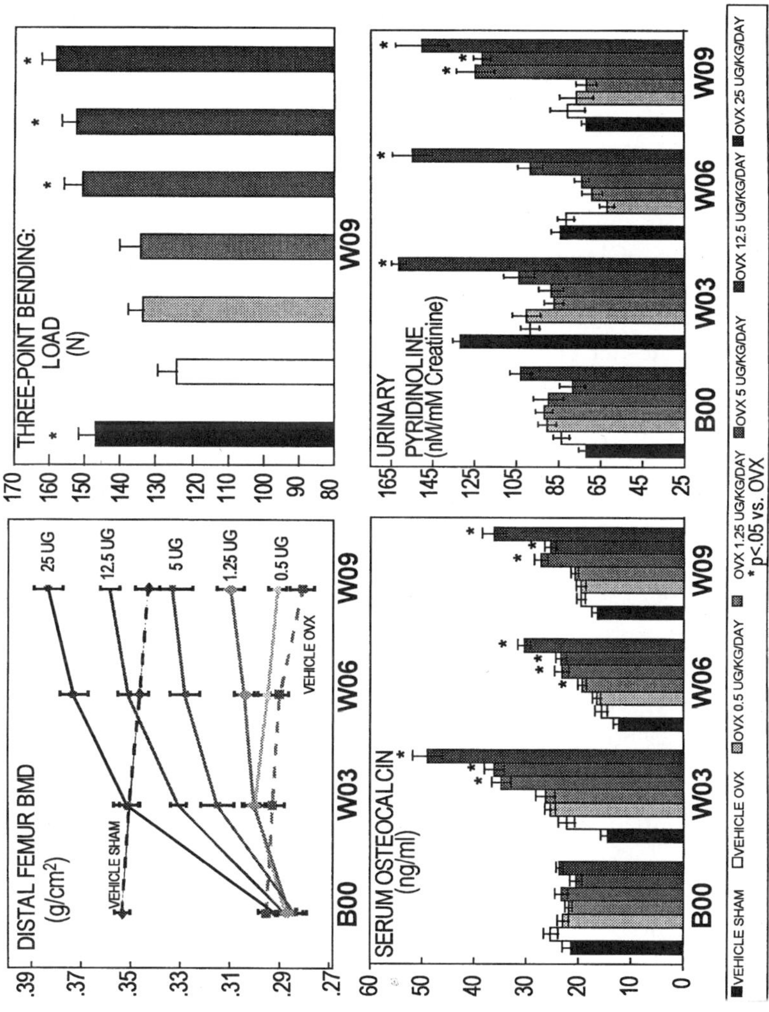

Figure 6.4
DEXA-determined BMD, biochemical markers, and mechanical strength in OVXed rats treated with various doses of RS-66271. B00, base values on week-0; W03, W06, W09, values by weeks 3, 6, and 9, respectively.

effect of the compound. Thus, in rats there was an obvious dose and temporal dissociation between increase in osteocalcin/bone density and any evidence of resorption. This appears to be the first demonstration of a clear uncoupling of bone formation from resorption, borne out by the histological picture of complete coverage of all trabecular surfaces by highly active osteoblasts with no detectable increase in resorptive surfaces.[56] That the receptors for PTH (and PTHrP) are located on cells of the osteoblastic lineage,[57,58] and activation of osteoclasts by PTH is mediated through osteoblasts,[59,60] suggests the existence of distinct and separable transduction pathways activating different early gene expression.[61,62]

B. Studies in Ovariectomized Monkeys

The results in rats suggested that there was a connection between the selective stimulation of bone formation by the MAP peptides and the magnitude and speed of increase in both trabecular and cortical bone mass. There was no "braking effect" of coupled resorption (increased turnover) slowing the net bone gain. However, it was pointed out that the rat is atypical in being a "modeling" rather than a "remodeling" species,[63-65] and that the extrapolability of these results to primates was therefore questionable. For this reason, further studies were carried out in the long-term ovariectomized cynomolgus monkey.[66,67]

Groups of recently captured, feral female cynomolgus monkeys, stratified on degree of epiphysial maturity, were assigned to sham or OVX groups. After ovariectomy or sham surgery, BMD and serum and urinary biochemical parameters were monitored for 12 months and then various daily sc doses of RS-66271 were administered for six months (Figure 6.5). BMD results at the end of this time revealed no response to doses at or below 1 μg/kg/day. Therefore, animals which had received 0.01–0.1 μg/kg/day were reassigned to receive a further six-month treatment with either placebo or 60 μg/kg/day.

There was a clear-cut increase in bone turnover in response to OVX in these animals, with increases in serum bone-specific alkaline phosphatase, osteocalcin, and urinary deoxypyridinolines (DPYD) (Figure 6.6). BMD decreased markedly for about six months in the OVX animals and then increased, but not to levels of the sham animals, between 9 and 12 months postovariectomy. From 12 to 18 months post ovariectomy BMD increased very slightly in the OVX animals, and generally in parallel to the sham animals. Eighteen months after ovariectomy, BMD seemed to stabilize in untreated OVX animals. These BMD excursions, which have also been noted by others,[68] could be due to continued growth because the animals had not yet reached peak bone mass and/or to relative prior calcium deprivation while they were in the wild.

RS-66271 at 10 and 60 μg/kg/day clearly increased serum levels of procollagen type 1 C-terminal peptide (C1CP) and osteocalcin, with no

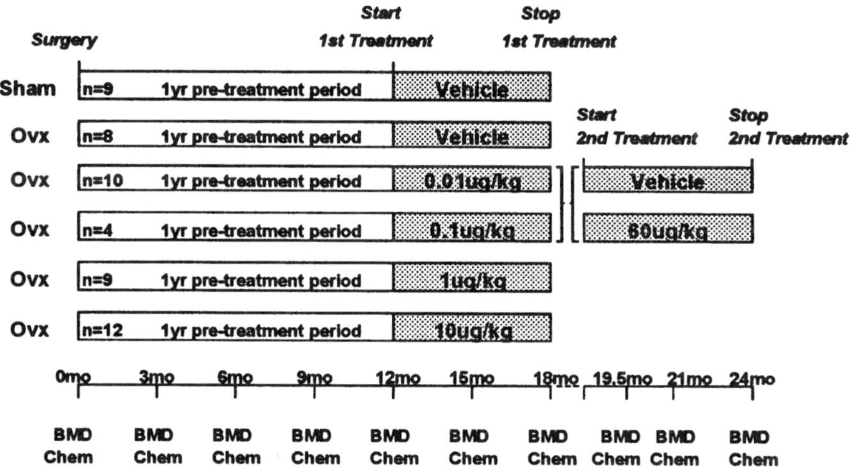

Figure 6.5
Schematic description of the monkey study.

elevation in urinary DPYD (Figure 6.7). These doses of RS-66271 also produced significant increases in BMD ranging from 2 to 7% for the whole body and 9 to 11% at the spine and hip (Figure 6.8), indicating efficacy at both trabecular and cortical sites, as seen in the rat studies. The increases in BMD could be detected after only three months of treatment. The total gain in BMD at all sites after six months of RS-66271 treatment resulted in BMD levels similar to those measured in the sham animals at 18 months (Figure 6.9).

A recent publication reviews a similar study performed with PTH(1-34) in cynomolgus monkeys.[69] Although the dosage schedule called for only three days of dosing per week for three months, the dose level of 10 μg/kg/day was comparable to the study using RS-66271. BMD data were similar but no markers were reported that can be used for comparison between RS-66271 and PTH-(1-34).

C. Studies in Corticosteroid-Treated Rabbits

The previous effects with the MAP analogs were generated in estrogen deprivation-induced osteoporosis, which is believed to be due to a combination of high bone turnover and resorption.[70,71] It might be hypothesized that it would be important for the action of the MAP analogs that the osteoblast population be in an activated state for the selective bone formative effects to be demonstrated. To test this hypothesis, further studies were undertaken in corticosteroid-dosed animals, in which osteopenia results principally from a suppression of osteoblast function, which may or may not be accompanied by increased osteoclastic activity. These es-

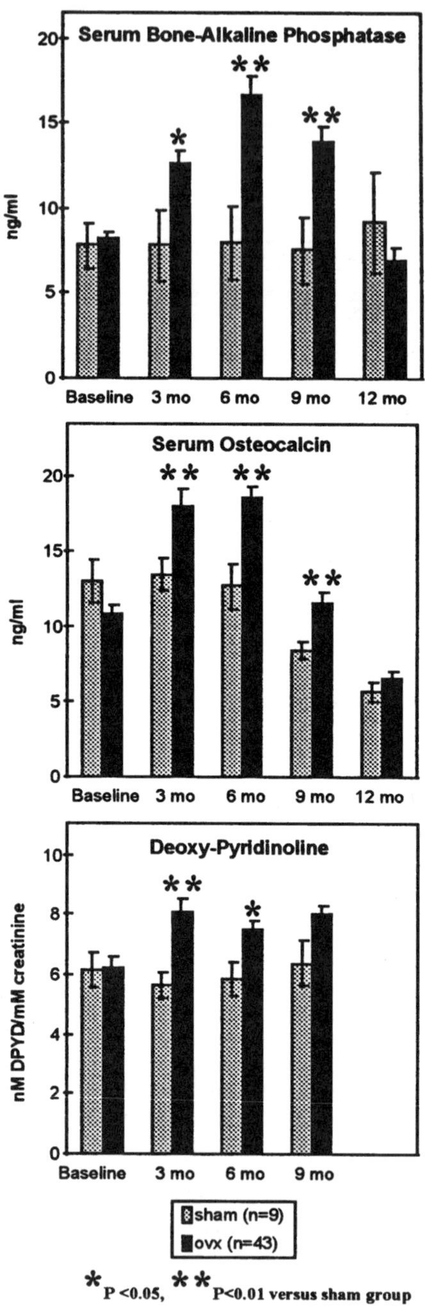

Figure 6.6
The effects of ovariectomy on three indices of bone formation and resorption in monkeys.

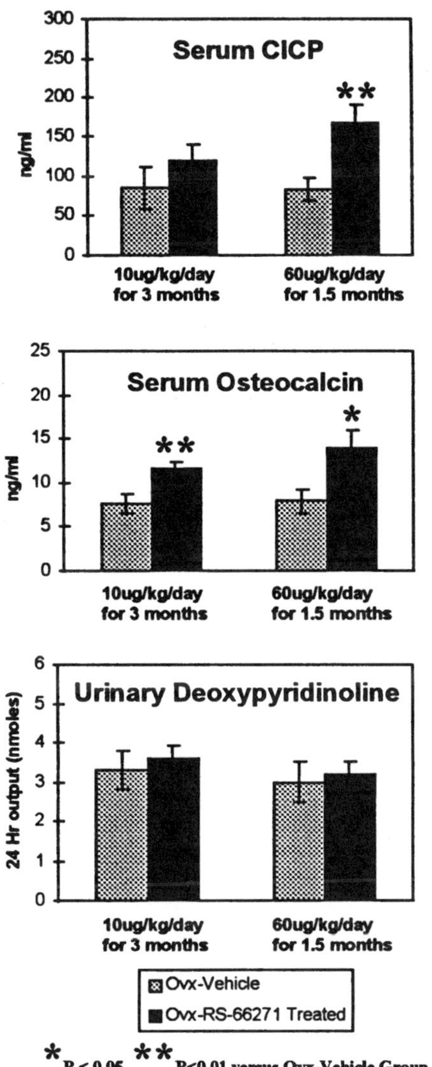

Figure 6.7
Serum and urinary indices of bone resorption (deoxypyridinoline) and formation (CICP and osteocalcin) in RS-66271-treated ovariectomized monkeys.

sential differences between the osteopenia resulting from OVX and corticosteroids are illustrated histologically by perforation of the trabeculae in the former compared to thinning of the trabeculae in the latter.[72-74]

There have been previous studies evaluating the effects of corticosteroids on bone in rats and in rabbits.[75-78] For unexplained reasons, rats do not consistently respond with bone loss except perhaps after gonadectomy.[79] On the basis of this literature and our own unpublished studies we elected to use rabbits. It was determined that a daily injected dose of

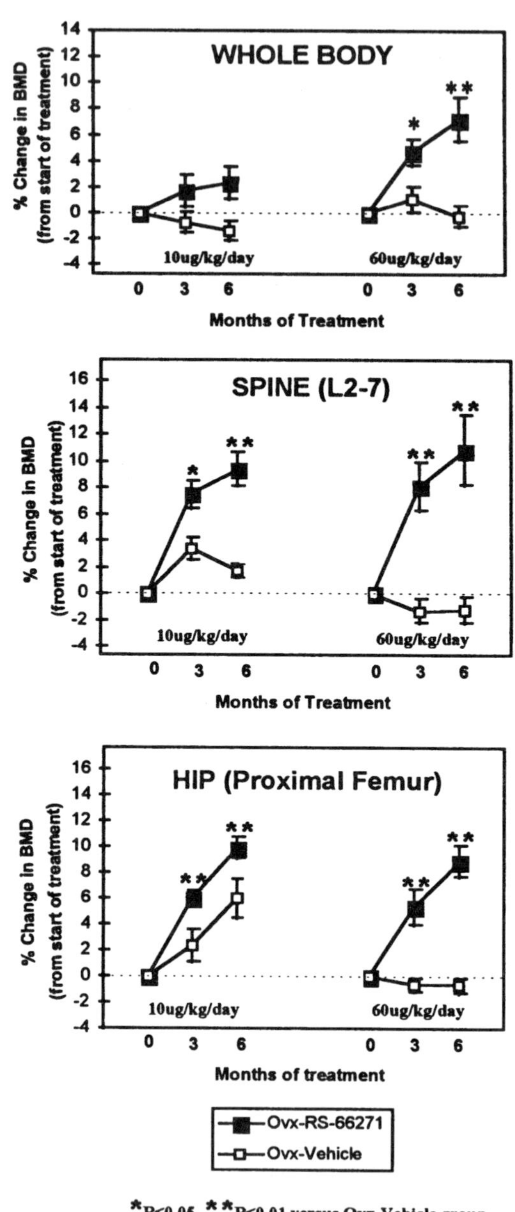

Figure 6.8
BMD increases at various parts of the skeletons of RS-66271-treated ovariectomized monkeys.

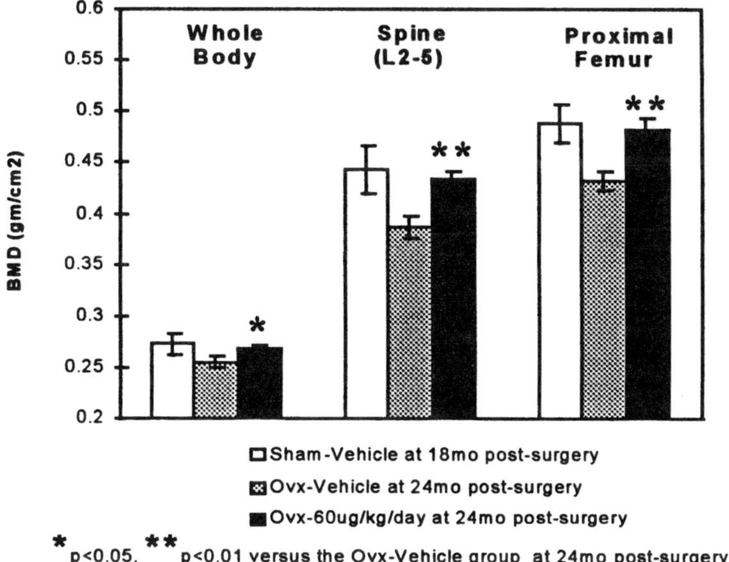

Figure 6.9
Comparison of raw BMDs of whole body, spine, and hip of ovariectomized monkeys after 6 months of RS-66271 treatment, beginning at 18 months post-ovariectomy, to those of sham monkeys.

0.15 mg/kg/day of prednisone resulted in a significant loss of bone at both trabecular and cortical sites, which peaked at six months.[80] This loss was associated with a very rapid (1 to 2 day) suppression of bone formation as indicated by circulating levels of osteocalcin but not with an increase (rather a decrease) in resorption on the basis of PYD levels, even after a one-year treatment. On this basis, and in contrast to some, but not all reports in man,[81,82] there does not appear to be an induction of a secondary hyperparathyroidism. (It has been suggested that the difference between the two species may lie in calcium metabolism/homeostasis.[83])

Administration of 10 µg/ kg/day of RS-66271 after stabilization of the osteopenia, 11 months into prednisone treatment and in the face of continued corticosteroid injection, rapidly reversed the deficit in BMD for both trabecular bone at the spine and femur (metaphysis) and cortical (femoral diaphysis) bone sites (Figure 6.10). The corticosteroid treatment was associated with decreases in both osteocalcin and PYD; RS-66271 induced major elevation in the former with little effect on the latter in these osteopenic animals after eight weeks of treatment (Figure 6.11). Even though this bone formation was extremely rapid, biomechanical testing showed that femoral 3-point bending load was returned to control levels. Additionally, the relationship between BMD and compressive and 3-point bending strength at vertebral and femoral sites, respectively, lay on the same regression line as for normal bone for all doses tested (Figure 6.12).

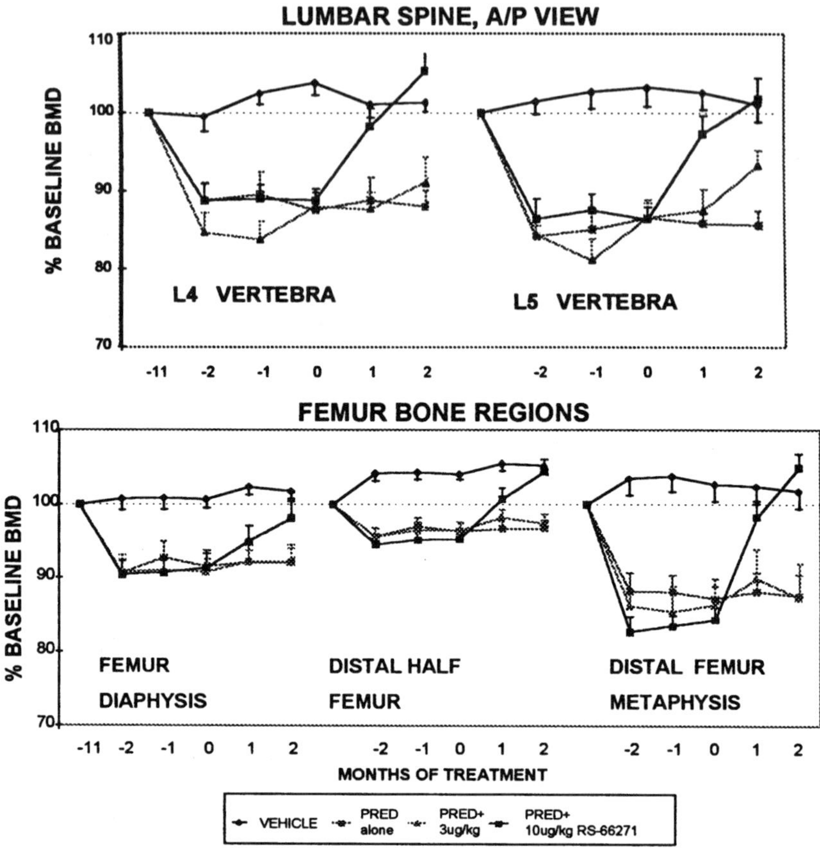

Figure 6.10
The effects of RS-66271 on BMD of trabecular and cortical bone regions in prednisone-treated rabbits.

Increases in resorptive markers in rabbits in response to RS-66271 have been noted only at higher doses than used in the above study; they were again associated with BMD which was higher than in the accompanying untreated control animals.[81] In addition, administration of 10 μg/kg/day of RS-66271 to otherwise untreated, nonosteopenic animals also caused an increase in PYD levels, but of course these animals started out with normal bone mass (Figure 6.13). Once again, in this new species, in a situation in which osteopenia resulted from a preferential suppression of osteoblastic function, bone formation was selectively stimulated versus bone resorption. On the other hand, increased resorption was observed if the compound effects were superimposed in a situation of normal bone mass, either by dosing normal animals or by continuing to dose osteopenic animals until after normal bone mass had been restored.

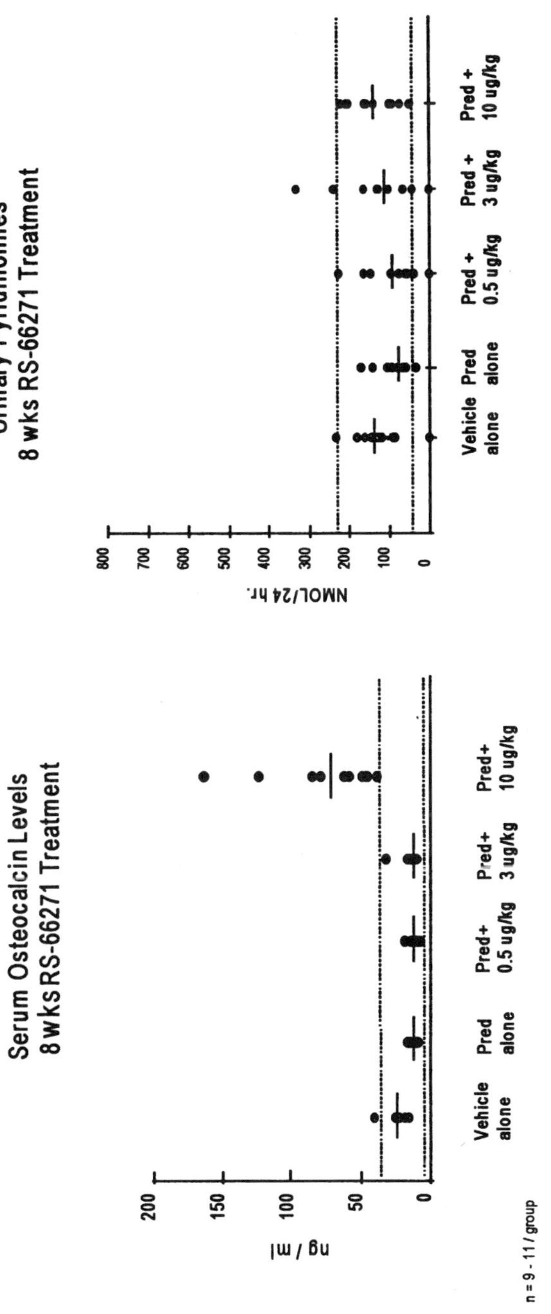

Figure 6.11
The effect of RS-66271 on serum osteocalcin and urinary pyridinolines in prednisone-treated rabbits.

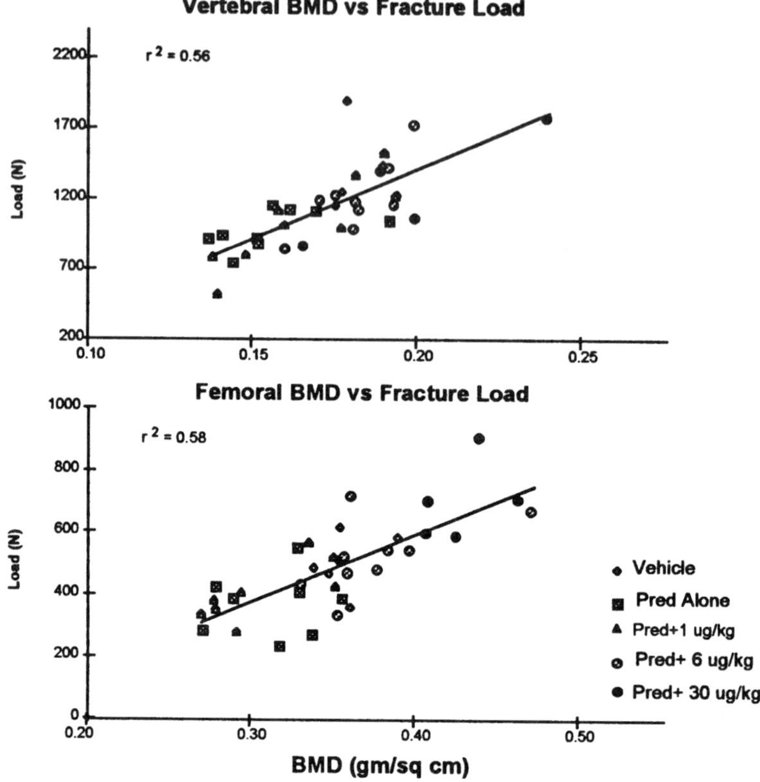

Figure 6.12
The correlation of BMD to fracture load of vertebrae and femurs in control rabbits, prednisone-treated rabbits, and rabbits treated with prednisone and different doses of RS-66271.

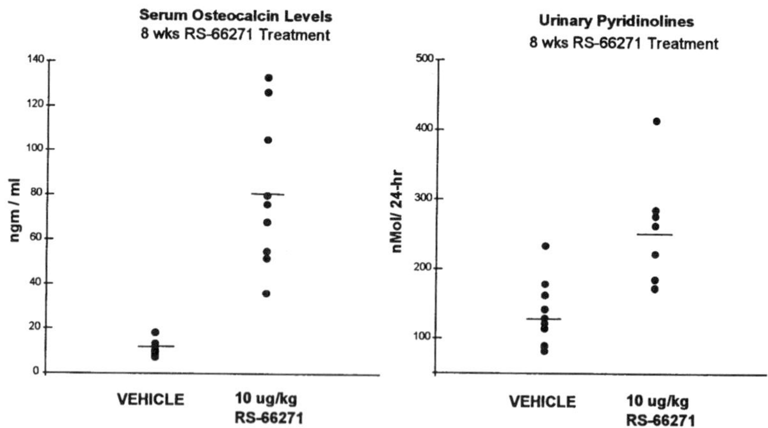

Figure 6.13
The RS-66271-induced increases in serum osteocalcin and urinary pyridinolines in otherwise untreated, nonosteoporotic rabbits.

IV. IMPLICATIONS OF THE OBSERVED EFFECTS OF THE MAP PEPTIDES IN OSTEOPENIA VERSUS NORMAL BONE MASS SITUATIONS

The experiments described above show the MAP analogs of hPTHrP-(1-34) to be bone anabolic agents causing an extremely rapid and high-magnitude gain in bone which is expressed at both trabecular and cortical sites regardless of gender in a range of both modeling and remodeling species and in osteopenia resulting from either increased or decreased turnover. It is suggested that the rapidity of this gain is due to a selective stimulation of osteoblast function which is dissociated from osteoclastic bone resorption. One explanation for the differences between the bone formation kinetics obtained with the MAP peptides and those obtained with PTH or PTHrP is that the latter agents do not uncouple the normally coupled responses of formation and resorption and thus only produce a small net gain.

However, one implication of the results obtained with RS-66271 is that, even if bone formation can be uncoupled from bone resorption in osteopenia, restoration of bone mass to normal or supranormal levels will activate another bone resorptive-stimulating mechanism. This suggests that the effect of anabolic agents will be self limiting and will tend to be lost as bone mass reaches normal levels; "normal" being defined by species and gender, but also by age and external forces such as muscle mass and contraction, weight bearing, etc. Thus, a more slow-acting anabolic agent such as PTH would be expected, and has been seen, to reach this diminishing return at a later time point.[84]

A second implication of these data is that studies in intact animals of either sex will not be predictive of the relative effects of these agents on bone formation and resorption and may give a false picture of induction of bone turnover as well as an underestimate of the potential magnitude and rapidity of ultimate gain in bone that can be achieved in an osteopenic situation. Carried to its logical conclusion, high-dose, long-term studies, epitomized by toxicology investigations, may in the case of this kind of agent give a false picture of the propensity to induce resorption and associated side effects. The preclinical studies recommended to be performed in osteopenic animals to assess the effects on bone quality,[85] may therefore also be pivotal in assessing efficacy and safety for the ultimate osteopenic patient population. Of course, in this population which may have as much as 25 to 40% bone loss, it is unlikely that any agent will be able to completely restore, or surpass, normal bone mass.

A final corollary of these experimental data is that the present regulatory guidelines for registration of drugs for treatment of osteoporosis, constructed with antiresorptive agents as models, may be inappropriate for judging bone anabolic agents. Bone restorative agents may restore bone at very different rates and probably should be discontinued after inducing an optimal return of bone mass. Although the question of maintenance treatment to retain the accreted bone once gained must be addressed,[86,87] imposition of arbitrary duration of primary drug treatment and follow-up in animal studies and human clinical trials is counter-intuitive. As with all previous drug categories, the clinical trial design should reflect the kinetics of response and intended/ recommended duration of treatment of the drug under consideration.

REFERENCES

1. Bauer, W., Aub, J. C., and Albright, F., Studies of calcium phosphorus metabolism: study of bone trabeculae as ready available reserve supply of calcium, *J. Exp. Med.*, 49, 145, 1929.
2. Selye, H., On the stimulation of new bone formation with parathyroid extract, irradiated ergosterol, *Endocrinology*, 16, 547, 1932.
3. Hefti, E., Trechsel, U., Bonjour, J.-P., Fleisch, H., and Schenk, R., Increase of whole-body calcium and skeletal mass in normal and osteoporotic adult rats treated with parathyroid hormone, *Clin. Sci.*, 62, 389, 1982.
4. Gunness-Hey, M. and Hock, J. M., Increased trabecular bone mass in rats treated with human synthetic parathyroid hormone, *Metab. Bone Dis. Rel. Res.*, 5, 177, 1984.
5. Habener, J. F., Rosenblatt, M., and Potts, J. T., Parathyroid hormone: biochemical aspects of biosynthesis, secretion, action, and metabolism, *Physiol. Rev.*, 64, 985, 1984.
6. Kemp, B. E., Moseley, J. M., Rodda, C. P., Ebeling, P. R., Wettenhall, R. E., Stapleton, D., Dieffenbach-Jagger, H., Ure, F., Michelangeli, V. P., Simmons, H. A., Raisz, L. G., and Martin, T. J., Parathyroid hormone-related protein of malignancy: active synthetic fragments, *Science*, 238, 1568, 1987.
7. Reeve, J., Meunier, P. J., Parsons, J. A., Bernat, M., Bijvoet, O. L., Courpron, P., Edouard, C., Klenerman, L., Neer, R. M., Renier, J. C., Slovik, D., Vismans, F. J. F. E., and Potts, J. T., Anabolic effect of human parathyroid hormone fragment on trabecular bone in involutional osteoporosis: a multicentre trial, *Br. Med. J.*, 280, 1340, 1980.
8. Slovik, D. M., Rosenthal, D. I., Doppelt, S. H., Potts, J. T., Daly, M. A., Campbell, J. A., and Neer, R. M., Restoration of spinal bone in osteoporotic men by treatment with human parathyroid hormone (1-34) and 1,25-(OH)2D, *J. Bone Min. Res.*, 1, 377, 1986.
9. Reeve, J., Davies, U. M., Hesp, R., McNally, E., and Katz, D., Treatment of osteoporosis with human parathyroid peptide and observations of the effect of sodium fluoride, *Br. Med. J.*, 301, 314, 1990.
10. Neer, M., Slovik, D. M., Daly, M., Potts, J. T., and Nussbaum, S. R., Treatment of postmenopausal osteoporosis with daily parathyroid hormone plus calcitriol, *Osteopor. Int.*, Suppl 1, S204, 1993.
11. Hori, M., Uzawa, T., Morita, K., Noda, T., Takahashi, H., and Inoue, J., Effect of human parathyroid hormone (PTH(1-34)) on experimental osteopenia of rats induced by ovariectomy, *Bone Miner.*, 3, 193, 1988.
12. Hock, J. M., Gera, I., Fonseca, J., and Raisz, L. G., Human parathyroid hormone (1-34) increases bone mass in ovariectomized and orchidectomized rats, *Endocrinology*, 122, 2899, 1988.
13. Wronski, T. J., Yen, C. F., Qi, H., and Dann, L. M, Parathyroid hormone is more effective than estrogen or bisphosphonates for restoration of lost bone mass in ovariectomized rats, *Endocrinology*, 132, 823, 1993.
14. Halloran, B. P. and Nissenson R. A., *Parathyroid Hormone-related Protein: Normal Physiology and its Role in Cancer*, CRC Press, Boca Raton, 1992.

15. Abou-Samra, A., Juppner, H., Force, T., Freeman, M. W., Kong, X. F., Schipani, E., Urena, P., Richards, J., Bonventre, J. V., Potts, J. J., Kronenberg, H. M., and Segre, G. V., Expression cloning of a common receptor for parathyroid hormone and parathyroid hormone-related peptide from rat osteoblast-like cells: a single receptor stimulates intracellular accumulation of both cAMP and inositol triphosphates and increases intracellular free calcium, *Proc. Natl. Acad. Sci., USA*, 89, 2732, 1992.
16. Caulfield, M. P., McKee, R. L., Goldman, M. E., Duong, L. T., Fisher, J. E., Gay, C. T., DeHaven, P. A., Levy, J. J., Roubini, E., Nutt, R. F., Chorev, M., and Rosenblatt, M., The bovine renal parathyroid hormone (PTH) receptor has equal affinity for two different amino acid sequences: The receptor binding domains of PTH and PTH-related protein are located within the 14-34 region, *Endocrinology*, 127, 83, 1990.
17. Chorev, M. and Rosenblatt, M., Structure-function analysis of parathyroid hormone and parathyroid hormone-related protein, in *The Parathyroids*, Bilezikian, J. P., Levine, M. A., and Marcus, R., Eds., Raven Press, New York, 1994, 139.
18. Hock, J. M., Fonseca, J., Gunness-Hey, M., Kemp, B. E., and Martin, T. J., Comparison of the anabolic effects of synthetic parathyroid hormone-related protein (PTHrP) 1-34 and PTH 1-34 on bone in rats, *Endocrinology*, 125, 2022, 1989.
19. Fraher, L. J., Hodsman, A. B., Jonas, K., Saunders, D., Rose, C. I., Henderson, J. E., Hendy, G. N., and Goltzman, D., A comparison of the *in vivo* biochemical responses to exogenous parathyroid hormone (1-34) and parathyroid hormone-related peptide (1-34) in man, *J. Clin. Endocrinol. Metab.*, 75, 417, 1992.
20. Inzucchi, S. E., Guinness-Henry, J., Mitnick, M. A., and Stewart, A. F., Parathyroid hormone -related protein (1-36) is equipotent with parathyroid hormone (1-34) in humans, *J. Clin. Endocrinol. Metab.*, 81, 199, 1996.
21. Reeve, J., Arlot, M., Bernat, M., Charhon, S., Edouard, C., Slovik, D., Vismans, F. J. F. E., and Meunier P. J., Calcium-47 kinetic measurements of bone turnover compared to bone histomorphometry in osteoporosis: the influence of human parathyroid fragment (hPTH1-34) therapy, *Metab. Bone Dis. Rel. Res.*, 3, 23, 1981.
22. Wronski, T. J. and Yen, C. F., Anabolic effects of parathyroid hormone on cortical bone in ovariectomized rats, *Bone*, 15, 51, 1993.
23. Mosekilde, L., Danielsen, C. C., Søgaard, C. H., McOsker, J. E., and Wronski, T. J., The anabolic effects of parathyroid hormone on cortical bone mass, dimensions and strength — Assessed in a sexually mature, ovariectomized rat model, *Bone*, 16, 223, 1995.
24. Neer, R., Slovik, D. M., Daly, M., Lo, C., Potts, J., and Nussbaum, S., Treatment of postmenopausal osteoporosis with daily parathyroid hormone plus calcitriol, in *"Osteoporosis 1990: Proceedings of the Third International Symposium on Osteoporosis"*, Christiansen, C. and Overgaard, K., Eds., Osteopress ApS, Copenhagen, 1990, Vol. 3, p. 1314.
25. Dempster, D. W., Feldman, F., Seldin, D., Jacobs, T. P., Siris, E., Cafferty, M., Parisien, M. V., Lindsay, R., Clemens, T. L., and Bilezekian, J. P., Skeletal disease in primary hyperparathyroidism, *J. Bone Min. Res.*, 4, 283, 1989.
26. Dobnig, H. and Turner, R. T., Evidence that intermittent treatment with parathyroid hormone increases bone formation in adult rats by activation of bone lining cells, *Endocrinology*, 136, 3632, 1995.
27. Gasser, J. A. and Jerome, C. P., Parathyroid hormone: A cure for osteoporosis? *Triangle*, 31, 111, 1992.
28. Raisz, L. G. and Niemann, I., Effect of phosphate, calcium and magnesium on bone resorption and hormonal responses in tissue culture, *Endocrinology*, 85, 446, 1969.
29. Howard, G. A., Bottemiller, B. L., Turner, R. T., Rader, J. I., and Baylink, D. J., Parathyroid hormone stimulates bone formation and resorption in organ culture: Evidence for a coupling mechanism, *Proc. Natl. Acad. Sci. USA*, 78, 3204, 1981.
30. Tam, C. S., Heersche, N. J. M., Murray, T. M., and Parsons, J. A., Parathyroid hormone stimulates the bone apposition rate independently of its resorptive action: Differential effects of intermittent and continual administration, *Endocrinology*, 110, 1982.

31. Dobnig, H. and Turner, R. T., Programmed intermittent sc infusion of parathyroid hormone (PTH) in sexually mature rats: Effects on bone and mineral metabolism, 10th Int Cong Endocrinology, San Francisco, Abstract #916, 1996.
32. Kitazawa, R., Imai, Y., Fukase, M., and Fujita, T., Effects of continuous infusion of PTH and PTH-related peptide on rat bone in vivo: comparative study by histomorphometry, *Bone Miner.*, 12, 157, 1991.
33. Avnur, Z., Krstenansky, J., Kimmel, D. B., and Vickery, B. H., Trabecular and cortical bone formative effects of RS-66271, a new highly potent agonist analogue of hPTHrP(1-34), IIIrd International Conference on New Actions of Parathyroid Hormone, Kyoto, Japan, April 18–21, Abstract 99, 1994.
34. Vickery, B. H., Avnur, Z., Cheng, Y., Chiou, S-S., Leaffer, D., Caulfield, J. P., Kimmel, D. B., Ho, T., and Krstenansky, J., RS-66271, a c-terminally substituted analog of human parathyroid hormone-related protein (1-34), increases trabecular and cortical bone in ovariectomized, osteopenic rats, *J. Bone Min. Res.*, 11, 1943, 1996.
35. Epand, R. M., Epand, R. F., Hui, S. W., He, N. B., and Rosenblatt, M., Formation of water-soluble complex between the 1-34 fragment of parathyroid hormone and dimyristoylphosphatidylcholine, *Int. J. Peptide Protein Res.*, 25, 594, 1985.
36. Klaus, W., Dieckmann, T., Wray, V., Schomburg, D., Wingender, E., and Mayer, H., Investigation of the solution structure of human parathyroid hormone fragment (1-34) by ^{1}H NMR spectroscopy, distance geometry and molecular dynamics calculations, *Biochemistry*, 30, 6936, 1991.
37. Barden, J. A. and Kemp, B. E., NMR solution structure of human parathyroid hormone(1-34), *Biochemistry*, 32, 7126, 1993.
38. Strickland, L. A., Bozzato, R. P., and Kronis, K. A., Structure of human parathyroid hormone(1-34) in the presence of solvents and micelles, *Biochemistry*, 32, 6050, 1993.
39. Barden, J. A. and Cuthbertson, R. M., Stabilized NMR structure of human parathyroid hormone(1-34), *Eur. J. Biochem.*, 215, 315, 1993.
40. Wray, V., Federau, T., Gronwald, W., Mayer, H., Schomberg, D., Tegge, W., and Wingender, E., The structure of human parathyroid hormone from a study of fragments in solution using ^{1}H NMR spectroscopy and its biological implications, *Biochemistry*, 33, 1684, 1994.
41. Barden, J. A. and Kemp, B. E., NMR study of a 34-residue N-terminal fragment of the parathyroid-hormone-related protein secreted during humoral hypercalcemia of malignancy, *Eur. J. Biochem.*, 184, 379, 1989.
42. Kaiser, E. T. and Kédzy, F. J., Amphiphilic secondary structure: Design of peptide hormones, *Science*, 223, 249, 1984.
43. Krstenansky, J. L., Trivedi, D., Johnson, D., and Hruby, V. J., Conformational considerations in the design of a glucagon analogue with increased receptor binding and adenylate potencies, *J. Am. Chem. Soc.*, 108, 1696, 1986.
44. Surewicz W. K., Neugebauer, W., Gagnon, L., MacLean, S., Whitfield, J. F., and Willick, G., Structure-function relationships in human parathyroid hormone: The essential role of the amphipathic α-helix, in *Peptides: Chemistry, Structure and Biology*, Hodges, R. S. and Smith, J. A., Eds., ESCOM, Leiden, 1994, 556.
45. Ösapay, G. and Taylor, J. W., Multicyclic polypeptide model compounds. 2. Synthesis and conformational properties of a highly α-helical uncosapeptide constrained by three side-chain to side-chain lactam bridges, *J. Am. Chem. Soc.*, 114, 6966, 1992.
46. Krstenansky, J. L., Owen, T. J., Yates, M. T., and Mao, S. J. T., Design, synthesis and antithrombin activity for conformationally restricted analogs of peptide anticoagulants based on the C-terminal region of the leech peptide, hirudin, *Biochim. Biophys. Acta*, 957, 53, 1988.
47. Neugebauer, W., Gagnon, L., Whitfield, J., and Willick, G. E, Structure and protein kinase C stimulating activities of lactam analogues of human parathyroid hormone fragment, *Int. J. Peptide Protein Res.*, 43, 555, 1994.

48. Krstenansky, J. L., Owen, T. J., Hagaman, K. A., and McLean, L. R., Short model peptides having a high α-helical tendency: design and solution properties, *FEBS Lett.*, 242, 409, 1989.
49. Kanellis, P., Romans, A. Y., Johnson, B. J., Kercret, H., Chioretti, R., Allen, T. M., and Segrest, J. P., Studies of synthetic peptide analogs of the amphipathic helix. Effect of charged amino acid residue topography on lipid affinity, *J. Biol. Chem.*, 255, 11464, 1980.
50. Fukushima, D., Kupferberg, J. P., Yokoyama, S., Kroon, D. J., Kaiser, E. T., and Kézdy, F. J., Synthetic amphiphilic helical docosapeptide with the surface properties of plasma apolipoprotein A-I, *J. Am. Chem. Soc.*, 101, 3703, 1979.
51. Pownall, H. J., Hu, A., Gotto, A. M., Albers, J. J., and Sparrow, J. T., Activation of lecithin:cholesterol acyl transferase by a synthetic model lipid-associating peptide, *Proc. Natl. Acad. Sci. USA*, 77, 3154, 1980.
52. Krstenansky, J. L., Ho, T. L., Pease, J. H. B., Park, J., Freedman, R., Chin, R., Avnur, Z., and Vickery, B. H., RS-66,271: dramatic improvement in the restoration of cortical and trabecular bone in osteopenic rats through the introduction of a decapeptide model amphipathic α-helix into human parathyroid hormone-related protein (1-34), submitted for publication, 1997.
53. Vickery, B. H., Avnur, Z., and Krstenansky, K. L., RS-66271, a new analog of hPTHrP(134), is a more potent bone anabolic agent in osteopenic rats than PTH(1-34), submitted for publication, 1997.
54. Hill, E. L., et al., Anabolic effect of RS-23581, a PTHrP analogue on bone in mature ovariectomized rats (in preparation).
55. Frost, H. M., The mechanostat: A proposed pathogenetic mechanism of osteoporosis and the bone mass: effects of mechanical and nonmechanical agents, *Bone Miner.*, 2, 73, 1987.
56. Leaffer, D., Sweeney, M., Kellerman, L. A., Avnur, Z., Krstenansky, L., Vickery, B., and Caulfield, J., Modulation of osteogenic cell ultrastructure by RS-23581, an analog of human parathyroid hormone (PTH)-related peptide-(1-34), and bovine PTH (1-34), *Endocrinology*, 136, 3624, 1995.
57. Rouleau, M. F., Warshawsky, H., and Goltzman, D., Parathyroid hormone binding in vivo to renal, hepatic, and skeletal tissues of the rat using an autoradiographic approach, *Endocrinology*, 118, 919, 1986.
58. Rouleau, M. F., Mitchell, J., and Goltzman, D., Characterization of the major parathyroid hormone target cell in the endosteal metaphysis of rat long bones, *J. Bone Min. Res.*, 5, 1043, 1990.
59. Rodan, G. A. and Martin, T. J., Role of osteoblasts in hormonal control of bone resorption: a hypothesis, *Calcif. Tissue Int.*, 33, 349, 1981.
60. Chambers, T. J., McSheehy, P. M. J., Thompson, B. M., and Fuller, K., The effect of calcium-regulating hormones, prostaglandins on bone resorption by osteoclasts disaggregated from neonatal rabbit bones, *Endocrinology*, 116, 234, 1985.
61. Fujimori, A., Cheng, S.-L., Avioli, L.V., and Civitelli, R., Dissociation of second messenger activation by parathyroid hormone fragments in cells, *Endocrinology*, 128, 3032, 1991.
62. Chiba, S., Un-no, M., Lee, K., Deeds, J. D., Neer, R. M., and Segre, G. V., Continuous versus intermittent PTH treatment effects on early gene expression in rat bone in vivo, *J. Bone Min. Res.*, 9 (Suppl. 1), S127, 1994.
63. Jee, W. S. S., The skeletal tissues, in *Cell and Tissue Biology*, Weiss, L., Ed., Baltimore: Urban & Schwartzenberg, 1988, 213.
64. Frost, H. M., Skeletal structural adaptations to mechanical usage (SATMU), 1. Redefining Wolff's law: the bone modeling problem, *Anat. Rec.*, 226, 403, 1990.
65. Frost, H. M., Skeletal structural adaptations to mechanical usage (SATMU), 2. Redefining Wolff's law: the bone remodeling problem, *Anat. Rec.*, 226, 414, 1990.
66. McRae, G. I., Avnur, Z., Tallentire, D., Zuber, Y., Sweeney, M., Kimmel, D. B., and Vickery, B. H., Time course of ovariectomy-induced osteopenia and increased bone turnover in the young adult cynomolgus monkey (submitted to *J. Bone Min. Res.*).

67. McRae, G. I., Avnur, Z., Tallentire, D., Shea, M., Kimmel, D. B., and Vickery, B. H., RS-66271, an analog of PTHrP(1-34), rapidly increases bone mineral density at spine and hip and bone strength of lumbar vertebrae in ovariectomized cynomolgus monkeys (in preparation).
68. Thompson, D. D., Seedor, J. D., Quartuccio, H., Solomon, H., Fioravanti, C., Davidson, J., Klein, H., Jackson, R., Clair, J., Frankenfield, D., Brown, E., Simmons, H. A., and Rodan, G. A., The bisphosphonate, Alendronate, prevents bone loss in ovariectomized baboons, *J. Bone Min. Res.*, 7, 951, 1992.
69. Jerome, C. P., Johnson, C. S., and Lees, C. J., Effect of treatment for 3 months with human parathyroid hormone (1-34) peptide in ovariectomized cynomolgus monkeys (*Macaca fascicularis*), *Bone*, 17, 415s, 1995.
70. Meunier, P. J. and Bressot, C., Endocrine influences on bone cells and bone remodeling evaluation by clinical histomorphometry, *Endocrinology of Calcium Metabolism*, 445, 1982.
71. Wronski, T. J., Walsh, C. C., and Ignaszewski, L. A., Histologic evidence for osteopenia and increased bone turnover in ovariectomized rats, *Bone*, 7, 119, 1986.
72. Bressot, C., Meunier, P. J., Chapuy, M. C., Lejeune, E., Edouard, C., and Darby, A. J., Histomorphometric profile, pathophysiology and reversibility of corticosteroid-induced osteoporosis, *Metab. Bone Dis. Rel. Res.*, 1, 303, 1979.
73. Dempster, D. W., Bone histomorphometry in glucocorticoid-induced osteoporosis, *J. Bone Min. Res.*, 4, 137, 1989.
74. Aaron, J., Francis, R. M., Peacock, M., and Makins, N. B., Contrasting micro anatomy of idiopathic and corticosteroid-induced osteoporosis, *Clin. Orthop.*, 243, 294, 1989.
75. Ortoft, G. and Oxlund, H., Reduced strength of rat cortical bone after glucocorticoid treatment, *Calcif. Tissue Int.*, 43, 376, 1988.
76. Thompson, J. S., Palmieri, G. M. A., Eliel, L. P., and Crawford, R. L., The effect of porcine calcitonin on osteoporosis induced by adrenal cortical steroids, *J. Bone Jt. Surg.*, 54A, 1490, 1972.
77. Thompson, J. S. and Urist, M. R., Effects of cortisone on bone metabolism in intact and thyroidectomized rabbits, *Calcif. Tissue Res.*, 13, 197, 1973.
78. Grardel, B., Sutter, B., Flautre, B., Viguier, E., Lavaste, F., and Hardouin, P., Effects of glucocorticoids on skeletal growth in rabbits evaluated by dual-photon absorptiometry, microscopic connectivity and vertebral compressive strength, *Osteoporosis Int.*, 4, 204, 1994.
79. Story, E., The effect of cortisone on normal and fractured bone in the rat, *Aust. New Zeal. J. Surg.*, 30, 36, 1960.
80. Waters, R., et al., Anabolic effects of RS66271 in a rabbit glucocorticosteroid osteopenia model (in preparation).
81. Cosman, F., Nieves, J., Herbert, J., Shen, V., and Lindsay, R., High dose glucocorticoids in multiple sclerosis patients exerts direct effects on the kidney and skeleton, *J. Bone Min. Res.* 9, 1097, 1994.
82. Paz-Pacheco, E., Fuleihan, G. E., and LeBoff, M. S., Intact parathyroid hormone levels are not elevated in glucocorticoid-treated subjects, *J. Bone Min. Res.*, 10, 1713, 1995.
83. Lindgren, J. U., DeLuca, H. F., and Mazess, R. B., Effects of 1,25 $(OH)_2D_3$ on bone tissue in the rabbit: studies on fracture healing, disuse osteoporosis, and prednisone osteoporosis, *Calcif. Tissue Int.*, 35, 591, 1984.
84. Mitlak, B. H., Burdette-Miller, P., Schoenfeld, D., and Neer, R. M., Sequential effects of chronic human PTH (1-84) treatment of estrogen-deficiency osteopenia in the rat, *J. Bone Min. Res.*, 11, 430, 1996.
85. Reginster, J. Y., Compston, J. E., Jones, E. A., Kaufman, J. M., Audran, M., Bouvenot, G., Frati, L., Mazzuoli, G., Gennari, C., and Lemmel, E. M., Recommendations for the registration of new chemical entities used in the prevention and treatment of osteoporosis, *Calcif. Tissue Int.*, 57, 247, 1995.

86. Jee, W. S. S., Ma, Y. F., and Chow, S. Y., Maintenance therapy for added bone mass or how to keep the profit after withdrawal of therapy of osteopenia, *Bone*, 17, 309S, 1995.
87. Ma, Y., Jee, W. S. S., Chen, Y., Gasser, J., Ke, H. Z., Li, X. J., and Kimmel, D. B., Partial maintenance of extra cancellous bone mass by antiresorptive agents after discontinuation of human parathyroid hormone(1-38) in right hind limb immobilized rats, *J. Bone Min. Res.*, 10, 1726, 1995.

Chapter 7

Commercial Exploitation of Parathyroid Hormone Therapy for the Treatment of Postmenopausal Osteoporosis

G. Marchand

CONTENTS

I. OSTEOPOROSIS — PREVALENCE AND IMPORTANCE

Osteoporosis is a disease characterized by low bone mass and structural deterioration of bone, leading to fragility and increased risk of fracture.[1] The most common osteoporotic fractures are those of the wrist, hip, and spine (vertebral crush fractures), but fractures can occur in all bones.[2] It is often called the silent disease because bone loss occurs without

0-8493-8556-3/98/$0.00+$.50

symptoms until fracturing begins. Everyone will experience some age-related bone loss, but not everyone will develop osteoporosis. The risk of developing the disease is increased by factors such as sex, race, age, diet, estrogen levels, exercise, smoking, alcohol, and the prolonged use of some medications, particularly glucocorticoids. Genetics is also important because maternal hip fracture is associated with a 100% increase in their daughters' fracture risk.[3] Typically, people may not know that they have osteoporosis until their bones become so weak that a sudden strain such as coughing or stepping out of a car, or a once-minor fall causes a bone to fracture or a vertebra to collapse.

Osteoporosis is recognized as a major health problem in the western world but may be even more prevalent in some third-world nations with widespread malnutrition. Postmenopausal Caucasian and Asian women are most at risk since they can lose up to 5% of their total bone volume per year[4] and up to 20% of their bone mass in the five to seven years following menopause.[5] It is less prevalent in black populations. The disease progresses with age, and as life expectancy increases, the prevalence of osteoporosis-related fractures also increases. Hence, osteoporosis has been identified by the World Health Organization as a disease that requires urgent attention.

Direct correlation of the disease to fracture incidence is difficult because of the lack of early diagnosis, unreported cases, the duration of the disease, tendency to attribute fractures to other causes, and inconsistent definition of the disease. The epidemiology has been the subject of numerous studies.[6-9] While the findings and assumptions vary from study to study, they consistently find that the prevalence of the disease is widespread and growing and that the impact on health costs will rise exponentially over the next 50 years.

It has been estimated that between 100 million and 200 million people worldwide, including 25 million Americans, are at risk of osteoporotic fracture,[10] that one of every two women and one of every eight men will have an osteoporosis-related fracture, and that by the age of 75 one third of all men will be affected by osteoporosis. It is estimated that 1.3 million to 1.5 million osteoporosis-related fractures occur in the U.S. annually and that of these 250,000 to 300,000 are hip fractures, 250,000 are wrist fractures, and more than 500,000 are vertebral fractures.[8,11,12] Hip fracture incidence is the measure used most often to demonstrate cost of osteoporosis since it always requires hospitalization and periods of rehabilitation. Hip fractures also represent an enormous burden in terms of morbidity and mortality, because 20% of patients who fracture a hip die within six months[10,13] and 50% of the survivors will be totally dependent on others.[14,15] The lifetime risk of osteoporotic hip fracture is 15% for white women and 5% for men. Measured by hip fractures alone, the cost to the U.S. healthcare system is estimated to be between $10 and $20 billion annually[16] and the cost to treat the three major types of osteoporotic fracture is $15 billion to $30 billion each year.[12] In older women or those with a decreased bone mass due to factors other than menopause, the incidence of vertebral fractures is 42%.[16]

The study most often cited as the benchmark for the prevalence of osteoporosis is the Rochester, Minnesota, study from the Mayo Foundation. Using data from this study and the accepted World Health Organization definition of established osteoporosis (bone density 2.5 SD below the mean for young normal women plus fracturing), it is projected that 30.3% of American women over the age of 50 have established osteoporosis.[9] Among women 80 years old and over, 27% have osteopenia in at least one skeletal site, and fully 70% have osteoporosis.[9]

While the impact of the disease today is a serious concern, the projections for its future consequences are even more dire. It is predicted that worldwide osteoporosis-related healthcare costs will rise to $60 billion by the year 2000; that hip fractures will more than double by the year 2050; and that annual direct healthcare costs of hip fractures alone in the U.S. will rise to $240 billion annually.[17,18] In Asia, the projections are even worse, because there may be a tenfold rise in osteoporotic fractures.[17]

These projections are based on trend experiences and on the aging population. The present world population of 325 million people who are 65 years and over will increase to more than 1,500 million by the year 2050.[18] In 2050, fully 22% of the world population will be over 65 and 5% over 85. The aging population doubles the cost estimates because incidence rates are higher and also because the cost of treating older patients (80 years and more) is more than twice the average cost of treating a younger patient.

Since all of the people in this category are already born, and since most of the people who will sustain osteoporotic fractures in the next 25 years already have established osteoporosis or at least osteopenia (1 SD below the mean of normal young women), the projections have a somewhat stronger basis. But, the projections do not include the possible impact of the introduction of more effective treatment or prevention.

The healthcare community has now awakened to the staggering economic and social burdens of osteoporosis. The 1990s have seen a significant increase in research initiatives by industry and publicly funded research institutions. Unfortunately, much needs to be done to educate the public about osteoporosis. In a recent study in Europe, only 22% of women over the age of 40 had discussed osteoporosis with their doctors, and only 17% had been tested for it.[14] New noninvasive techniques for monitoring bone density are now available which will enable clinicians to diagnose osteoporosis before fractures occur. Although prevention of osteoporosis is a compelling idea, the deficit-ridden economies of most countries make nation-wide routine monitoring and treatment with preventive agents unlikely.

II. OSTEOPOROSIS THERAPY — TODAY'S MARKET

The single aim of current treatments for osteoporosis is to maintain normal bone and hence reduce the risk of fractures. This includes exercise and calcium supplementation and drugs to inhibit bone resorption. Three classes of antiresorptive drug are currently being used, estrogen, calcitonin, and bisphosphonates.[19] The osteoporosis therapy market is expected to be worth $3.5 billion in 1997.

The market is currently dominated by HRT (hormone replacement therapy) which accounted for $1.5 billion in 1994 and was growing by 10 to 15% per year. Estrogens lower the rate of bone remodeling and thus reduce postmenopausal bone loss. This translates into a significant reduction of vertebral fractures with long-term HRT.[20,21] The positive effects of estrogens on bone and cardiovascular disease need to be balanced against the periodic bleeding and increased risk of cancers of breast and uterus with long-term use.[22] The side effects and fear of cancer together produce a poorly compliant patient population with some estimates of compliance as low as 16%.[23] Currently, two tissue-specific estrogens, raloxifene and droloxifene, are in development. These compounds preserve the beneficial effects of estrogens on bone without affecting breast and uterus.

Two other kinds of antiresorptive product, calcitonin accounts for just under $800 million (1994), and the newer family of bisphosphonates account for most of the remainder of the market. Calcitonin reduces bone turnover which slows bone loss and can be delivered intranasally.[24] Calcitonin is not widely used in North America because of its cost, but it has large markets in Japan and Italy. The launch of new bisphosphonates (some of which are 5000 times more effective than the original Didronel®) including Merck's alendronate (Fosamax®) will change this product mix somewhat. Bisphosphonates are analogs of pyrophosphate which slow bone loss by binding to hydroxyapatite and inhibiting osteoclast activity as well as directly promoting osteoclast death by apoptosis (see Chapter 5). Clinical studies have shown alendronate to increase bone mineral density and significantly reduce the incidence of vertebral fractures during a three-year study period.[25] Although they are poorly absorbed, these agents are active orally and should be a significant advance in the treatment of osteoporosis. Other products including vitamin D products and ipriflavone, which have a minor anabolic activity, enjoy a smaller share of the market. The overall market is expected to continue to grow at a 10 to 15% annual rate until the year 2000 and should reach more than $5 billion dollars by that time.

Market growth is being driven by emphasis on early diagnosis and increased patient awareness in response to concerted education programs. In spite of this recent growth, the current level of treatment for women at risk when combined with the low compliance is still below 10% and in most cases treatment is started only after osteoporosis is established.

This would indicate much room for continued growth in the market for preventative therapies for osteoporosis.

At $3.5 billion, the total market pales beside the direct cost of fractures related to osteoporosis. Educational programs aimed at increasing the use of preventative therapies are cost effective for the healthcare system in spite of the relatively low reduction in risk factor provided by the current treatments.

III. ANABOLIC THERAPY — MARKET OPPORTUNITY

None of the antiresorptive products on the market today is a cure for osteoporosis nor does any reestablish bone mass already lost to the disease. They can only slow the progression of the disease, and their effects wear off when treatment is discontinued. The questionable efficacy coupled with the asymptomatic nature of all but the more advanced stages of the disease and the real and perceived side effects of the current treatments will continue to lower the level of treatment and compliance. This means that there will be a continuing high number of patients who will develop an established osteoporosis and remain with a high fracture risk.

It is evident that the market offers opportunity and indeed a need for a safe and effective treatment that would *restore* lost bone. The introduction of anabolic agents will create an entirely new kind of product. Such "anabolic therapeutics" will be targeted initially and primarily at the patients who have already progressed to osteopenia and established osteoporosis, usually the over-65 age group.

In this market segment, the anabolic products will have a clear advantage when compared to the current antiresorptive products which will be seen by the medical community as being ineffective once the disease has reached an advanced stage. The pharmacoeconomic advantage of an effective anabolic treatment for this very large market segment will be evident to healthcare regulators and to the insurers and managers of healthcare programs. The ability of PTH to compete in the preventive treatment market will depend on its cost and its potential to form better quality bone than that formed by antiresorptive treatments.

While bone resorption-inhibiting drugs are currently the only therapeutic option for treating osteoporosis, stimulators of bone formation are in development. The current list of experimental anabolic agents include fluoride, IGF-I (insulin-like growth factor I), and PTH.

The ability of fluoride to stimulate bone formation through a direct stimulation of osteoblasts has been known for many years (see Chapter 9). The results of early studies using high doses of fluoride indicated that the ion significantly increased bone mineral density, but this was accompanied by serious gastrointestinal side effects and was not associated with a decreased fracture incidence.[26,27] Newer, slow-release fluoride formulations are better tolerated, significantly increase bone mineral density, and most important, reduce fracture incidence.[28] Fluoride therapy will remain controversial until the issues of side effects and biomechanical strength are resolved. However, since fluoride is not patentable the costly studies to determine its efficacy may never be conducted.

IV. PTH ADVANTAGES

In the past, the development of PTH as an anabolic drug to treat postmenopausal osteoporosis was hindered by reservations about injection being its only route of administration, the difficulty of producing large amounts of the peptide economically, and the inability of pharmaceutical companies to patent it.[29] With the emergence of solutions to these problems, PTH is becoming the agent of choice for several academic and pharmaceutical research initiatives in the development of anabolic treatments for osteoporosis. Today, at least five major pharmaceutical companies have initiated PTH programs, mostly based on the PTH-(1-34) analog or the native molecule, PTH-(1-84). A recent survey of academic experts in osteoporosis found that 100% of the respondents thought that anabolic agents for bone would be developed and 60% felt this would happen within the next 10 years.[30] Of the agents currently in development, over 50% of the respondents selected PTH-like agents and IGF as the anabolic therapies with the greatest promise.[30]

As discussed in Chapter 5, new, small, potently anabolic, patented analogs of PTH are now available. In addition to the patent protection of molecules such as hPTH-(1-31)NH_2 and its cyclic lactam derivatives, these novel PTH analogs can have significant advantages over the natural hormone, hPTH-(1-84), and the PTH-(1-34) fragment in animal trials. Their improved efficacy should provide the opportunity for a lower dosage and the obvious product safety and regulatory advantages that follow from that.

With a further understanding of the mechanism by which PTH and its fragments stimulate bone growth will come further improved low molecular weight compounds which can mimic the anabolic action of PTH when delivered by mouth or aerosol. In the meantime, the available small PTH analogs will be platforms for the development of nonpeptide PTH mimetics. The novel, small PTH analogs with potent bone building capabilities enable a wide range of research options for the delivery of this drug and therefore a wider range of products for osteoporosis treatment. One option currently being investigated is to deliver PTH in an aerosol. Indeed, the pulmonary epithelium is the best for allowing the passage of small peptides such as hPTH-(1-34), but not hPTH-(1-84), into the circulation.[31] However, it has yet to be shown that the resulting intermittent PTH pulses are sufficient for triggering and driving the bone-building mechanism.

While side effects have not been an issue in PTH administration to humans to date, no patients have been on PTH therapy for the years that may be required to restore the severely depleted bone in an established osteoporotic patient, and hence the potential side effects that may be associated with long-term administration are not known. hPTH-(1-31)NH_2's uni-signalling mechanism, targeting only adenylyl cyclase, may provide an added advantage of not frequently and supranormally activating the family of phospholipase Cβ-mediated processes that are additionally turned on by both hPTH-(1-34), and hPTH-(1-84) some of which, such as increased protein kinase C activity, are well-known tumor-promoters.[32] The simpler signaling of these molecules will also provide advantages in seeking regulatory approval.

The issue of large-scale, economically viable production of PTH has also been addressed. There have now been many reports of the large-scale production of biologically active recombinant parathyroid hormone. For example, *Escherichia coli* bacterial expression systems for [Pro^{-1}]-hPTH-(1-84)[33-36] and hPTH-(1-38)[37] can produce hormones whose biological activity is indistinguishable from that of chemically produced hPTH-(1-84), despite the N-terminal proline residue.[33]

The first of the PTHs for treating osteoporosis, recombinant native hPTH-(1-84) which can only be delivered by injection, is in development by Allelix Biopharmaceuticals Inc. and Astra. Their phase II clinical trial has been completed and the phase III trial should begin later in 1997. This should pave the way for the new, very small PTH analogs, such as hPTH-(1-31)NH_2 or its cyclic analogs (see Chapter 5) which will be the next generation of better, safer, and possibly noninjectable anabolic products. They will be economically produced by solid-phase synthesis rather than by recombinant technology.

REFERENCES

1. Anonymous, Consensus development conference: Osteoporosis, *Am. J. Med.*, 90, 107, 1991.
2. Lindsay, R., The menopause and osteoporosis, *Obstet. Gynecol.*, 87, 16S, 1996.
3. Cummings, S. R., Nevitt, M. C., Browner, W. S., Stone, K., Fox, K. M., Ensrud, K. E., Cauley, J., Black, D., and Vogt, T. M., Risk factors for hip fracture in white women. Study of Osteoporotic Fractures Research Group, *N. Engl. J. Med.*, 332, 767, 1995.
4. Riggs, B. L. and Melton, L. J. III, Involutional osteoporosis, *N. Engl. J. Med.*, 314, 1676, 1986.
5. Riggs, B., Wahner, H., Dunn, W., Mazess, R., Offord, K., and Melton, L., Differential changes in bone mineral density of the appendicular and axial skeleton with aging, *J. Clin. Invest.*, 67, 328, 1981.
6. Dennison, E., The epidemiology of osteoporosis, *Br. J. Clin. Pract.*, 50, 33, 1996.
7. Rungby, J., Hermann, A. P., and Mosekilde, L., Epidemiology of osteoporosis. Implications for drug therapy, *Drugs & Aging*, 6, 470, 1995.

8. Nevitt, M. C., Epidemiology of osteoporosis, *Rheum. Dis. Clin. North Am.*, 20, 535, 1994.
9. Melton, L. J. III, How many women have osteoporosis now?, *J. Bone Min. Res.*, 10, 175, 1995.
10. Cummings, S. R., Kelsey, J. L., Nevitt, M. C., and O'Dowd, K. J., Epidemiology of osteoporosis and osteoporotic fractures, *Epidemiol. Rev.*, 7, 178, 1985.
11. Cummings, S. R., Rubin, S. M., and Black, D., The future of hip fractures in the United States, *Clin. Orthop. Rel. Res.*, 252, 163, 1990.
12. Melton, L. J. III, Lane, A. W., Cooper, C., Eastell, R., O'Fallon, W. M., Riggs, B. L., Prevalence and incidence of vertebral deformities, *Osteop. Int.*, 3, 113, 1993.
13. Keene, G., Parker, M., and Pryor, G., Mortality and morbidity after hip fractures, *Br. Med. J.*, 307, 1248, 1993.
14. Rowe, R., COMMENT: Preventive strategies: is current clinical practice effective for bones?, *Br. J. Clin. Pract.*, 50, 47, 1996.
15. Melton, L. J. III, Epidemiology of fractures, in *Osteoporosis: Etiology, Diagnosis and Management*, Riggs, B. L. and Melton, L. J. III, Eds., Raven Press, New York, 1988, 113.
16. Melton, L. J. III, Kan, S. H., Frye, M. A., Wahner, H. W., O'Fallon, W. M., and Riggs, B. L., Epidemiology of vertebral fractures in women, *Am. J. Epidemiol.*, 129, 1000, 1989.
17. Cooper C., Campion, G., and Melton, L. J. III, Hip fractures in the elderly: A world-wide projection, *Osteop. Int.*, 2, 285, 1992.
18. Lindsay, R., The burden of osteoporosis: cost, *Am. J. Med.*, 98 (Suppl. 2A), 2A-9S, 1995.
19. Adachi, J. D., Current treatment options for osteoporosis, *J. Rheumatol.*, 23 (Suppl. 45), 11, 1996.
20. Lindsay, R., Hart, D. M., Forrest, C., and Baird, C., Prevention of spinal osteoporosis in oophorectomized women, *Lancet*, ii, 1151, 1980.
21. Tohme, J., Cosman, F., and Lindsay, R., Osteoporosis, in *Principles and Practices of Endocrinology and Metabolism*, 2nd ed., Becker, K. L., Ed., J. B. Lippincott, New York, 1995, 567.
22. Lips, P., Prevention of hip fractures: Drug therapy, *Bone*, 18 (Suppl. 3), 159S, 1996.
23. Wallace, W. A., Price, V. H., Elliot, C. A., MacPherson, M. B. A., and Scott, B. W., Hormone replacement therapy acceptability to Nottingham postmenopausal women with a risk factor for osteoporosis, *J. Roy. Soc. Med.*, 83, 699, 1990.
24. Gennari, C. and Avioli, L. V., Calcitonin therapy in osteoporosis, in *The Osteoporotic Syndrome*, 2nd ed., Avioli, L. V., Ed., Grune and Stratton, New York, 1987, 121.
25. Liberman, U. A., Weiss, S. R., Broll, J., Minne, H. W., et al., Effect of oral alendronate on bone mineral density and the incidence of fractures in postmenopausal osteoporosis, *N. Engl. J. Med.*, 333, 1437, 1995.
26. Riggs, B. L., O'Fallon, W. M., Lane, A., Hodgson, S. F., Wahner, H. W., Muhs, J., Chao, E., and Melton, L. J. III, Clinical trial of fluoride therapy in postmenopausal osteoporotic women: extended observations and additional analysis, *J. Bone Min. Res.*, 9, 265, 1994.
27. Bilezikian, J. P., Current and future nonhormonal approaches to the treatment of osteoporosis, *Int. J. Fertil.*, 41, 148, 1996.
28. Pak, C. Y. C., Sakhaee, K., Adams-Huet, B., Piziak, U., Peterson, R. D., and Poindexter, J. R., Treatment of postmenopausal osteoporosis with slow-release sodium fluoride, *Ann. Int. Med.*, 123, 401, 1995.
29. Kimmel, D. B., Slovik, D. M., and Lane, N. E., Current and investigational approaches for reversing established osteoporosis, *Rheum. Dis. Clin. N. Am.*, 20, 735, 1994.
30. Gruber, H. E., Farley, S. M., and Baylink, D. J., Predictions on future diagnosis and treatment of osteoporosis: Results and discussion of a recent opinion poll, *Calcif. Tissue Int.*, 57, 83, 1995.
31. Patton, J. S., Trinchero, P., and Platz, R. M., Bioavailability of pulmonary delivered peptides and proteins: α-interferon, calcitonins and parathyroid hormones, *J. Controlled Rel.*, 28, 79, 1994.
32. Whitfield, J. F., *Calcium in Cell Cycles and Cancer*, CRC Press, Boca Raton, 1995.

33. Paulsen, J., Ochs, D., Harder, M., Duvos, C., Mayer, H., and Wigender, E., Large-scale preparation and biological activity of recombinant human parathyroid hormone, *J. Biotechnol.*, 39, 129, 1995.
34. Harder, M. P. F., Sanders, E. A., Wingender, E., and Deckwer, W.-D., Production of human parathyroid hormone by recombinant *Escherichia coli* TG1 on synthetic medium, *J. Biotechnol.*, 32, 157, 1994.
35. Harder, M. P. F., Sanders, E. A., Wingender, E., and Deckwer, W.-D., Studies on the production of human parathyroid hormone by recombinant *Escherichia coli*, *Appl. Microbiol. Biotechnol.*, 39, 329, 1993.
36. Wingender, E., Bercz, G., Blocker, H., Frank, R., and Mayer, H., Expression of human parathyroid hormone in *Escherichia coli*, *J. Biol. Chem.*, 264, 4367, 1989.
37. Gram, H., Ramage, P., Memmert, K., Gamse, R., and Kocher, H. P., A novel approach for high level production of a recombinant human parathyroid hormone fragment in *Escherichia coli*, *Biotechnology*, 12, 1017, 1994.

Chapter **8**

The Insulin-Like Growth Factors: Potential Anabolic Agents for The Skeleton

Anna Johansson and Clifford J. Rosen

CONTENTS

0-8493-8556-3/98/$0.00+$.50

I. INTRODUCTION: THE ROLE OF INSULIN-LIKE GROWTH FACTORS IN BONE DISEASE

Insulin-like growth factors (previously called somatomedins) are ubiquitous polypeptides produced, secreted, and degraded by various tissues.[1] In mammalian species, IGF-I and IGF-II are found in large concentrations bound to a family of IGF-specific binding proteins (IGFBPs). Because they circulate in the blood, the IGFs have traditionally been considered endocrine "effectors" performing two distinct physiologic roles: 1) mediating growth hormone's activity on the cartilaginous growth plate (hence the term somatomedins), and 2) exerting insulin-like action on target cells (hence the name insulin-like growth factors). IGF-I is essential for linear bone growth. This is best illustrated by single point mutations in the growth hormone receptor gene which result in a short stature phenotype despite high levels of circulating growth hormone (GH).[2] Also, it is clear that under specific circumstances, IGFs can lower serum glucose and act directly on the insulin receptor. But the IGFs also have potent paracrine and autocrine effects on cell growth and differentiation that are independent of GH. It is this fine balance between local and systemic activities of these unique growth factors that permit their consideration as possible treatment options for several metabolic disorders.

The advent of recombinant gene technology in the mid 1980s spurred tremendous interest in the pharmacologic application of the IGFs. Besides the obvious diseases, such as diabetes mellitus and GH resistance syndromes, musculoskeletal and neurodegenerative disorders were also identified as being amenable to treatment with the IGFs. However, some of that enthusiasm has waned in recent years as the role IGFs play in cell growth, neoplastic behavior, and apoptosis has become more apparent. Notwithstanding those considerations, the skeleton has been proposed as an ideal target organ for treatment with the IGFs. The rationale for using IGFs to increase bone mass includes the following: 1) IGF-I and IGF-II are found in very high concentrations within the skeletal matrix and are synthesized by bone-forming cells;[3,4] 2) both IGFs are modest mitogens but strong differentiation factors for osteoblasts;[5] 3) all components of the IGF regulatory system (IGFs, IGFBPs, IGF receptors, IGFBP-specific proteases) are part of the remodeling process;[1] and 4) the aging skeleton, which is characterized by low bone mass, also features a significant decline in osteoblastic activity and reduced skeletal IGFs, thereby making it potentially amenable to "replacement" therapy.[6] In fact, the growth- and differentiation-promoting properties of the skeletal IGFs have made these proteins high-profile candidates for anabolic treatments in adult metabolic bone disorders.

The prevalence of osteoporosis and the heightened awareness of this disorder has focused attention on newer treatment options which focus on building bone mass rather than preventing bone loss. The hope that skeletal growth factors can reverse the skeletal fragility and fractures associated with osteoporosis has served to accelerate experimental studies with these peptides in animals and humans. Such studies have not been limited to the family of IGFs. Rather, other skeletal growth factors, including fibroblast growth factor (FGF), platelet-derived growth factor (PDGF), and transforming growth factor-β (TGF-β), have been examined in great detail to determine their potential role in modulating bone formation. Although these growth factors could become important therapeutic modalities for bone disorders, this chapter will focus solely on IGF-I, primarily because of all the above-named peptides, IGF-I has been the one which has been the most extensively studied with both cell and animal models.

II. OVERVIEW OF THE IGFs AND THE IGF REGULATORY SYSTEM WITH PARTICULAR FOCUS ON THE SKELETON

A. Circulating IGFs and Their Regulation

If the IGFs are to be considered as anabolic agents for disorders such as osteoporosis, a thorough understanding of the systemic as well as skeletal IGF regulatory systems is essential. As noted previously, IGF-I and IGF-II circulate in high concentrations in serum bound to six IGFBPs.[7] Serum IGF-I comes primarily from the liver where it is produced in response to pulses of GH secretion from the pituitary. Although GH is the principal regulator of systemic IGF-I, other factors, acting on the hepatocyte, can regulate expression of GH receptors and the messages from the activated receptors that induce IGF-I synthesis. Nutritional determinants (e.g., protein or calorie intake) and insulin can also modulate serum IGF-I levels via hepatic interactions.[8] Aging, exercise, and certain drugs also modulate GH-induced IGF-I expression in the liver.[9]

Besides affecting the absolute concentration of IGF-I (or IGF-II) in serum, several other factors determine the precise amount of IGF bioavailability for tissue utilization. These factors include the IGFBPs, IGFBP-specific proteases, and IGF receptors. The IGFBPs are a family of highly conserved binding proteins which exhibit strong affinity for IGF-I or -II, but not for insulin.[10] Six IGFBPs have currently been identified. These proteins are synthesized in virtually every tissue and are also present in high concentrations in the serum (total amounts of IGFBPs exceed those of the two IGFs by one third, thereby leaving little or no free IGF in the circulation).[10] The presence of excess IGFBPs in serum is probably protective under normal physiologic conditions since excess free IGF-I could produce hypoglycemia and prolonged stimulation of cell proliferation. Indeed, after exogenous IGF-I administration there is a transitory period where total IGF concentrations can exceed the binding capacity of the IGFBPs and have side effects such as significant hypoglycemia.[11] The IGFBPs are carrier proteins for the IGFs, proverbial shuttles moving IGF-

I and -II in and out of the circulation. However, the IGFBPs are also local modulators of IGF bioactivity and regulate the tissue activity for their specific growth factor.

The largest of the six IGFBPs is IGFBP-3, a 42-kDa protein induced by GH and fully saturated with IGF-I and IGF-II. It is the predominant serum IGFBP with a concentration of approximately 150 nM (the total serum IGF concentration (IGF-I+IGF-II) is approximately 100 nM).[12] IGFBP-3 binds both to the IGFs and another GH-dependent protein, the acid-labile subunit (ALS).[13] This fully saturated circulating ternary complex (ALS · IGFBP-3 · IGF-I or -II) serves as the major reservoir for IGFs in plasma. Its large size also precludes its escape into the interstitium. However, proteolysis of portions of the IGFBP-3 molecule can lead to impaired binding to the ALS and dissociation of IGFs from the complex.[14] In general, the IGFBPs bind IGFs with a far higher affinity than do IGF receptors. Therefore, excess molar concentrations of IGFBPs mean that there has to be an *in vivo* way of separating these fairly tenacious IGFBPs from the IGFs in order to ensure tissue activity. In fact there are IGFBP-3 proteases in human serum which are active at physiologic pH and likely serve to detach the IGFs from their transport vehicle.[15] Regulation of these circulating proteases is not well defined, but as pregnancy proceeds toward parturition, serum IGFBP-3 proteolysis becomes nearly complete.[15] This may be a critical mechanism which permits IGF-I to be more bioavailable during states of accelerated growth and anabolism. Finally, it should be noted that IGFBP-3 can also be produced locally and serve as an agonist or antagonist for autocrine or paracrine secreted IGF-I. A putative IGFBP-3 receptor has recently been identified suggesting that IGFBP-3 can have IGF-independent activity on cell replication.[16] Recent studies have also shown that the p53 tumor suppressor protein can regulate IGFBP-3 synthesis, further supporting a critical role for this binding protein in the regulation of cell growth.[17] Since IGFBP-3 is constitutively expressed by osteoblasts, its role in regulating bone cell function remains an area of intense investigation.[18]

The other five IGFBPs (IGFBP-1,-2,-4,-5,-6) are present in relatively low concentrations (3 to 18 nM) in serum, are unsaturated, and can translocate into the interstitium.[19] IGFBP-4 (24 kDa) and IGFBP-5 (32 kDa) are produced by skeletal cells and are regulated by analogs that stimulate cyclic AMP synthesis (e.g., PTH, forskolin).[19] Skeletal IGFBP-4 message is also controlled by 1,25 dihydroxyvitamin D3.[20] *In vitro* studies have shown that in every cell system IGF activity is inhibited by adding IGFBP-4 either before, during, or after administration of IGF-I or -II. IGFBP-4 can also undergo proteolysis, and recent studies have shown that IGF-I itself can control the rate of IGFBP-4 proteolysis.[21]

IGFBP-5 has the unique property of binding to extracellular matrices and can store IGFs within the interstitium or in skeletal tissues.[22] In bone, IGFBP-5 has been shown to enhance the bioactivity of IGF-I and to bind avidly to calcium hydroxyapatite.[19] IGFBP-1, -2, and -6 have also been detected in calcified tissues. IGFBP-1, which is acutely regulated by insulin, can be expressed in bone cells and can inhibit IGF-stimulated osteoblastic activity. Skeletal IGFBP-1 message is suppressed by insulin and enhanced by glucocorticoids.[23] The roles of IGFBP-2 and IGFBP-6 in the skeleton have not been clearly defined. In fact, most studies have focused on three skeletal IGFBPs (IGFBP-3, -4, -5), their relationship to bone turnover, and their regulation by calciotropic hormones.

Whether in the interstitium or in the circulation, the IGF regulatory system is composed of four basic elements: 1) the *ligands* (IGF-I, or II); 2) the *carrier proteins*, IGFBPs (1-6); 3)IGFBP-specific *proteases* which function to cleave the IGFBPs, thereby allowing the IGFs to dissociate from their transport carriers; and 4) the *receptors* which mediate IGF cellular actions (the Type I and the Type II IGF receptor). The Type I receptor is a dimeric structure which closely resembles the insulin receptor and is composed of intracellular and extracellular domains).[24] Signaling pathways, including intrinsic tyrosine kinase activity, are similar to those of insulin, which at high concentrations can occupy the Type I receptor (just as IGF-I at high concentrations can activate the insulin receptor).[25] The Type II receptor, on the other hand, is a monomeric structure which bears no resemblance to the insulin receptor, cannot bind insulin, and has a higher affinity for IGF-II than IGF-I.[26] It has no intrinsic kinase activity, but is structurally very similar to the mannose 6-phosphate receptor.[26]

B. Skeletal IGFs, IGFBPs and Their Role in Bone Turnover

Not unlike the circulatory IGF regulatory system, the skeletal IGF circuit is composed of both IGFs, IGFBPs 1-6, the Type I and Type II IGF receptor, and certain IGFBP-specific proteases (IGFBP-4 and -5 proteases). The principal origin of these IGF elements is the osteoblast, although the circulation can contribute to the overall skeletal pool of IGFs and IGFBPs.[1] In addition to osteoblastic production of IGF-I, both IGF receptors have been reported on osteoclasts, and there is some suggestion that preosteoclasts can differentiate under the influence of IGF-I or IGF-II.[27,28]

The IGFs act on bone cells in the same way they act on the cells in noncalcified tissues. Both IGF-I and IGF-II stimulate bone formation via osteoblasts although IGF-I is slightly more potent than IGF-II.[29] Both can enhance preosteoblast replication and stimulate Type I collagen synthesis.[29,30] In addition, both IGFs inhibit collagen degradation by suppressing the synthesis of certain collagenases and metalloproteinases.[30] Most important, though, IGFs are essential for the maintenance of the differentiated osteoblast phenotype.[31]

Both IGF receptors are found on bone cells (osteoblasts and osteoclasts), but the Type I receptor appears to mediate most of the anabolic effects of IGF-I.[32] IGF-II, but not IGF-I, can bind to the Type II receptor, while insulin, IGF-I, and IGF-II can bind to the Type I receptor. Following binding of the IGFs to their receptor, there is activation of protein tyrosine kinases which results in phosphorylation of an insulin receptor substrate (IRS-1) that can influence cell growth and replication.[33] Several calciotropic hormones (e.g., PTH, 1,25 dihydroxyvitamin D) and local skeletal growth factors (e.g., PDGF) can regulate IGF binding to its receptor as well as IRS-I activation.[34]

Besides the control exerted by IGF ligands and their receptors at the level of the osteoblast, another set of regulatory factors for skeletal IGF bioactivity are the expression and production of IGFBPs and IGFBP-specific proteases. As noted previously, all six IGFBPs are produced by osteoblasts, although IGFBP-3, -4, -5 are the most abundant.[1] The calciotropic hormone, PTH, as well as other adenylyl cyclase stimulators, stimulate production of these IGFBPs even though each IGFBP may have a different role in regulating IGF's activity in the skeleton. As noted previously, 1,25 dihydroxyvitamin D3, another calciotropic hormone, can induce IGFBP-4 synthesis in bone cells.[20] Overall, the expression sequence for each IGFBP can be related to the development of the osteoblast phenotype. IGFBP-4 for example, may be an early differentiation switch which slows proliferation of the preosteoblasts and permits expression of specific functional phenotypes. 1,25 dihydroxyvitamin D3, a hormone with strong differentiation-enhancing activity, has long been recognized as a key element in the osteoblastic differentiation scheme.[35] Since 1,25 dihydroxyvitamin D3 is a potent regulator of IGFBP-4 production in skeletal cells, it seems likely that part of the antiproliferative effects of 1,25 dihydroxyvitamin D3 on bone cells could be mediated through induction of this IGFBP.

In general, the IGFBPs either augment or inhibit IGF bioactivity depending on the physiologic milieu in which they are operating. Proteolysis of the IGFBPs, however, can enhance IGF bioactivity by limiting IGFBP binding. IGFBP-specific proteases are active in the skeleton and have recently been described although their precise function is still unclear. One well-known IGFBP-3 specific protease is prostate-specific antigen (PSA), an enzyme produced by prostate cells, which under proper circumstances can support metastatic prostatic growth in bone.[36] An IGFBP-4 specific protease, active at very low pH, can be induced by IGF-I itself.[21] Similarly, IGF-I has been shown to prevent IGFBP-5 proteolysis *in vitro*.[37] Thus, the IGFs can regulate their own IGFBPs through posttranslational modifications. This sets up a cycle whereby the IGFBPs control IGF bioactivity but the IGFs can, in turn, regulate their own IGFBPs. This level of redundancy and control serves to both promote and check the activities of these potent growth factors.

The skeletal regulatory circuit is further complicated by multihormonal control. For example, PTH regulates not only IGFBP production but also induces IGF-I synthesis in osteoblasts. This action may have major pharmacologic significance since anti-IGF-I antibodies prevent PTH induction of collagen matrix synthesis in calvarial cells.[38] Growth hormone can also enhance skeletal IGF-I production in osteoblasts even though it has traditionally been considered as working on chondrocytes at the growth plate. On the other hand, 1,25 dihydroxyvitamin D3 and glucocorticoids both suppress IGF-I expression in normal and transformed osteoblasts.[20] As noted previously, PTH, GH, and insulin also regulate expression of skeletal IGFBPs (IGFBP-1, -4, and-5) and probably the IGFBP proteases necessary for liberating IGFs from their binding proteins.[1] Thus, the bone turnover process, orchestrated by calciotropic hormones and local growth factors, is intimately associated with various IGF regulatory components (see Figure 8.1). Since the IGFs can stimulate bone formation, investigators have begun to consider ways to manipulate components of the IGF regulatory circuit to enhance bone mass in various metabolic bone disorders.

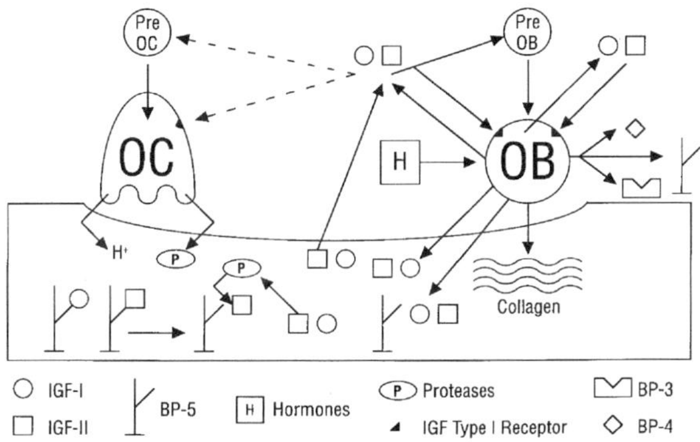

Figure 8.1
This schematic represents the basic multicellular unit (BMU) and its relationship to the IGF regulatory system. Each component of this system plays an integral role in the process of bone remodeling. Osteoblasts (OB) produce IGF-I, IGF-II, and at least three IGFBP-s (-3, -4, -5). The IGFs are liberated from bone matrix (after being bound to IGFBP-5) during the process of bone resorption as osteoclasts (OC) release H^+ and proteolytic enzymes (P). These proteases serve to break down the organic bone matrix but, under the influence of growth factors (including IGF-I/-II), could promote dissociation of the IGFBPs from their IGFs. Both IGFs can act in a paracrine fashion to enhance further production of IGF-I/II or the IGFBPs from OBs. IGFs can also contribute to the circulating pool of growth factors or become dissociated from their respective IGFBPs and act on bone cells. The effects of IGFs on OCs remain somewhat controversial, although it seems likely that some form of OC recruitment can occur under the influence of IGF-I. Systemic hormones (H) (e.g., PTH, 17β-estradiol, vitamin D, thyroid hormone, etc.) can regulate OB synthesis and release of IGFs and IGFBPs. The IGFBPs serve to promote or antagonize the action of the IGFs. In addition, both Type 1 and the Type 2 IGF receptor (Type 2 not shown) are present on OBs and possible OCs. The IGF can promote mitogenesis of OB precursors as well as differentiated functions of mature OBs (collagen synthesis). Therefore, it seems likely that the IGFs are another set of unique polypeptides which may couple the processes of resorption with formation. The reader should be cautioned that the picture is overly simplistic and that many other cytokines and growth factors are involved in the intercellular communication network necessary for the bone remodeling process to occur.

III. APPLICATION OF THE IGFs TO SKELETAL DISORDERS IN ANIMALS

A. General Principles of Targeting Skeletal IGFs

Although it has already been pointed out that the IGFs are logical candidates for anabolic therapy in skeletal diseases, it also clear from the previous discussion that the IGF system in bone and the circulation is complex and redundant. Several layers of control could enhance or prevent locally or systemically administered growth factors from exerting their effects on bone cells. This has led to experimental strategies in animals where the dose, the mode of administration, the vehicle for transport, and the frequency of IGF-I treatment have varied. This discussion will focus on the use of rhIGF-I in various animal models. However, it is important to remember that any strategy to directly administer IGFs to enhance skeletal activity is fraught with potentially serious side effects. Therefore, other experimental approaches which indirectly activate the skeletal IGF system have been considered. The two most common modalities which enhance local IGF-I production are GH and PTH. Each can induce IGF-I production in the skeleton and therefore provide some target specificity. But as noted previously, the major skeletal action of GH is on the growth plate. Its effects on the remodeling unit are generally modest and include activation of both resorption and formation.[39] For example, in hypophysectomized rats, GH is less anabolic to the skeleton than PTH.[40] Moreover, GH raises serum IGF-I levels more than skeletal concentrations, can induce insulin resistance, and may be associated with water retention. PTH, on the other hand, works almost exclusively on skeletal IGF-I (rather than circulatory IGF-I), has been shown to be anabolic when administered intermittently, and can effect change in the remodeling sequence without dramatically altering other aspects of the IGF regulatory system.[41,42] But it is still not clear that all the anabolic properties of PTH are mediated through IGF-I, and long-term studies with this agent have only just begun. In lieu of those considerations, this section will focus on administration of IGF-I to experimental animals.

B. Types of Administration and Experimental Models

The experimental paradigms in which IGF-I administration has been utilized to effect skeletal changes are quite varied. In general, though, studies with rhIGF-I have included: 1) administration to GH-deficient or GH-resistant animals, and 2) treatment of specific skeletal conditions in which IGF-I may positively affect bone formation, such as diabetes, ovariectomy (OVX), immobilization, or aging. In each study, the mode of administration and the length of the studies have also varied, making interpretation of data from these *in vivo* studies somewhat difficult.

Early studies reported that rhIGF-I profoundly affected linear growth in hypophysectomized animals.[43] But besides increasing skeletal length, it was clear that parenterally administered IGFs also increased body weight and organ size.[44] In particular, lymph tissue, the spleen and the thymus, hypertrophied in response to rhIGF-I.[44] This effect was not nearly as pronounced when rhGH was administered although weight gain and water retention in animals were common features of both these types of treatment. Still, IGF-I dramatically affected linear growth. Using a murine GH knockout model which was manipulated to over-express IGF-I, Behringer et al. convincingly demonstrated that IGF-I can compensate for complete absence of GH by promoting linear growth and weight gain.[45]

Although the effects of rhIGF-I on linear growth in GH-deficient animals were clear cut, IGF-I activity on other skeletal parameters and in other conditions has been somewhat inconsistent. For example, Tobias found opposing effects of IGF-I on formation of trabecular bone compared to cortical bone in adult female rats.[46] In genetically GH-deficient mice *(lit/lit)* given rhIGF-I for two weeks, body weight increased, but bone mineral content did not.[47] Similarly, Rosen et al. administered a high dose of rhIGF-I to normal 12-week-old rats and found that although linear growth was stimulated, bone mineral density actually declined.[48] In each case, the effects of IGF-I on the cartilaginous growth plate differed from its actions on the modeling process.

Another complicating factor in terms of skeletal responsiveness (bone mineral content, bone density, histomorphometric indices, and cellular parameters) to rhIGF-I has been the status of the IGF regulatory system in the experimental model. For example, GH-deficient animals have low levels of IGFBP-3, therefore administration of IGF-I may lead to more bioavailable IGF-I at a dose lower than conventional therapy would predict. On the other hand, starving rats have more IGFBP-1 (and possibly more IGFBP-4) in the circulation, may have greater peripheral resistance to parenterally administered IGFs (via alterations in receptor number or postreceptor messengers), and therefore require higher doses of IGF-I to induce a significant skeletal effect. Since the goal of IGF therapy in skeletal disorders is to enhance bone formation, knowledge of the perturbations in the IGF regulatory system of the model being tested is essential for understanding potential end points of efficacy.

This principle is exemplified by application of rhIGF-I therapy in two experimental systems, diabetic osteopenia and immobilization-induced osteoporosis. In both conditions, the pathophysiologic problem is reduced bone formation. Therefore, a therapy which would enhance osteoblastic activity (e.g., IGF-I) would be ideal. However, administration of rhIGF-I to spontaneously diabetic BB rats with low bone formation and osteopenia did not change epiphyseal width, osteoblast surface, or osteocalcin concentrations.[49] Similarly, Bickle et al.[50] treated hindlimb-immobilized male rats with very high doses of rhIGF-I and failed to find changes in bone formation parameters. Undoubtedly, in both models, there was either resistance at the receptor level to IGF-I, or increased amounts of inhibitory IGFBPs which interfered with IGF coupling to its receptor. These studies are further evidence that a full understanding of the IGF regulatory system both in the skeleton and in the circulation of the experimental model is critical when considering the results of treatment with IGF-I.

Although IGF-I treatment in those two conditions has been somewhat disappointing, rhIGF-I has been successfully used in models of low bone mass associated with ovariectomy. Since postmenopausal changes in bone mass are the most common cause of increased skeletal fragility and fractures in humans, experimental studies have focused on the application of rhIGF-I in ovariectomized (OVX) animals. Kalu et al.[51] were the first to report that subcutaneous injections of rhIGF-I to adult OVX rats led to partial restoration of femoral calcium content and trabecular bone volume compared to vehicle-treated OVX animals. However, IGF-I did not increase the actual number of osteoblasts (or osteoclasts) beyond OVX control levels. This may be due to the fact that OVX in rats itself leads to short-term increases in serum levels of IGF-I and IGFBP-3 as well as a transient rise in linear growth and osteoblast number.[52] Ammann et al.[53] also demonstrated that continuous infusions of rhIGF-I to OVX rats for six weeks enhanced periosteal bone apposition and midshaft tibial and lumbar bone mineral density. However, bone strength and stiffness were not affected by this treatment. More recently, Mueller et al.[54] proved that daily subcutaneous treatment with rhIGF-I (0.2-0.8 mg/kg/d) to adult OVX animals increased osteoid and triple tetracycline labeled surfaces as well as mineral apposition rates and trabecular bone volume. The highest doses of rhIGF-I also increased osteoclast number on bone biopsy.

Major changes in osteoclast number and activity associated with rhIGF-I treatment are not totally unexpected when the role of IGF-I as a coupling agent in remodeling is considered. As noted earlier, both IGF receptors have been found on osteoclasts, and IGF-I can directly enhance recruitment and activation of preosteoclasts.[28] These *in vitro* data are reinforced by human studies with rhIGF-I and rhGH which have confirmed that these treatments can lead to dose-dependent increases in bone resorption.[55] Thus, some of the variability in bone responsiveness to IGFs can be accounted for by differential activation of osteoclast activity.

Systemically administered IGF-I can also cause hypoglycemia as well as weight gain and organ hypertrophy. Two alternative approaches have been considered: 1) direct infusion of IGF-I into bone, and 2) complexing IGF-I to carrier proteins. In the former case, Spencer et al.[56] demonstrated that intra-arterial infusion of rhIGF-I into the right hindlimb of ambulatory rats for 14 days led to increased cortical and trabecular bone formation, along with increased osteoblast number. However, no other studies using this approach have been published. Therefore it is likely that this method will not turn out to be practical. On the other hand, the complexing of IGF-I to IGFBP-3 has tremendous potential. As noted earlier, IGFBP-3 is the largest IGFBP and the principal carrier of IGFs in the circulation.

When bound to IGF-I and the ALS, it serves as a circulating storage depot for the IGFs and to protect the organism against the hypoglycemic effects of the IGFs. Moreover, IGFBP-3 is produced by osteoblasts, and under the right *in vitro* conditions can augment IGF's stimulatory activity. Coupling of IGF-I to IGFBP-3 in equimolar concentrations could theoretically prolong the half-life of circulating IGF-I as well as promoting IGFs skeletal activity.

The use of rhIGF-I/IGFBP-3 to stimulate bone formation has been accomplished in rats. In the initial studies, Bagi et al.[57] treated 16-week-old OVX rats with diluent, rhIGF-I (0.9 and 2.6 mg/kg/day) or rhIGF-I/IGFBP-3 in a 1:1 molar ratio (0.9, 2.6 and 7.5 mg/kg/day) for eight weeks. At the end of the treatment periods, measures of bone growth and turnover were studied by fluorochrome labeling. Not unexpectedly both IGF-I and IGF-I/IGFBP-3 increased linear growth to the same extent, and these changes were associated with marked enhancement in lean body mass. However the complex of IGF-I/IGFBP-3 more markedly increased bone formation than rhIGF-I (see Figure 8.2). This was best exemplified in trabecular areas (e.g., the lumbar vertebrae) where bone thickness increased significantly in both IGF-I- and IGF-I/IGFBP-3 treated groups although the highest doses of the complex provided the greatest stimulus to new bone formation. In addition to structural trabecular changes, femoral bone mineral density and content were also increased as were periosteal, modeling-dependent bone surfaces on the endocortical envelope. This resulted in a greater increase in cortical thickness in animals treated with IGF-I/IGFBP-3 than in those treated with IGF-I alone. Along with enhanced thickness, connectivity was preserved post-OVX when IGF-I/IGFBP-3 was administered.[58] These structural changes were also associated with increases in the mechanical strength of the bone.[59]

Thus, in several studies, the IGF-I/IGFBP-3 complex appears to be superior to IGF-I in modulating changes in both cortical and trabecular architecture. Almost certainly this is a result of delivering higher doses of rhIGF-I by way of the IGF-I/IGFBP-3 complex. This can be successfully accomplished because there are few side effects associated with high doses of IGF-I when administered complexed to IGFBP-3. On the other hand, at the highest dose of rhIGF-I alone nearly half the animals developed severe hypoglycemia, but no hypoglycemia was noted in any animal treated with the 7.5 mg/kg/day dose of rhIGF-I/IGFBP-3.[57-60] Thus the complex can deliver high circulating levels of IGF-I without the side effects associated with increased free concentrations of this growth factor. This alone has raised the possibility that this complex may be particularly useful in managing certain bone disorders associated with low bone mass in humans. However, some caution should be used in interpreting these data. First, it should be noted that these studies were done in rats, animals which differ significantly from humans in their skeletal modeling–remodeling processes. Second, these are short-term studies in animals. Long-term safety and efficacy in humans remain to be established. Third, it is

(a)

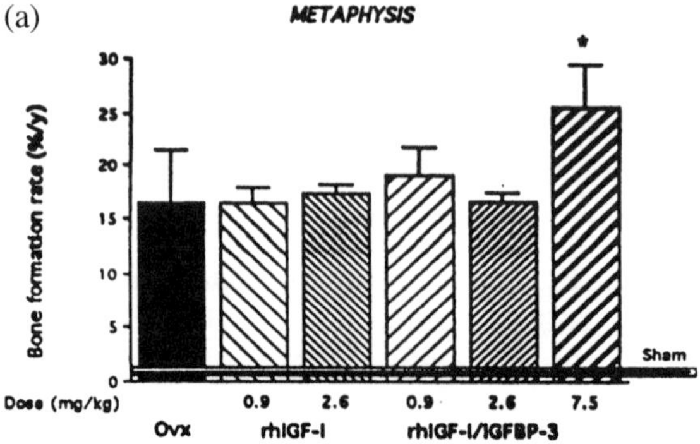

(b)

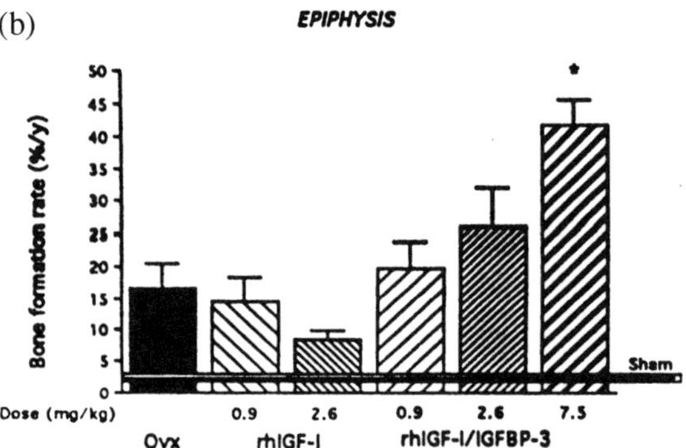

(c)

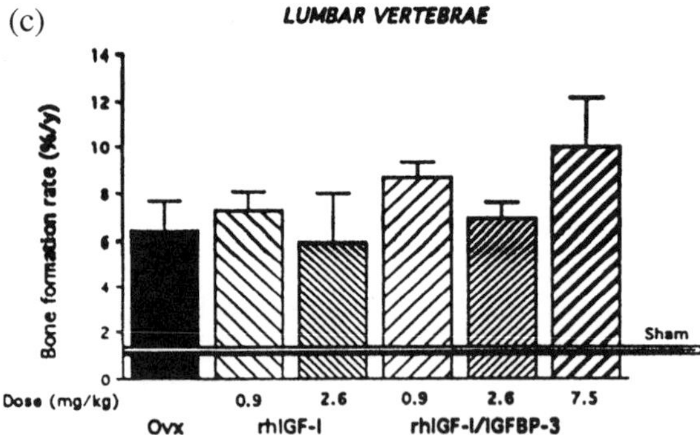

Figure 8.2
Dose-related effects of rhIGF-I and rhIGF-I/IGFBP-3 complex on bone formation rate in metaphyses (A), epiphyses (B), and lumbar vertebral bodies (C) after 8 weeks of treatment. Each column shows the mean ± SEM; *p <0.05 versus OVX group by analysis of variance followed by Dunnett's test. Data for sham group are included for comparison only. (From Bagi, C. M., Brommage, R., Deleon, L., Adams, S., Rosen, D., and Sommer, A., *J. Bone Min. Res.*, 9, 1301, 1994. With permission.)

unclear how much bone resorption is stimulated during treatment with the complex and whether long-term therapy will result in a new remodeling balance without significant increases in bone mass. However, despite these potential uncertainties, data from the IGF/IGFBP-3 trials are certainly promising and do warrant further studies.

In summary, animal studies designed to use rhIGF-I to enhance skeletal mass provide a mixed picture. At relatively high doses, bone formation can be stimulated and linear growth is generally accelerated. Changes in bone resorption occur, but they are not as great as the increases in bone formation. However, organ hypertrophy, fluid retention, and hypoglycemia are potential limiting factors. In addition, not all animal models of reduced bone formation respond to rhIGF-I treatment. On the other hand, ovariectomized animals respond positively to rhIGF treatment by enhancing bone mass and connectivity. Treatments which include IGF-I complexed to IGFBP-3 may provide higher local doses of IGF-I while limiting systemic side effects.

IV. HUMAN STUDIES WITH rhIGF-I

A. Introduction

The central role of IGF-I in the bone remodeling process implied by experimental studies has inspired clinical investigations with rhIGF-I. The major issue has been to establish whether there is a potential use for rhIGF-I as an anabolic agent in osteoporosis.[60] So far, only short-term controlled trials have been performed with treatment periods between 6 and 42 days. Therefore, the effects on bone metabolism have been estimated by biochemical markers in serum and urine. These so-called biomarkers are proteins and enzymes released from bone cells or bone matrix during the remodeling process and are assumed to reflect the activity of the osteoblasts and the osteoclasts. Bone cell activity estimated by biomarkers is considered to reflect ongoing bone formation and resorption. However, it is difficult to estimate the net effect on bone mass and bone structure from studies of changes in biomarkers in response to a specific therapy. Nevertheless, the use of biomarkers provides a tool for detecting effects on bone metabolism by a specific treatment and finding out whether the treatment enhances or inhibits the remodeling process.

B. Studies with rhIGF-I

The first study which examined the effect of rhIGF-I on bone metabolism was performed in a single patient, a 59-year-old man with idiopathic osteoporosis who received 80 μg/kg of rhIGF-I subcutaneously twice per day for one week.[61] Potent effects were seen on both bone formation and bone resorption during the treatment week according to the changes in bone biomarkers (osteocalcin, PICP [procollagen type I C-terminal peptide], bone-specific alkaline phosphatase, cross-linked collagen type I telopeptide, and fasting urinary excretion of hydroxyproline and calcium). During a follow-up period of several weeks, there was a sustained increase in indices of bone formation in serum, whereas the urinary excretion of calcium was reduced. These skeletal stimulatory effects were recently confirmed in several other controlled studies.[62-68]

Ebeling et al.[62] treated 18 healthy postmenopausal women for six days with different doses of rhIGF-I (30, 60, 120, or 180 μg/kg/day). All doses resulted in increased serum levels of PICP, a peptide released during the synthesis of procollagen type I, in a dose-dependent manner with mean percentage increase ranging from 20 to 79% of baseline values. Increased urinary levels of deoxypyridinoline, a bone-specific crosslink of mature collagen type I released during bone resorption, were seen in the higher dose groups, ranging from 31 to 59%. There was no significant effect on bone resorption in the group receiving 30 μg/kg, indicating that a low dose of rhIGF-I selectively enhanced bone formation.

Stimulation of bone formation without enhancement of bone resorption was also seen in the lowest dose group from a study of 24 men with idiopathic osteoporosis who received 20, 40, or 80 μg/kg of rhIGF-I daily for six weeks.[63] In this trial, sustained stimulation of bone metabolism was present after six weeks of daily injections with rhIGF-I. The effects were most pronounced on the indices of collagen turnover, with dose-dependent increases in serum levels of PICP ranging from 12 to 34% of baseline values, and urinary levels of deoxypyridinoline ranging from 4 (not significant) to 39%.

The possibility of stimulating bone formation selectively with a low dose of rhIGF-I is appealing. Histomorphometric studies in rats suggest that increased resorption is present when higher doses of IGF-I are used, whereas lower doses lead to a sustained increase in bone mass.[54] Furthermore, in humans, doses higher than 40 to 60 μg/kg/day of rhIGF-I were accompanied by frequent side effects such as tachycardia, nausea, and headache.[62-64] All side effects subside when treatment is discontinued or the dose is reduced. In a study of young healthy women, a glucose infusion was given concomitantly with a relatively high dose of rhIGF-I (100 μg/kg/twice/day) and no side effects were seen during six days of treatment.[65] Hypoglycemia is the most feared side effect due to the insulin-like action of IGF-I but interestingly was not noted in this particular study.

Injecting relatively high doses of rhIGF-I into fasting healthy young women for six days resulted in a substantial elevation of indices of bone formation without affecting bone resorption.[65] The discrepancy between the dose-dependent increase in both resorption and formation in the studies on postmenopausal women and osteoporotic men, and the stimulation of bone formation but not resorption in fasting premenopausal women could be due to several factors. Besides the presence of estrogen and the younger age of the women studied by Grinspoon et al.,[65] all subjects had fasted for four days before treatment with placebo or rhIGF-I and continued to do so during the entire study. During the four-day fasting period, indices of bone metabolism in serum and urine dropped by approximately 50%, and when the rhIGF-I treatment was completed at day 10, the serum levels of both osteocalcin and PICP were increased compared to the levels in placebo-treated patients, whereas resorption indices were not. This could indicate that bone resorption was inhibited by a mechanism that could not be overcome by IGF-I.

Another effect of fasting is that serum levels of IGF-I decrease considerably, while IGFBP-1 levels rise dramatically. This particular IGFBP is inversely related to insulin, and, under experimental conditions, inhibits IGF action. Furthermore, IGFBP-3 levels in serum were reduced following treatment with rhIGF-I. Changes in systemic and local levels of one or more IGFBPs could have important regulatory effects on the skeletal action of IGF-I.

All these studies indicate that systemic IGF-I profoundly affects bone metabolism. The exact mechanism is not known, but direct actions on bone cells are likely according to the previously described experimental studies *in vitro* and *in vivo*. It has also been shown that IGF-I acts to increase the 1α-hydroxylation of 25-hydroxyvitamin D3 in the kidney,[69] which is another way IGF-I may affect skeletal calcium balance.

C. Studies with rhGH and/or rhIGF-I

Growth hormone is secreted from the pituitary throughout life, although in diminishing amounts in the 7th decade and beyond. GH exerts many of its effects via increased local and systemic levels of IGF-I. GH treatment in adults can result in increased bone turnover, both in GHD (growth hormone deficient) patients, and in subjects with normal GH secretion.[70,71] A few studies have evaluated the differences in bone metabolism between rhIGF-I and rhGH. In a double-blind crossover study with twelve weeks of wash-out and follow-up between treatments, the effects of rhIGF-I were compared to those of rhGH in men with idiopathic osteoporosis, aged 32 to 57 years.[64] The doses used (80 μg/kg/day of rhIGF-I and 2 U/m^2 of rhGH) resulted in 30% higher circulating IGF I levels during treatment with rhGH than with rhIGF-I. Both treatments resulted in increased bone turnover according to changes in biochemical indices, especially osteocalcin where there was a 20% increase in both treatment groups after only four days of rhIGF-I and seven days of rhGH. There was a mean increase of 29% in type I collagen synthesis (as measured by PICP) and a 44% increase in urinary deoxypyridinoline (reflecting breakdown of type I collagen) following rhGH treatment compared to a 43% increase in PICP and a 29% increase in deoxypyridinoline excretion after seven days of rhIGF-I injections. The increase in PICP was seen after four days of rhIGF-I and after seven days of rhGH, whereas the enhancement of bone resorption was detected after four days of rhGH and not until day seven of rhIGF-I. Thus, there was a more pronounced elevation in PICP during rhIGF-I ($p < 0.05$) than during rhGH treatment. These differences could reflect contrasts in study design or unequivalent doses, but could also represent difference in their basic mechanism of skeletal action.

Ghiron et al.[66] studied 16 healthy elderly women of mean age 72 years who received rhGH (25 µg/kg/day) or rhIGF-I in a high (60 µg/kg twice daily)- or low (15 µg/kg twice daily)-dose regimen for 4 weeks. After three weeks of treatment, the increases in bone biomarkers reached their maximum. High dose rhIGF-I and GH stimulated both bone formation and bone resorption, whereas there was only enhanced bone formation in the group receiving the low dose of rhIGF-I. Qualitatively, the difference between GH and rhIGF-I with regard to the effects on bone and calcium metabolism may also be related to the effects on the handling of phosphate in the kidney. Similar results have been obtained in healthy men by Bianda et al.[67]

There is one report concerning long-term treatment with rhIGF-I in a postmenopausal woman with the Werner's syndrome, osteoporosis, and a low serum IGF-I concentration.[68] Along with estrogen substitution therapy, rhIGF-I was given in increasing doses from 30 to 75 µg/kg/day but was reduced to 60 µg/kg/day when side effects occurred and supraphysiological serum concentrations of IGF-I were detected. She was treated with rhIGF-I for 26 weeks, and along with clearly increased biomarker levels in serum and urine, bone mineral density of the spine increased by 3% compared to baseline after three and six months of therapy.

D. Conclusions Concerning the Use of rhIGF-I in Humans

According to these studies, subcutaneous injections with rhIGF-I have significant effects on the bone-remodeling process in doses which are tolerable to patients. Whether this presumed activation of remodeling can be used as an anabolic treatment for osteoporosis is yet to be determined. Several authors have reported that a low dose of rhIGF-I, 20 to 30 µg/kg/day, increased the levels of formation indices despite little effects on bone resorption. This suggests a direct effect on the osteoblast. Theoretically, repeated low doses of rhIGF-I could be used to support differentiated osteoblastic function. This would be of special benefit in syndromes of osteopenia where bone formation is impaired, e.g., idiopathic osteoporosis in young individuals and glucocorticoid-induced osteoporosis. However, much longer studies which include estimates of bone mass, strength, and structure will be necessary before conclusions regarding the anabolic potentials of rhIGF-I can be drawn.

V. FUTURE PROSPECTS

In order for a prospective anabolic agent to be effective on the skeleton in humans several criteria must be met. These include: 1) the ability to stimulate bone formation over bone resorption; 2) maximal skeletal activity with minimal actions on noncalcified tissues; 3) enhancement in bone strength as well as density; and 4) absence of serious side effects. rhIGF-I has been shown to stimulate new bone formation and to be anabolic for the skeleton in animal and human studies. However, it is still not clear if the long-term effects of rhIGF-I on remodeling will permit a continual increase in bone mass over time. IGF-I is a ubiquitous polypeptide expressed in many tissues. Thus, systemic administration of rhIGF-I may not permit selective targeting to bone, and therefore may lead to unwanted side effects. Finally, there are few studies of bone strength and mechanical capacity in IGF-I treated animals. Hence, a final judgment about the efficacy of rhIGF-I as an anabolic agent in the treatment of metabolic bone diseases has yet to be written. It is clear though that skeletal IGFs represent an important final common pathway for hormonal regulation of remodeling. It remains to be seen whether hormonal agents which enhance skeletal IGF-I selectively may prove more beneficial in clinical trials than systemic administration of the intact peptide, or the peptide bound to a carrier protein. However, this is not to say that there may be limited utility for rhIGF-I in catabolic states such as anorexia nervosa or after hip fractures. Additional studies will be able to address the effect of rhIGF-I in those conditions. In the meantime, a better understanding of the skeletal IGF regulatory system may provide investigators with other therapeutic options (including recombinant IGFBPs or protease inhibitors) in the future to treat the syndromes of low bone mass.

ACKNOWLEDGMENT

This work was supported in part by a grant from the National Institutes of Aging RO 10942-02.

REFERENCES

1. Rosen, C. J., Donahue, L. R., and Hunter, S. J., IGFs and bone: the osteoporosis connection, *Proc. Soc. Exp. Biol. Med.*, 206, 83, 1994.

2. Blum, W. F., Hall, K., Ranke, M. B., and Wilton, P., Growth hormone insensitivity syndromes: a preliminary report on changes in IGFs and their binding proteins during treatment with recombinant IGF-I, *Acta Pediatr. Suppl.*, 391, 15, 1993.
3. Bautista, C. M., Mohan, S., and Baylink, D. J., IGFs are present in the skeletal tissues of vertebrates, *Metabolism*, 39, 96, 1990.
4. Mohan, S. and Baylink, D. J., Autocrine and paracrine aspects of bone metabolism, *Growth Genet. Hormone*, 6, 1, 1990.
5. Canalis, E., Pash, J., and Varghese, S., Skeletal growth factor, *Crit. Rev. Eukaryot. Gene Express.*, 3, 155, 1993.
6. Nicholas, V., Prewett, A., Bettica, P., Mohan, S., Finkleman, R. D., Baylink, D. J., and Farley, J. R., Age-related decreases in IGF-I and transforming growth factors-beta in femoral cortical bone from both men and women: implications for bone loss with aging, *J. Clin. Endocrinol. Metab.*, 78, 1011, 1994.
7. Clemmons, D. R., Hubner, C. C., Jones, J. I., McCusker, R. H., and Busby, W. H., IGFBPs: mechanisms of action at the cellular leve, in *Modern Concepts of IGF*, Spencer, E. M., Ed., Elsevier, New York, 1991, 475.
8. Clemmons, D. R., Smith-Banks, A., and Underwood, L. E., Reversal of diet induced catabolism by infusion of IGF-I in humans, *J. Clin. Endocrinol. Metab.*, 75, 234, 1992.
9. Rosen, C. J., Donahue, L. R., and Hunter, S. J., Age-related changes in insulin-like growth factor binding proteins, *J. Clin. Endocrinol. Metab.*, 71, 575, 1990.
10. Jones, J. I. and Clemmons, D. R., IGFs and their binding proteins: biological actions. *Endocrine Revs.*, 3, 1995.
11. Bondy, C. A., Clinical Uses of IGF-I, *Ann. Intern. Med.*, 120, 593, 1994.
12. Martin, J. L. and Baxter, R. C., IGFBP-3: Biochemistry and physiology, *Growth Regul.*, 2, 8, 1992.
13. Blum, W. F., Albertsson-Wikkland, K., Rosberg, S., and Ranke, M. B., Serum levels of IGF-I and IGFBP-3 reflect spontaneous GH secretion, *J. Clin. Endocrinol. Metab.*, 76, 1610, 1993.
14. Holly, J. M. and Wass, J. A., IGFs: Autocrine, paracrine or endocrine new perspectives of the somatomedin hypothesis in the light of recent developments, *J. Endocrinol.*, 122, 611, 1989.
15. Binoux, M., Hossenlopp, P., Lassarre, C., and Segovia, B., Degradation of IGFBP-3 by proteases: physiological implications, in *Modern Concepts of the IGFs*, Spencer, E. M., Ed., Elsevier, New York, 1991, 327.
16. Valentis, B., Bhala, A., and De Angelis, T., The human IGFBP-3 inhibits the growth of fibroblasts with a targeted disruption of the IGF-I receptor gene, *Mol. Endocrinol.*, 9, 361, 1995.
17. Buckbinder, L., Talbott, R., Velasco-Miguel, S., Takenaka, I., Faha, B., Seixinger, B. R., and Kley, N., Induction of the growth inhibitor IGFBP-3 by p53, *Nature*, 377, 646, 1996.
18. Schmid, C., Ernst, M., Zapf, J., and Froesch, E. R., Release of IGFBPs by osteoblasts: stimulation by estradiol and GH, *Biochem. Biophys. Res. Commun.*, 160, 788, 1989.
19. Mohan, S., IGFBPs in bone cell regulation, *Growth Regulation*, 3, 67, 1993.
20. Scharla, S. H., Strong, D. D., Mohan, S., Baylink, D. J., and Linkhart, T. A., 1,25 dihydroxyvitamin D differentially regulates the production of IGF-I and IGFBP-4 in mouse osteoblasts, *Endocrinology*, 129, 3139, 1991.
21. Durham, S. K., Riggs, B. L., and Conover, C. A., IGFBP-4 IGFBP-4 protease system in normal human osteoblast-like cells, *J. Clin. Endocrinol. Metab.*, 79, 1752, 1994.
22. Conover, C. A., Bale, L. K., Clarkson, J. T., and Torring, O., Regulation of IGFBP-5 mRNA expression and protein availability in rat osteoblast-like cells, *Endocrinology*, 132, 2525, 1993.
23. Conover, C. A., Lee, P. D. K., Riggs, B. L., and Powell, D. L., IGFBP-1 expression in human bone cells: regulation by glucocorticoids and insulin, *Endocrine Society Meeting*, 1996, p. 730.
24. Humbel, R. E., IGF-I and IGF-II, *Eur. J. Biochem.*, 190, 445, 1990.

25. LeRoith, D., Werner, H., Beitner-Johnsson, D., and Roberts, C. T., Molecular and cellular aspects of the IGF-I receptor, *Endocrine Revs.*, 16, 143, 1995.
26. Zapf, J., Schmid, C., and Froesch, E. R., Biological and immunological properties of IGF-I and IGF-II, *Clin. Endocrinol. Metab.*, 13, 3, 1984.
27. Slootweg, M. C., Most, W. W., Van Beek, E., Schot, L. P. C., Papapuculs, S. E., and Löwik, C. W. G. M., Osteoclast formation together with IL-6 production in mouse long bones is increased by IGF-I, *J. Endocrinol.*, 132, 432, 1992.
28. Mochizuki, H., Hakeda, Y., Wakatsuki, N., Usui, N., Akashi, S., Sato, T., Tanaka, K., and Kumegawa, M., IGF-I supports formation and activation of osteoclasts, *Endocrinology*, 131, 1075, 1991.
29. Canalis, E., Centrella, M., and McCarthy, T. L., Regulation of IGF II production in bone cultures, *Endocrinology*, 129, 2457, 1991.
30. McCarthy, T. L., Centrella, M., and Canalis, E., Regulatory effects of IGF-I and IGF-II on bone collagen synthesis in rat calvarial cultures, *Endocrinology*, 124, 301, 1989.
31. Canalis, E., Skeletal growth factors, in *Osteoporosis*, Marcus, R., Feldman, D., and Kelsey, J., Eds., Academic Press, San Diego, 1996, 266.
32. Centrella, M., McCarthy, T. L., and Canalis, E., Receptors for IGF-I and IGF-II in osteoblast-enriched cultures from fetal rat bone, *Endocrinology*, 126, 39, 1990.
33. Meyers, M. G., Sun, X. J., Cheatham, B., Jachna, B. R., Glasheen, E. M., Backer, J. M., and White, M. F., IRS-1 is a common element in insulin and IGF-I signalling to the phosphatidylinositol 3′ kinase, *Endocrinology*, 132, 1421, 1993.
34. Rubini, M., Werner, H., Gandini, E., Roberts, C. T., LeRoith, D., and Baserga, R., PDG increases the activity of the promoter of the IGF-I receptor gene, *Exp. Cell Res.*, 211, 374, 1994.
35. Lian, J. B. and Stein, G. S., Osteoblast biology, in *Osteoporosis*, Marcus, R., Feldman, D., and Kelsey J., Eds., Academic Press, San Diego, 1996, 23.
36. Cohen, P., Graves, H. C., Peehl, D. M., Kamarei, L., Giudice, L. C., and Rosenfeld, R. G., PSA is an IGFBP3 protease found in seminal plasma, *J. Clin. Endocrinol. Metab.*, 75, 1046, 1992.
37. Kanzaki, S., Hilliker, S., Baylink, D. J., and Mohan, S., Evidence that human bone cells in culture produced IGFBP-4 and -5 proteases, *Endocrinology*, 134, 383, 1994.
38. Canalis, E., Centrella, M., Burch, W., and McCarthy, T. L., IGF-I mediates selective anabolic effects of PTH in bone cultures, *J. Clin. Invest.*, 83, 60, 1989.
39. Holloway, L., Butterfield, G., Hintz, R. L., Gesundheit, N. M., and Marcus, R. M., Effects of human GH on metabolic indices, body composition and bone turnover in healthy elderly women, *J. Clin. Endocrinol. Metab.*, 79, 470, 1994.
40. Dobnig, H. and Turner, R. T., Evidence that intermittent treatment with PTH increases bone formation in adult rats by activation of bone lining cells, *Endocrinology*, 136, 3632, 1995.
41. Mosekilde, L. and Reeve J., Treatment with PTH peptides, in *Osteoporosis*, Marcus, J., Feldman, D., and Kelsey, J., Eds., Academic Press, San Diego, 1996, 1293.
42. Watson, P., Lazowski, D., Han, V., Fraher, L. J., Steer, B., and Hodsman, A. B., PTH restores bone mass and enhances osteoblast IGF-I gene expression in ovariectomized rats, *Bone*, 16, 357, 1995.
43. Schoenle, E., Zapf, J., Humbel, R. E., and Froesch, E. R., IGF-I stimulates growth in hypophysectomized rats, *Nature*, 296, 252, 1982.
44. Guler, H. P., Zapf, J., Scheweiller, E., and Froeach, E. R., Recombinant IGF-I stimulates growth and has distinct effects on organ size in hypophysectomized rats, *Proc. Natl. Acad. Sci. USA*, 85, 4889, 1988.
45. Behringer, R. R., Lewin, T. M., Quaife, C. J., Palmitier, R. D., Brinster, R. I., and D'Ercole, A. J., Expression of IGF-I stimulates normal somatic growth in GH deficient mice, *Endocrinology*, 123, 1033, 1990.
46. Tobias, J. H., Chow, J. W. M., and Chambers, T. J., Opposite effects of IGF-I on the formation of trabecular and cortical bone in adult female rats, *Endocrinology*, 131, 2387, 1992.

47. Donahue, L. E., Watson, G., and Beamer, W. G., Regulation of metabolic water and protein compartments by IGF-I and, testosterone in GH deficient lit/lit mice, *J. Endocrinol.*, 139, 431, 1993.
48. Rosen, H. N., Chen, V., Cittadini, A., Greenspan, S. L., Douglas, P. S., Moses, A. C., and Beamer, W. G., Treatment with rhGH and IGF-I in rats increases bone mineral content but not bone density, *J. Bone Min. Res.*, 10, 1352, 1995.
49. Verhage, J., Duiker, A. M. H., Visser, W. J., van Herck, E., Van Bree, R., and Bouillon, R., The effects of systemic insulin, IGF-I and GH on bone growth and turnover in spontaneously diabetic BB rats, *J. Endocrinol.*, 134, 173, 1992.
50. Bickle, D. D., Harris, J., Halloran, B. P., and Morey-Holton, E. R., Skeletal unloading induces resistance to IGF-I, *J. Bone Min. Res.*, 9, 1789, 1994.
51. Kalu, D. N., Liu, C. C., Salerno, E., Salih, M., Echon, R., Ray, M., and Hollis, B. W., IGF-I partially prevents ovariectomy-induced bone loss: a comparative study with PTH, *J. Bone Min. Res.*, S1, 548, 1991.
52. Kalu, D. N., Arjmandi, B. H., Liu, C. C., Salih, M. A., and Birnbaum, R. S., Effects of ovariectomy and estrogen on the serum levels of IGF-I and IGFBP-3, *Bone Miner.*, 25, 135, 1994.
53. Ammann, P., Rizzoli, R., Meyer, J. M., Slosman, D., and Bonjour, J. P., IGF-I and pamidronate increase bone mineral density in ovariectomized adult rats, *Am. J. Physiol.*, 265, E770, 1993.
54. Mueller, K., Cortesi, R., Modrowski, D., and Marie, P. J., Stimulation of trabecular bone formation by IGF-I in adult ovariectomized, *Am. J. Physiol.*, 267, E1, 1994.
55. Eberling, P. R., Jones, J. D., O'Fallon, W. M., Janes, C. H., and Riggs, B. L., Short term effects of recombinant hIGF-I on bone turnover in normal women, *J. Clin. Endocrinol. Metab.*, 77, 1384, 1993.
56. Spencer, E. M., Liu, C. C., Si, E. C. C., and Howard, G. A., In vivo actions of IGF-I on bone formation and resorption in rats, *Bone*, 12, 1991.
57. Bagi, C. M., Brommage, R., Deleon, L., Adams, S., Rosen, D., and Sommer, A., Benefit of systemically administered rhIGF-I and rhIGF-I/IGFBP-3 on cancellous bone in ovariectomized rats, *J. Bone Min. Res.*, 9, 1301, 1994.
58. Bagi, C., Meulen, M. V., Brommage, R., Rosen, D., and Sommer, A., The effect of systemically administered rhIGF-I/IGFBP-3 complex on cortical bone strength and structure in ovariectomized rats, *Bone*, 16, 559, 1995.
59. Bagi, C. M., DeLeon, E., Brommage, R., Rosen, D., and Sommer, A., Treatment of ovariectomized rats with the complex of rhIGF-I/IGFBP-3 increases cortical and cancellous bone mass and improves structure in the femoral neck, *Calcif. Tissue Int.*, 57, 40, 1995.
60. Johannson, A. G. and Rosen, C. J., IGF-I as potential therapy in metabolic bone diseases, in *Bone Biology of Bone*, Raisz, L. G., Rodan, G., and Bilezikian, J., Eds., Academic Press, San Diego, 1996, chapter 79.
61. Johansson, A. G., Lindh, E., and Ljunghall, S., IGF-I stimulates bone turnover in osteoporosis, *Lancet*, 339, 1619, 1992.
62. Ebeling, P. R., Jones, J. D., O'Fallon, W. M., Janes, C. H., and Riggs, B. L., Short term effects of recombinant human IGF-I on bone turnover in normal women, *J. Clin. Endocrinol. Metab.*, 77, 1384, 1993.
63. Johansson, A. G., Lindh, E., Kollerup, G., and Ljunghall, S., Dose dependent effects of IGF-I on the metabolism of collagen type I in male osteoporosis, *J. Bone Min. Res.*, 10, S249, 1995.
64. Johansson, A. G., Lindh, E., Blum, W. F., Kollerup, G., Sorensen, O. H., and Ljunghall, S., Effects of growth hormone and IGF-I in men with idiopathic osteoporosis, *J. Clin. Endocrinol. Metab.*, 81, 44, 1996.
65. Grinspoon, S. K., Baum, H. B. A., Peterson, S., and Klibanski, A., Effects of rhIGF-I administration on bone turnover during short-term fasting, *J. Clin. Invest.*, 96, 900, 1995.

66. Ghiron, L. J., Thompson, J. L., Holloway, L., Hintz, R. L., Butterfield, G. E., Hoffman, A. R., and Marcus, R., Effects of recombinant IGF-I and growth hormone on bone turnover in elderly women, *J. Bone Min. Res.*, 10, 1844, 1995.
67. Bianda, T. L., Schmid, C., Hussain, M. A., Keller, A., Glatz, Y., Bouillon, R., and Froesch, E. R., Effects of short term IGF-I or growth hormone treatment on bone turnover, renal phosphate reabsorption and calcitriol production in healthy man, *J. Bone Min. Res.*, 10, S192, 1995.
68. Rubin, C. D., Reed, B., Sakhaee, K., and Pak, C. Y. C., Treating a patient with the Werner syndrome and osteoporosis using recombinant IGF-I, *Ann. Intern. Med.*, 121, 665, 1994.
69. Nesbitt, T. and Drezner, M. K., IGF-I regulation of renal 25 hydroxyvitamin D-1-hydroxylase activity, *Endocrinology,* 132, 133, 1993.
70. Brixen, K., Nielsen, H. K., Mosekilde, L., and Flyvbjerg, A., A short course of recombinant human growth hormone treatment stimulates osteoblasts and activates bone remodeling in normal human volunteers, *J. Bone Min. Res.*, 5, 609, 1990.
71. Binnerts, A., Swart, G. R., Wilson, J. H. P., Hoogerbrugge, N., Pols, H. A. P., Birkenhager, J. C., and Lamberts, S. W. J., The effect of growth hormone administration in growth hormone deficient adults on bone, protein, carbohydrate and lipid homeostasis as well as on body composition, *Clin. Endocrinol.*, 37, 79, 1992.

Chapter **9**

Osteogenic Actions of Fluoride: Its Therapeutic Use for Established Osteoporosis

K.-H. William Lau, Kristina Åkesson, Cesar R. Libanati, and David J. Baylink

CONTENTS

0-8493-8556-3/98/$0.00+$.50

I. INTRODUCTION

Fluoride ion is an important trace element in humans and, at minute concentrations, plays important roles in modulating cellular functions of various tissues and organs by regulating the activity of a number of enzymes. Fluoride is widely distributed throughout the environment, and high fluoride concentrations can be found naturally in water in various regions of the world. Fluoride is used extensively in industry. Airborne fluoride can be absorbed through the respiratory tract in people living or working in areas where air contains dusts rich in fluoride.[1] Thus, humans can be exposed to fluoride at a wide range of concentrations from various environmental sources. Earlier studies in the 1930s have revealed that: 1) prolonged industrial exposure to excessive doses of fluoride led to the development of skeletal fluorosis, a condition characterized by osteosclerosis and calcification of ligaments and tendons, particularly of the vertebral column, and 2) the severity of skeletal fluorosis correlated with the extent and duration of exposure to fluoride.[2,3] Skeletal fluorosis is characterized by an unbalanced coupling in favor of bone formation. These observations prompted Rich and co-workers, in 1961, to advance the concept that lower doses of fluoride may be used therapeutically in humans to increase bone formation and thereby strengthen the skeleton without development of severe osteosclerosis and other skeletal side effects.[4-6] They found that low doses of fluoride did increase calcium balance,[4,5] and subsequently bone morphometric evidence has revealed that the effects of fluoride to increase bone mass was due to an increase in bone formation and not to a reduction in bone resorption, and that the increase in bone formation was mediated through a fluoride-dependent increase in the osteoblast number.[7,8] These findings led to intense investigations into the potential application of fluoride therapy for osteoporosis.

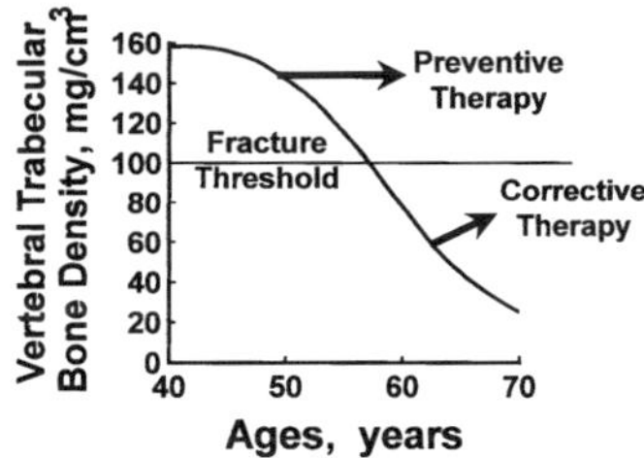

Figure 9.1
Schematic plot of the relationship between vertebral trabecular bone density and age. The fracture threshold line represents the putative bone density value (i.e., 100 mg/cm^3) above which the incidence for osteoporotic spinal fractures is low and below which spinal fractures are likely to occur. By definition, the occurrence of an osteoporotic spinal fracture can be prevented by maintaining the bone density above the fracture threshold (as with preventive therapies). When the bone density has decreased to a value below the fracture threshold (i.e., established osteoporosis), a corrective (restorative) anabolic therapy is required to correct the bone density deficit. (From Libanati, C., Lau, K.-H. W., and Baylink, D. J., *Osteoporosis*, 1996, 1259. With permission.)

Osteoporosis is a disease characterized by the decrease in bone mass and the deterioration of microarchitectural integrity of bone tissues, which leads to impaired bone strength. The two common forms of primary osteoporosis are senile osteoporosis and postmenopausal osteoporosis. When the bone mass decreases below the putative "fracture threshold" level, the susceptibility to fragility fractures is increased.[9] Bone mass is determined by the balance of bone resorption and bone formation rates. In the normal skeleton, a compensatory increase in bone formation follows an increase in bone resorption, i.e., bone formation is coupled to bone resorption, and thus, no net bone is gained or lost during the bone turnover process. In osteoporotic patients, this bone coupling process is defective in that the balance favors bone resorption, leading to the loss of bone mass.[10] The therapeutic strategy for those patients whose bone density is still above the fracture threshold (Figure 9.1) is to treat with an antiresorptive drug in order to maintain bone mass and prevent fractures (i.e., preventive therapy). There are several effective antiresorption drugs, i.e., bisphosphonates, calcitonin, and estrogen, approved for treatment of osteoporosis. For those patients with established osteoporosis whose bone mass has decreased to a level below the fracture threshold and who have already suffered from fragility fractures, antiresorption therapy alone is unlikely to eliminate the risk for new fractures. Accordingly, a rational therapy for these patients would be to treat with an anabolic agent that would increase bone mass to a level above the fracture threshold (i.e., corrective therapy). There are several anabolic agents that stimulate bone formation. These include androgens, fluoride, growth factors, and PTH. Of these agents, fluoride is the only orally active drug that is currently in clinical trials. Thus, fluoride increases spinal bone density and is relatively inexpensive.

This chapter, which will focus on the anabolic actions of fluoride on bone cells and its clinical application for treatment of established osteoporosis, is divided into three sections. The first section deals with the *in vitro* anabolic effects of fluoride on bone cells and bone organ cultures. Because the knowledge of the mechanism of action of a drug is important for its proper use, a discussion of the potential molecular mechanism(s) of fluoride's osteogenic action is also included. The second section reviews the *in vivo* actions of fluoride in animal models with respect to the pharmacokinetics, toxicity, and osteogenic actions of fluoride on the various laboratory animal models. The effects of fluoride incorporation into bone matrix on bone quality in the experimental animal models will also be discussed. The third section addresses the clinical use of fluoride for established osteoporosis. This section will focus on the fluoride pharmacokinetics, therapeutic serum fluoride level, dosage regimen, skeletal response to fluoride therapy, side effects, and efficacy on reduction of fracture rate in patients with established osteoporosis.

II. *IN VITRO* ANABOLIC ACTIONS OF FLUORIDE ON BONE AND BONE CELLS

A. Effects of Fluoride on Bone Cell Proliferation *In Vitro*

Although it has been recognized for over half a century that fluoride stimulates bone formation *in vivo*, it was not until 1983 that the first conclusive evidence for a direct anabolic action of fluoride on bone cells became available. Then, it was demonstrated *in vitro* that fluoride acts directly on primary chicken bone cells to stimulate cell proliferation and differentiation.[11] The *in vitro* bone cell mitogenic action of fluoride was subsequently confirmed by a number of laboratories[12-23] and extended to bone cells of various species, including humans, as shown in Figure 9.2, which indicates that fluoride at clinically relevant concentrations (i.e., 5-15 μM)[24] increased the [^{3}H]thymidine incorporation and cell doubling in normal human bone cells. These *in vitro* anabolic observations are consistent with the past morphometric findings of a fluoride-dependent increase in bone cell number *in vivo*, raising the possibility that the *in vitro* mitogenic action of fluoride is relevant to clinical situations.

B. Effects of Fluoride on Bone Cell Activities *In Vitro*

In addition to its effect on bone cell proliferation, fluoride at the mitogenic doses *in vitro* increased mature osteoblastic activities, i.e., alkaline phosphatase specific activity,[11-13,19-21] collagen synthesis,[11,13,19,20] and the $1,25(OH)_2D_3$-dependent osteocalcin synthesis and secretion[13,19,20] in bone cell monolayer cultures. In addition, the *in vitro* fluoride treatment in-

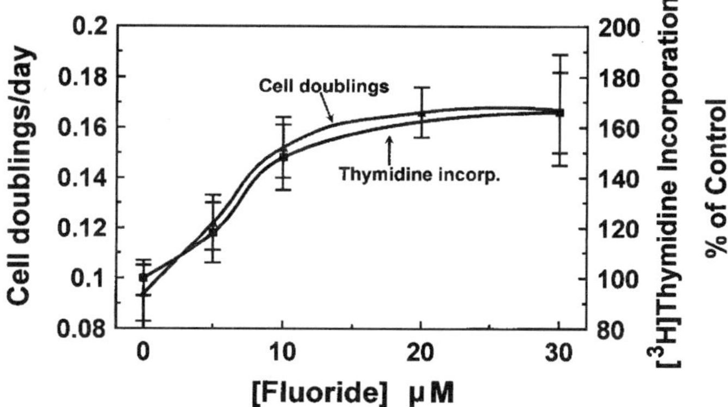

Figure 9.2
Fluoride increases human bone cell proliferation *in vitro*. Normal human bone cells were isolated from the trabecular bone of femoral head samples obtained during hip replacement surgery with collagenase digestion. Human bone cell proliferation was measured by [^{3}H]thymidine incorporation into DNA and by the number of cell population doublings/day. Points are the mean of six replicates. Bars represent the SEM. (From Wergedal, J. E., Lau, K.-H. W., and Baylink, D. J., Fluoride and bovine bone extract influence cell proliferation and phosphatase activities in human bone cell cultures, *Clin. Orthop. Rel. Res.*, 233, 274, 1988. With permission.)

creased transient calcium uptake[25,26] and sodium-dependent phosphate transport[22,27] in bone cell monolayer cultures, suggesting that fluoride may also act directly on bone cells to stimulate osteoblastic activities. These observations support the conclusion that the stimulation of bone formation is a consequence of fluoride's direct stimulation of bone cell proliferation and activities, which ultimately increase the number of active osteoblasts. Consistent with the hypothesis that it can promote the progression of the proliferation and differentiation of osteoprogenitor cells leading to increased bone formation, fluoride has been shown to stimulate bone nodule formation (an index of *de novo* bone formation) in bone cell monolayer cultures.[14-16]

C. Effects of Fluoride on Bone Organ Cultures *In Vitro*

Fluoride at mitogenic doses significantly increased [^{3}H]thymidine incorporation, alkaline phosphatase activity, [^{3}H]hydroxyproline incorporation, *de novo* collagen synthesis, and [^{45}Ca] incorporation in embryonic calvarial or tibial organ cultures *in vitro*, indicating that it can stimulate bone formation in bone organ cultures.[11,28,29] In support of the conclusion that fluoride has anabolic actions on bone organ cultures, it was found that the *in vitro* incubation of fetal mouse tibiae in cultures with a clinically relevant concentration of fluoride for six days also significantly increased the bone calcium deposition and thickened the compacta.[30]

D. Molecular Mechanism of Action of Fluoride on Bone Cells

Information regarding the characteristics of the fluoride-mediated stimulation of bone cell proliferation should provide important insights into the molecular mechanism of the osteogenic action of fluoride. In this regard, recent studies have disclosed three unique properties of the *in vitro* bone cell mitogenic activity of fluoride for which any potential model of the molecular mechanism of osteogenic action of fluoride must account: 1) consistent with the *in vivo* observations that fluoride's anabolic effect is specific for the skeletal tissues, the *in vitro* mitogenic activity of fluoride is specific for cells of skeletal origin;[11,12,31] 2) fluoride requires the presence of bone cell growth factor(s) to stimulate bone cell proliferation;[16,17,32] and 3) fluoride's osteogenic action is sensitive to changes in medium phosphate concentrations.[25,32]

Regarding the molecular mechanism of the osteogenic action of fluoride, a recent model involving the regulation of the Ras-Raf-MAP kinase (MAPK) signal transduction pathway through a specific inhibition of an osteoblastic phosphotyrosyl protein phosphatase (PTPP) activity has been advanced (Figure 9.3).[31,33] This model is based on recent discoveries regarding the Ras-Raf-MAPK mitogenic signal transduction pathway. In this pathway, the binding of a growth factor (e.g., IGF-I) to its cell surface receptor activates the receptor's intrinsic tyrosyl kinase activity through

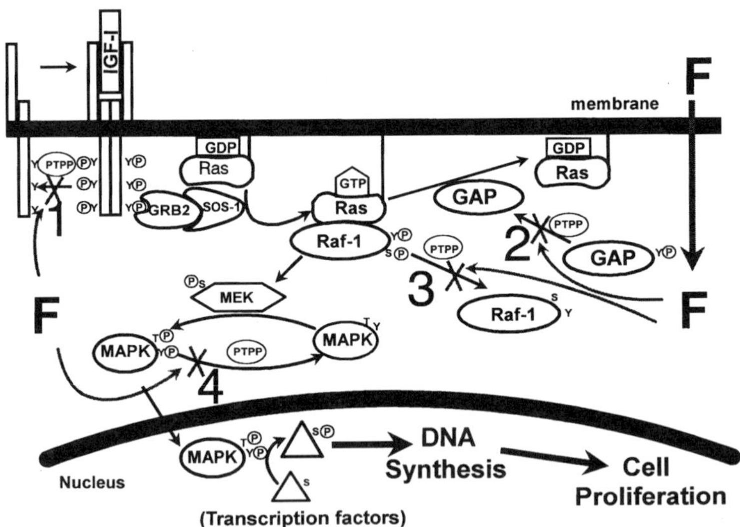

Figure 9.3
A proposed molecular mechanism for the mitogenic action of fluoride on bone cells. The model is described in detail in the text. (From Libanati, C., Lau, K.-H. W., and Baylink, D. J., Fluoride therapy for osteoporosis, in *Osteoporosis*, Marcus, R., Feldman, D., and Kelsey, J., Eds., Academic Press, San Diego, 1996, 1259. With permission.)

autophosphorylation, which triggers a cascade of phosphorylation reactions, subsequently leading to the tyrosyl phosphorylation of a number of cellular signaling proteins.[34,35] In particular, the activated receptor recruits and phosphorylates docking proteins, such as Grb2.[36] Grb2 then targets Sos-1 to the membrane to catalyze the exchange of GDP to GTP on Ras.[37] Upon the binding of GTP, Ras is activated, which leads to activation of Raf-1.[38] The inactivation of Ras is mediated by rasGAP, which catalyzes the hydrolysis of the protein-bound GTP.[37] Tyrosyl phosphorylation of rasGAP leads to dissociation of rasGAP and Ras and thereby inhibits the GTP hydrolysis of the Ras and maintains Ras in the activated state, which results in an activation of Raf-1.[38-40] The activated Raf-1 phosphorylates and activates MEK,[41] which phosphorylates, and activates MAPK on both a threonyl and a tyrosyl residue.[41,42] The activated MAPK migrates into the nucleus, phosphorylates and activates a number of transcription factors and proto-oncogenes,[43,44] actions which collectively lead to increased gene expression, DNA synthesis, cell proliferation, and/or differentiation.[40-42]

In the Ras-Raf-MAPK pathway, at least four components, i.e., growth factor receptor, rasGAP, Raf-1, and MAPK, are regulated by tyrosyl phosphorylation. An overall increase in the tyrosyl phosphorylation level of these proteins leads to an activation of this mitogenic signal transduction pathway and cell proliferation. The model postulates that fluoride, upon its entry into the bone cells, inhibits the activity of the fluoride-sensitive PTPP, which leads to the reduction of the dephosphorylation of one or more of these four proteins (identified in Figure 9.3 as 1 through 4). As a consequence, their overall tyrosyl phosphorylation status will rise, which subsequently leads to the potentiation of bone cell proliferation initiated by the bone cell growth factor.

The mechanism as to how fluoride enters the cell is unknown. Because 1) the uptake of fluoride into cells is rapid and occurs in minutes,[45] 2) the uptake of fluoride is enhanced by chloride deficiency,[46] and 3) fluoride, like chloride, is a halide, and it is reasonable to speculate that cellular uptake of fluoride is mediated through the chloride channel.

This proposed model is attractive in that it appears to account for each of the aforementioned three characteristics of the fluoride-induced bone cell mitogenesis. First, there is a fluoride-sensitive, acid PTPP activity in osteoblasts but not in other cells and tissues.[31] Thus, the effect of fluoride on this enzyme (and the consequent effect on cell proliferation) should be specific for bone cells. Second, a fluoride-dependent inhibition of the dephosphorylation of a phosphotyrosyl protein can increase its overall phosphorylation level. However, it is effective only when the basal level of phosphorylation has been increased in response to activation of a tyrosyl kinase. Accordingly, this model predicts that the optimal mitogenic effect of fluoride requires the presence of a bone cell growth factor to increase basal cellular tyrosyl phosphorylation rate. Third, fluoride can act as a transition state analog of phosphate.[47] Thus, as predicted by the proposed model, transition state analogs of phosphate, such as vanadate and molybdate, which are potent inhibitors of PTPPs at concentrations that inhibited the fluoride-sensitive PTPP activity, also stimulated bone cell proliferation to the same extent as fluoride.[29,31] In addition, if fluoride functions as a transition state analog of phosphate to stimulate bone cell proliferation through its inhibition of the fluoride-sensitive PTPP, it follows that the *in vitro* mitogenic action of fluoride would be sensitive to changes in medium phosphate concentrations.

In further support of this model, a fluoride-sensitive PTPP has been identified in bone cells and shown to be inhibited by mitogenic concentrations of fluoride, molybdate, or vanadate *in vitro*.[31,48-51] More important, fluoride and vanadate each at doses that inhibit this fluoride-sensitive PTPP activity significantly increased tyrosyl phosphorylation levels of at least 13 cellular proteins in human bone cells with a time course that is consistent with an inhibition of dephosphorylation.[52] These findings are consistent with the hypothesis that the mitogenic action of fluoride is mediated through an increase in the tyrosyl phosphorylation level of cellular signaling proteins resulting from an inhibition of PTPP activities. Most important, there is preliminary evidence that some of these cellular proteins, whose overall tyrosyl phosphorylation level and activity were stimulated by fluoride or vanadate, are MAPK, rasGAP, and Raf-1.[52,53] Thus, these findings together afford compelling, albeit circumstantial, evidence for the proposed model in Figure 9.3.

Bonjour and co-workers[22,54] have proposed a competing model which also involves tyrosyl phosphorylation of MAPK. In contrast to the model in Figure 9.3, their proposed mechanism focuses on the concept that fluoride stimulates bone cell proliferation by increasing the activity of a tyrosyl kinase (as opposed to inhibiting a PTPP). These investigators proposed that fluoride forms an aluminum fluoride complex, which activates a Gi protein. Accordingly, they predict that fluoride is ineffective, unless aluminum ion is also present.[54] The activation of this Gi protein would lead to stimulation of a tyrosyl kinase activity, which consequently results in tyrosyl phosphorylation and activation of MAPK and subsequently increased bone cell proliferation.

While some of the existing data on the fluoride-mediated bone cell proliferation are also consistent with this model (e.g., increased tyrosyl phosphorylation of MAPK), the model fails to reconcile several important discrepancies. This model does not explain the cell/tissue specificity, the requirement of growth factor(s), or the sensitivity to phosphate, of the osteogenic action of fluoride. Moreover, the effective doses of aluminum and fluoride in their studies (50 μM and 0.75 mM, respectively) were at least one order of magnitude higher than the serum concentrations of these ions in fluoride-treated patients. There is also evidence that fluoride inhibits, rather than stimulates, receptor tyrosyl kinase activities,[55] and that aluminum and fluoride appear to act through different and independent pathways to stimulate human bone cell proliferation,[56] findings which are not compatible with the proposed model.

In summary, although the exact molecular mechanism of the osteogenic action of fluoride has not been established, current evidence is consistent with the involvement of the activation of the Ras-Raf-MAPK signal transduction pathway through increased tyrosyl phosphorylation level of key signaling proteins in this pathway (e.g., MAPK, Raf-1, and rasGAP). The most likely explanation for the increase in the tyrosyl phosphorylation level of these signaling proteins is an inhibition of a specific osteoblastic fluoride-sensitive PTPP by osteogenic doses of fluoride. Nevertheless, further studies are required to definitively resolve the molecular mechanism of action of fluoride on bone cells.

III. *IN VIVO* ACTIONS OF FLUORIDE IN ANIMAL MODELS

An appropriate animal model would be very useful in addressing mechanistic issues of the *in vivo* osteogenic actions of fluoride. A suitable animal model for investigations of clinically relevant issues should be one that displays skeletal responses to fluoride that resemble those seen in humans, i.e., increased cancellous bone formation, increased osteoblast number, and a large increment in trabecular bone density. Unfortunately, there is currently no good laboratory animal model that mimics all of the skeletal changes seen in humans.

A majority of animal work with fluoride was performed with the rat model. Unfortunately, rats are resistant to the mitogenic action of fluoride. This can be explained in part by the fact that intestinal absorption of fluoride in the rat is 4 to 5 times less than in humans.[57] However, even large doses of fluoride in rats do not produce a large osteogenic effect.[57-61] Although many other animal models (e.g., mice, dogs, pigs, chicken, rabbits, and sheep) have been studied, none show the large osteogenic effect that is seen in humans. Accordingly, there is currently no suitable animal model that can be used to evaluate osteogenic responses to fluoride therapy, and extrapolation of animal studies to humans should be done with caution. Nonetheless, useful information on fluoride toxicity and other issues have been obtained in animal studies.

Accordingly, in this section, we will review several aspects of the *in vivo* fluoride actions in the various laboratory animal models; namely, fluoride pharmacokinetics, toxicity, osteogenic actions, and effects on bone formation and bone quality.

A. Fluoride Pharmacokinetics in Laboratory Animals

A detailed knowledge of fluoride's pharmacokinetics is essential if its pharmacologic and toxicologic effects are to be adequately understood.

Thus, fluoride pharmacokinetics have been evaluated in several animal models, including rats,[62-66] pigs,[67,68] dogs,[69] cats,[69] rabbits,[69] and hamsters.[69] Ingested fluoride in each animal species is rapidly and extensively absorbed from the gastrointestinal tract into the circulation.[62-69] While the majority of ingested fluoride is absorbed through the small intestine,[70] it is unique among the halides in that a significant amount is absorbed in the stomach.[63] The rate of gastric absorption of fluoride is pH-dependent and is inversely proportional to the pH of the gastric contents.[63,70] The fecal fluoride typically accounts for 10 to 30% of the ingested fluoride.[63] The rate and extent of fluoride absorption in the rat can be significantly reduced by calcium, magnesium, and several other di- or trivalent cations in the gastrointestinal tract.[68] This effect has been attributed to the formation of insoluble fluoride compounds (e.g., CaF_2) which are poorly absorbed. Long-term balance studies indicated that net secretion of fluoride into the gastrointestinal tract (i.e., fecal excretion > dietary intake) could occur when plasma fluoride concentrations were high.[63] This raises the possibility that a small component of the absorbed fluoride can be resecreted into the gastrointestinal tract.

The clearance of plasma fluoride by the kidney and skeletal tissues in the rat is rapid.[62,63,66] The shape of the serum fluoride curve after readily soluble NaF administration indicates a distribution half-life of about one hour and an elimination half-life of approximately six hours. The clearance of plasma fluoride in growing pigs decreased with age from >8 to <1.5 ml/min/kg.[67,68] The renal clearance rate of fluoride is a function of urinary pH.[69,71,72] The rate of renal and skeletal clearance of fluoride is different among various animal species. The renal clearance varied from 1.5 ml/min/kg in the dog and rabbit to 3.5 ml/min/kg in the rat and hamster,[69] and the skeletal clearance rate ranged from 2.1 ml/min/kg in the dog to >4.5 ml/min/kg in the cat, rabbit, and hamster.[69] These indicate that the fluoride pharmacokinetics (and bioavailability) are different among different animal species.

The plasma concentration of absorbed fluoride and the amount of fluoride incorporated into bone matrix in each animal species, including humans, depend on the dose of fluoride and the duration of treatment.[62,63,66] Changes in renal excretion and/or gastrointestinal absorption would influence plasma fluoride levels which, in turn, would alter fluoride uptake into the skeleton. Accordingly, acidosis decreases renal excretion of fluoride in the rat, which subsequently results in increased serum and bone fluoride levels.[73] Aluminum, magnesium, and strontium ions which reduce gastrointestinal fluoride absorption, decrease serum and bone fluoride levels in rats.[70,74]

On the basis of the above findings, it is concluded that the bioavailability of fluoride in a given animal species would depend not only on the amount of fluoride ingested and the duration of treatment, but also on the efficiency of gastrointestinal fluoride absorption, kidney function, as well as the rate of fluoride deposition into the skeleton.[66,75,76]

B. Toxicity, Teratogenicity, and Carcinogenicity of Fluoride

Data on the toxicity of high fluoride doses in large mammals, including humans, are scarce. Most available toxicity studies were performed in small animals, such as rats, mice, and rabbits. Acute exposure to a very high dose of fluoride (e.g., >10 mg NaF/kg, ip injection) is toxic to the rodents and damages the kidneys.[77-80] Intake of even larger doses of fluoride has been reported to induce pulmonary damage in rabbits[81] and dogs,[82] and inhibited insulin secretion in rats.[83] Long-term oral administration of a large dose of fluoride dramatically reduces blood flow in the gastrointestinal mucosa, and as a result, significantly harms the gastric mucosa in rats and humans.[84,85] The fluoride-induced gastric mucosal lesions regress after cessation of the fluoride administration.[85] High fluoride intakes have been associated with the development of hypocalcemia and secondary hyperparathyroidism in laboratory animals.[86,87] The oral fluoride LD_{50} is 80 to 114 mg/kg for rats and 97 mg/kg for mice, with NaF as the fluoride source.[88] Thus, it seems that large doses of fluoride are toxic for many animal species.

A question as to whether high intakes of fluoride are teratogenic, mutagenic, or carcinogenic in animals has been raised in the past. While some *in vitro* cytogenetic studies have reported cytotoxic and mutagenic effects of high doses of fluoride on mammalian cells,[89-91] the most recent studies have found no effects.[92-95] It should be emphasized that the fluoride doses used in *in vitro* studies are much higher than either therapeutic or lethal blood fluoride levels and that therapeutically relevant levels (i.e., 5-15 μM) of fluoride have no *in vitro* cytogenic or mutagenic effects in various mammalian, including human, cells. There is also no evidence that long-term administration of large doses of fluoride in the rat have teratogenic or carcinogenic effects *in vivo*,[96,97] nor is there evidence that administration of a large dose of fluoride for six weeks causes cytogenetic damage in mice *in vivo*.[98]

In summary, it is now generally considered that therapeutic doses of fluoride (i.e., 5 to 15 μM serum level) are not teratogenic, mutagenic, or carcinogenic in laboratory animals or humans.[96,99,100]

C. Osteogenic Effects in Animal Models

The osteogenic actions of fluoride have been investigated in a number of animal models, including small (rat, mouse, rabbit, chicken) and large (pig, dog, sheep, monkey) animals.[101,102] The efficacy for bone formation in these studies was assessed by increases in bone density, histomorphometric, or biochemical bone formation parameters. These studies used varying fluoride compounds, doses (i.e., from therapeutic doses to toxic), treatment duration (i.e., from several days to several years), and routes of administration. These important variables would significantly influence the fluoride bioavailability and pharmacokinetics. Thus, it has been difficult to compare and extrapolate the results of animal work to humans. In addition, while fluoride treatment markedly increases spinal bone density and bone formation in humans, many animal species do not show increases in bone density and histomorphometric bone formation parameters in response to the fluoride treatment. More important, the increases in bone formation and density in animal models are smaller than in humans. Thus, the currently used animal models are not ideal for evaluation of clinically relevant issues regarding the osteogenic actions of fluoride.

The following summarizes the osteogenic effects of fluoride in the various laboratory animal models with respect to bone density, histomorphometry, and serum biochemical markers.

1. Bone Density

Early radiologic studies have provided some evidence that fluoride treatment increases bone density in several animal species. Treatment with fluoride (along with a sufficient dietary calcium supplementation) for 2 to 6 months increased cortical bone density and thickness in kittens[103] and young pigs.[104] Sheep treated with 1.9 to 4.7 mg/kg/day of NaF for 33 months developed exostoses on long bones.[105] These findings are consistent with an anabolic action of fluoride on the skeleton. However, there is also radiologic evidence that fluoride may reduce bone density in certain species. In this regard, rats treated with 120 ppm (2.86 mM) of NaF in drinking water for four weeks had decreased trabecular thickness compared to control rats.[106] Treatment of lambs with 2 to 4 mg/kg/day of NaF for 15 weeks led to a slight reduction in cortical thickness.[101] The bone calcium content in mice treated with 0.8 mg NaF/kg/day for four weeks was also significantly lower than in controls.[107]

2. Bone Histomorphometry

Treatment of rats with 30 to 100 ppm (0.71 to 2.38 mM) of NaF in drinking water for up to 35 days increased periosteal cancellous bone formation in rats.[18,58-61,106,108] Fluoride treatment has also been shown to increase the osteoid and bone formation parameters in cancellous bones in mice,[107] pigs,[109,110] ewes,[111,112] and chickens.[113] These findings indicate that fluoride treatment increases cancellous bone formation indices *in vivo* in several animal species. Fluoride treatment increased the number of osteoblasts and osteoblast-covered surface in rats[18,106] and lambs.[112] Thus, the increase in bone formation is most likely due to fluoride-induced stimulation of osteoblast proliferation. However, there are also studies showing that fluoride treatment not only failed to increase, but also significantly decreased, several bone formation parameters in dogs and rats. Daily administration of 0.7 mg/kg/day of NaF for six months significantly decreased several cancellous bone formation indices in beagle dogs.[114]

Rats on a high dose (8 mg NaF/kg/day) of fluoride for three months also had a significantly reduced cancellous bone volume.[60] Treating rats with therapeutically relevant doses of fluoride also did not increase histomorphometric indices of bone formation *in vivo*, even though a significant amount of fluoride had been incorporated into the bone.[113,115]

Results of studies on the effect of fluoride treatment on cortical bone are conflicting.[116] Pigs fed 2 mg NaF/kg/day for six months showed a significant increase in femoral cortical bone porosity.[117] In contrast, treatment of ovariectomized beagle dogs with fluoride for six months showed a significant reduction in cortical bone porosity in the ribs.[60] In humans, fluoride therapy increases endocortical bone formation and cortical width of the ileum.[118] The reason for the lack of an osteogenic response at cortical bone sites in some animals is unclear.

One possible explanation for this discrepancy is that the skeletal fluoride response in animals is dose dependent. A biphasic response in histomorphometric indices of bone formation was observed with 14-day-old chickens fed 0 to 8.4 mM NaF daily for two weeks. Bone formation indices increased with fluoride doses up to about 5 mM and then decreased with the higher dose.[113] A biphasic response in the indices of tibial metaphyseal bone formation was also observed in rats.[59] If dose is a partial explanation for some of the species variation, it seems likely that the species-dependent variation in fluoride bioavailability (see Section III.A) would also contribute to the interspecies variation in the osteogenic response. Another possibility is that there may be a resistance to fluoride at the molecular level. This is suggested by the results of studies of human osteoporotic patients, according to which some patients have a very small osteogenic response to fluoride despite having adequate serum levels of fluoride (see Section IV.D.4.a).

Some laboratory animals, e.g., beagle dogs,[119] pigs,[120] rats,[121,122] and lambs,[112] after treatment with fluoride, displayed histomorphometric evidence of mineralization defects, such as reduced mineral apposition rate and increased mineralization lag time. The mineralization defect occurs in cortical[120] and periosteal,[121,122] as well as cancellous,[119] bone. Because the fluoride-induced mineralization defect appears to be prevented by high dietary calcium intakes,[103] the mineralization defect might be associated with a calcium deficiency resulting from a rapid increase in bone formation. Alternatively, it could be due to a direct action of fluoride on mineralization by osteoblasts. Additional work is required to determine the cause of the fluoride-induced mineralization defect.

3. *Serum Biochemistry*

Most studies showed that administration of low doses of fluoride did not significantly affect serum calcium, phosphorus, and vitamin D metabolites in most animal species,[59,101,123] with the exception of ewes, which showed a significant decrease in serum calcium and phosphorus levels.[111]

Fluoride increases serum markers of bone formation, such as alkaline phosphatase and osteocalcin, in rats,[123] chickens,[113] and sheep.[101,111,112] These findings further support the conclusion of an anabolic effect of fluoride on bone formation in some animal species.

However, it should be noted that administration of high doses of fluoride in the rat,[58,108] rabbit,[124] sheep,[101,125] and ewe[101] caused a transient decrease in serum calcium, which could lead to the development of secondary hyperparathyroidism. But, because fluoride treatment effectively increases bone formation parameters in thyroparathyroidectomized rats,[108] the *in vivo* osteogenic effects of fluoride are probably unrelated to the circulating PTH level.

In summary, relatively low doses of fluoride have anabolic actions on the skeletons of several animal species, though there is considerable interspecies variation in the magnitude of the skeletal response. None of the responses observed so far in animals equals the large osteogenic response seen in humans. This limits the usefulness of animal models for probing the mechanism for the osteogenic response. However, animal models can be useful for other studies of fluoride, such as the effect of fluoride on bone quality, which is discussed below.

D. Effects on Bone Quality and Strength

Fracture risk is determined by the bone biomechanical strength, which is determined by bone quality as well as bone mass. Fluoride treatment stimulates the incorporation of fluoride into bone mineral crystals, which has been shown to alter the bone mineral physiochemical properties. Accordingly, the incorporation of fluoride into bone mineral crystals may be an important issue concerning the effects of fluoride on bone mineral quality.

1. Effect of Fluoride Incorporation on Bone Mineral

Fluoride treatment significantly increases the bone fluoride content in all animal species, and the amount of fluoride incorporation is directly proportional to fluoride dose and duration of treatment.[101,126,127] Fluoride treatment produces a number of changes in the mineral phase of bone. Normal bone mineral exists in the form of hydroxyapatite crystals. Incorporation of fluoride substitutes fluoride for the hydroxyl group in apatite to form fluorohydroxyapatite crystals.[128] X-ray diffraction studies indicate that fluoride treatment improves apatite crystallinity of bone minerals, increases crystal size, and decreases the degree of lattice distortion.[129] Consistent with this conclusion, fluoride administration in rodents increased the mineral crystal size in cortical bones *in vivo*.[130,131] The effect of fluoride was confined almost entirely to increases in width and thickness of the mineral crystal and not to changes in crystal length.[128] The fluoride ion does not diffuse in large amounts into preformed hydroxyapatite crystals in highly mineralized bone, but it is incorporated into fluorohydroxyapatite crystals during new bone mineralization. Thus, most of the fluoride is deposited in actively mineralizing bone.[132]

In vivo administration of fluoride also increases bone mineral density (calcium content per unit bone weight) and microhardness in cortical bones of laboratory animals.[131,133,134] When finely ground rat or chicken bone powders were fractionated according to specific density, the percent by weight of powders having a higher specific density (i.e., >2.1 g/ml) was significantly greater in fluoridated bones than in control bones.[102,135] The increased mineral density is the result of fluoride-induced increases in bone mineral maturation and hypermineralization of the cortical bone[135] and, as such, may in part account for the observed increase in microhardness in fluoridated bones.[130-134] Accordingly, fluoride treatment produces areas of high mineral density in cortical bones of many animal species, including humans.[129,133,136,137]

In addition to high mineral density areas, fluoride treatment also produces areas of under-mineralized matrix. This results in a picture of mottled bone with zones of low mineral density (but well-organized matrix) and hypomineralized halos around mottled lacunae.[138-140] The reason for this hypomineralization is unclear, but it could be in part due to calcium deficiency and the consequent mineralization defect brought on by the increased calcium demand to mineralize the new bone formed during the fluoride treatment.[141] The increased variability of bone mineral content with areas of high as well as low mineral density could weaken the bone integrity and may be an important contributor to decreased quality of the fluoride-treated bone.[142]

2. Effects of Incorporation of Fluoride on Bone Strength

Most of the studies on bone strength have been performed with the rat model by measuring the biomechanics in cortical bone.[57,115,143-149] With the exception of a single report showing a positive effect of fluoride on breaking strength,[147] the overwhelming majority of the studies with the rat indicate that fluoride treatment either decreased,[143,144,147,148] or did not affect, the mechanical strength of cortical bones.[57,145,146] However, a biphasic relationship between bone strength and bone fluoride content was noted in a recent study,[57] wherein fluoride had a positive effect on femoral bending strength at low fluoride intake (peak bone strength occurred at an intake of 16 ppm of fluoride), and a negative effect at higher doses. Nevertheless, it is generally accepted that the incorporation of high levels of fluoride in bone mineral leads to reduction in bone strength and that the deleterious effects of fluoride on cortical bone quality is seen once the bone fluoride level reaches about 0.5% (i.e., 5,000 to 10,000 ppm).[57,144]

It appears that the dosage and duration of the fluoride treatment are both important factors determining whether fluoride treatment would weaken cortical bone.[150,151] Accordingly, while treating rats with low doses of fluoride (i.e., <50 ppm) for 3 to 6 months did not significantly affect femoral bone strength, treatment with the same doses for 12 to 18 months increased bone fluoride content to >10,000 ppm (i.e., by 1%) and reduced femoral bone strength by more than 20%.[144] There is also a marked reduction of cortical bone strength in rabbits at high doses, but low doses of fluoride tend to increase bone strength.[150] A similar biphasic effect of fluoride on cortical bone strength has been observed in fluoridated rat femurs.[57] These effects may be related to the amount of fluoride incorporation which is related to dosage and duration of the treatment.

Information concerning vertebral bone strength in laboratory animals is limited. A recent study showed that high intakes of fluoride (100 and 150 ppm NaF for 90 days) reduced the biomechanical competence of vertebral body in the rat, in spite of a significant increase in trabecular bone volume.[127] These findings suggest that fluoride treatment in the rat may not beneficially affect bone quality and that the increase in bone mass during fluoride treatment in the rat does not translate into an improvement of bone strength.[127,145]

Studies of the effects of fluoride on bone strength in other animal models have also yielded confusing results. Merkey has noted that NaF at doses between 100 and 200 ppm significantly increased breaking strength and bone ash volume of humeri and tibiae of White Leghorn pullets[152] and coop-reared broilers,[153,154] but other investigators found either a significant reduction in breaking strength[148,155] or no effects.[156] Several other animal studies (dogs, calves, and pigs) focusing on fluoride-induced changes in cortical bone biomechanics have also yielded conflicting results. No significant increase of biomechanical strength was noted after prolonged treatment with fluoride in calves,[157] domestic pigs,[110] and dogs,[158] even though there were significant increases in bone fluoride content.

In summary, it is generally accepted that incorporation of a high level of fluoride in bone mineral has a deleterious effect on bone quality and strength. It is now clear that the level of fluoride incorporation is proportional to fluoride dosage and treatment time. Accordingly, in order to avoid harmful effects on bone quality and strength, it may be necessary to reduce the amount of fluoride incorporated without a significant reduction in its osteogenic action by adjusting the dosage and/or treatment duration of the fluoride therapy.

IV. CLINICAL USE OF FLUORIDE FOR ESTABLISHED OSTEOPOROSIS

While fluoride remains an investigational drug for osteoporosis in the U.S., it has been approved for many years in several European countries for treating osteoporosis. Accordingly, there is a large amount of information regarding the use of fluoride therapy in humans. This section will review and summarize some of the key findings of the fluoride therapy of established osteoporosis in humans.

A. Fluoride Pharmacokinetics and Metabolism in Humans

Good fluoride responders (those who show an increased spinal bone density of at least 13 mg/cc per year) were characterized by increased extrarenal clearance (i.e., bone deposition) and decreased renal fluoride clearance.[159] A positive correlation between urinary fluoride level and lumbar bone mineral content was also noted in good responders.[160] In addition, a larger increase in bone mineral content was reported to be associated with the age-related decrease in renal functions.[161] Thus, fluoride pharmacokinetics and bioavailability are important factors of skeletal response to fluoride therapy in humans. In addition to dosage and body size, four additional factors are important in determining serum fluoride level in humans: 1) fluoride salts and forms, 2) gastrointestinal absorption, 3) fluoride tissue deposition, and 4) renal clearance. This section will address each of these factors.

1. Fluoride Salts and Forms

Two types of fluoride compound, i.e., NaF and sodium monofluorophosphate (MFP), are currently available for use in humans. Like NaF, MFP stimulates osteoblast proliferation and bone formation *in vitro*[162] and *in vivo*.[163] An earlier study suggested that the bioavailability of fluoride was greater for MFP than for NaF in osteoporotic patients.[164] A more recent study, however, showed that NaF and MFP had a comparable fluoride bioavailability in postmenopausal women.[165] MFP appears to have two major advantages over NaF: 1) unlike NaF, which frequently causes gastric irritation due to gastric absorption and formation of hydrofluoric acid with HCl in the stomach, MFP has much less harmful gastrointestinal effects, because MFP is hydrolyzed in the small intestine by alkaline phosphatase to release free fluoride ion for rapid absorption in the duodenum;[162] and 2) while the intestinal absorption of NaF is significantly reduced by calcium,[166] calcium and other divalent cations have no effect on intestinal absorption of MFP.[167] Thus, MFP can be taken simultaneously with calcium without concern of decreased absorption.

Both NaF and MFP are also available in enteric-coated and slow release forms. Enteric-coated forms of fluoride salts would minimize potential gastrointestinal irritations. The use of slow-release forms enables the maintenance of a patient's serum fluoride concentration at the therapeutic level without sharp postabsorption peaks, which are not required to increase bone formation but could increase fluoride deposition in bone. As an example, Figure 9.4 shows that a large acute peak in serum fluoride level was obtained after plain MFP was administered, which did not occur with the 12-hour slow-release MFP (MFP-SR) therapy.

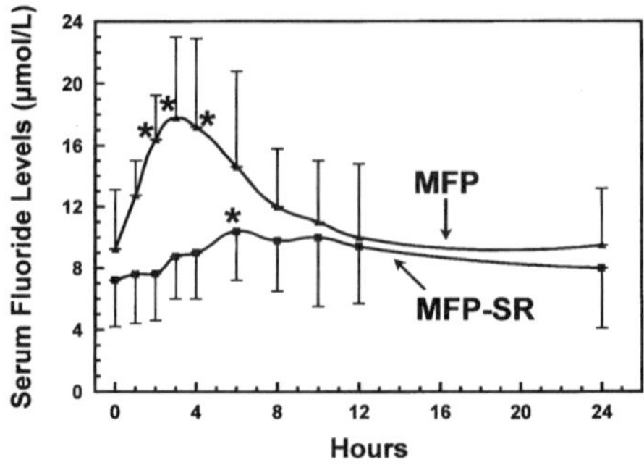

Figure 9.4
Serum fluoride levels (mean and SD) over 24 hours in six osteoporotic patients following a single 76-mg dose of either plain monofluorophosphate (MFP) or 12-hour slow-release monofluorophosphate (MFP-SR). *$p < 0.05$. (From Resch, H., Libanati, C., Talbot, J., Tabuenca, M., Farley, S., Bettica, P., Tritthart, W., and Baylink, D.J., Pharmacokinetic profile of a new fluoride preparation: sustained-release monofluorophosphate, *Calcif. Tissue Int.*, 54, 7, 1994. With permission.)

2. *Fluoride Absorption in Humans*

The mechanism of fluoride absorption in humans is similar to that in laboratory animals. Under fasting conditions, almost 100% of the orally ingested fluoride salts in humans are absorbed in the gastrointestinal tract through passive mechanisms.[168,169] The fluoride absorption is low in the stomach, very high in the duodenum, and slightly lower in the jejunum.[1] As in animals, the efficiency of fluoride absorption in humans is influenced by three key factors: 1) the type of fluoride salts; 2) the presence of other compounds that would influence fluoride absorption (e.g., Ca^{++}, Mg^{++}, Al^{+3}, other di- or trivalent cations, and Cl^{-}); and 3) the physiological and pathological state of patients (e.g., age, body acid–base equilibrium, gastric and urine pH, renal function).[170]

3. *Tissue Distribution of Fluoride in Humans*

In humans, absorbed fluoride enters the circulation and is distributed between two major compartments: extracellular fluids and soft tissue, where it has a half-life of a few hours; and the hard tissues (bone, calcified cartilages, and teeth), where it has a much longer half-life (up to several years). The main deposition site for fluoride ions is the bone. Fluoride ions are not homogeneously distributed in bone, but are deposited primarily in areas that are actively mineralizing during fluoride treatment.[138] Thus, the amount of fluoride deposited in bone is determined by the bone formation rate, the serum concentration of fluoride (which is influenced by the dosage), and the exposure time (which is related to the treatment duration). Fluoride deposited in the skeleton is removed by osteoclastic resorption during remodeling. Part of the released fluoride is probably recycled into new bone matrix, while the rest is excreted in the urine. Therefore, the fluoride content in bone would drop slowly, but progressively, once the fluoride therapy is stopped.[171]

4. *Renal Clearance*

In humans, 75% of the total excreted fluoride is in the urine, 12 to 20% is in feces, and 5 to 13% is in sweat.[172] Fluoride is freely filtered in the kidney.[173] The amount of fluoride excreted depends on the filtered load (i.e., the glomerular filtration rate × blood fluoride concentration) and free water clearance: the greater the free water clearance, the greater the fluoride excretion.[174] Since diet can influence urinary pH, vegetarian diets, which are alkaline, could lead to greater fluoride retention.[174] Even a moderate impairment of renal function would predispose to excessive fluoride retention during fluoride therapy.[175] Increased fluoride retention would increase the risk of skeletal fluorosis. Therefore, fluoride should only be used as a therapeutic agent with great caution in patients with renal insufficiency.[176,177]

B. Therapeutic Serum Level of Fluoride

The serum fluoride level is probably the most important index for monitoring the therapeutic dose, because fluoride acts directly on bone cells to increase bone formation *in vitro*.[11,12] Serum fluoride levels in patients receiving fluoride should be monitored to detect abnormally high or subtherapeutic fluoride levels. The timing of serum fluoride measurements is an important issue since oral intakes of fluoride often produce acute peaks which are usually three times the morning predose level. We measure the serum fluoride concentration just before the morning fluoride dose.[24] The morning predose concentration would most likely represent the steady-state serum fluoride concentration and would be an acceptable representation of the mean serum level throughout the 24-hour dosing period.

The optimum serum fluoride concentrations for osteogenic actions in humans have not been convincingly established. Taves[178] in 1970 proposed that fasting serum fluoride levels be maintained between 5 and 10 μM for an osteogenic response in humans. These proposed limits have frequently been referred to as the therapeutic window for fluoride therapy. While this putative therapeutic window was based solely on theoretical considerations which have not been confirmed, there is circumstantial evidence supporting such a window. In this regard, in agreement with the lower limit of the theoretical therapeutic window, anecdotal data indicate that serum fluoride concentrations below 5 μM rarely produce a significant increase in bone formation in humans. The determination of the upper limit for serum fluoride has been more difficult. *In vitro* studies reveal that the dose-dependent stimulation of human osteoblast proliferation and differentiation persists at fluoride concentrations of 10 to 15 μM (Figure

9.2).[12] It is conceivable that serum fluoride levels of 10 to 15 μM will produce greater increases in bone formation than 5 μM in humans. However, it is also conceivable that the greater increases in bone formation by higher fluoride doses (e.g., 15 μM) would be offset by a greater incidence of harmful side effects (e.g., osteomalacia and reduced bone strength due to increased fluoride incorporation). Consequently, the benefit-to-risk ratios of higher fluoride doses will determine the upper optimum limit. Unfortunately, the relationship between benefit-to-risk data and serum fluoride concentrations is lacking. The rationale for assigning 5 to 10 μM serum fluoride as a safe and effective concentration is based on two findings: 1) a consistent stimulation of bone formation was observed in patients when fasting serum fluoride levels were maintained at 5 to 10 μM;[24,179] and 2) no serious side effects were observed at a serum fluoride concentration of 5 to 10 μM. Until more information concerning the efficacy and toxicity of fluoride in humans becomes available, a morning predose serum fluoride concentration of 5 to 10 μM would seem to be a reasonable therapeutic serum concentration for adults with established osteoporosis.

C. Dosage and Regimen of Fluoride Therapy

Three recent randomized, prospective, placebo-controlled studies seem to indicate that the dosage and scheduling of fluoride therapy significantly influence therapeutic efficacy.[180-184] Studies from the Mayo Clinic, Rochester, Minnesota,[180] and Henry Ford Hospital, Detroit, Michigan,[181] showed that postmenopausal women treated with 75 mg NaF/day (34 mg/day elemental fluoride) for four years showed no significant reduction in vertebral fracture rate compared to placebo controls, despite a 35% increase in the spinal bone density. A subsequent extended analysis by the Mayo Clinic group on 50 of the patients who, because of side effects, took lower fluoride doses and who had a smaller increase in spinal bone density (<17%) and a lower serum fluoride concentration (<8 μM), showed moderate but significant decreases in spinal fracture rate.[182] This *post hoc* analysis, while lacking the rigor of a controlled study, suggests that patients who showed very rapid increases in bone density or a large augmentation in serum fluoride levels did not have a decrease in fracture rate. A potential explanation, from histomorphometric evidence, of the lack of a beneficial effect on vertebral fracture rate in patients with larger fluoride dose may be the development of a statistically significant osteomalacia, even though these patients had received daily supplementation of 1500 mg calcium carbonate.[118] Accordingly, if the assumption that higher serum fluoride concentrations would elicit a larger increase in bone formation is valid, it follows that the higher the serum fluoride level, the greater the demand for calcium. If so, patients with a lower serum fluoride concentration would have a smaller increase in bone formation and would show less tendency toward osteomalacia.

Another prospective, randomized, controlled study from Southwestern University in Dallas, Texas,[183,184] which used an intermittent slow release form of NaF with a dosage regimen consisting of 14-month cycles (12 months receiving fluoride and 2 months off therapy) at 50 mg NaF/day (23 mg/day of elemental fluoride) with 800 mg/day calcium citrate supplementation for four years, showed a marked decrease in vertebral fracture rate. This study has four major differences compared to those of the Mayo Clinic and the Henry Ford Hospital: 1) it used a lower fluoride dose (23 mg/day vs. 34 mg/day) given with calcium, thus further decreasing fluoride absorption; 2) it used a slow-release form of NaF rather than plain NaF; 3) the regimen contained a two-month "off" fluoride period; and 4) patients were supplemented with calcium citrate instead of calcium carbonate. The time "off" fluoride during the intermittent regimen could facilitate the resolution of any degree of osteomalacia that might have occurred during the fluoride therapy. In addition, calcium citrate is more soluble and more readily absorbed than calcium carbonate.[185] Thus, the use of calcium citrate may reduce the risk of fluoride-induced osteomalacia. Indeed, these investigators found no histomorphometric evidence for secondary hyperparathyroidism or osteomalacia in their fluoride-treated patients.[183,184] Although this intermittent regimen had smaller increases in spinal bone density than the plain NaF regimen, it showed a greater reduction in risk for new vertebral fractures. Thus, these observations raise the possibility that moderate, intermittent doses of fluoride may have a favorable benefit-to-risk ratio. Such a theoretical advantage of intermittent over continuous fluoride treatment merits further evaluation.

The usual dosage of fluoride for established osteoporosis is 20 to 30 mg of elemental fluoride daily.[24] This dosage range is used to achieve a morning predose serum concentration of 5 to 10 μM. However, the required fluoride dose that would achieve serum fluoride concentrations within the therapeutic range is influenced by age, renal function, and other clinical factors[186] and may vary from one individual to another. There is a strong correlation between fluoride and creatinine clearances.[160] As renal function declines, as in old age (most patients with established osteoporosis are in their seventh and eighth decades), serum fluoride concentrations would rise. As a result, the dosage of fluoride in each patient may require some adjustments in order to maintain serum fluoride concentration within the putative "therapeutic window."

D. Clinical Skeletal Response of Fluoride Treatment

The clinical osteogenic responses to fluoride therapy in humans are assessed by means of serum biochemical markers, bone histomorphometric parameters, and bone density measurements.

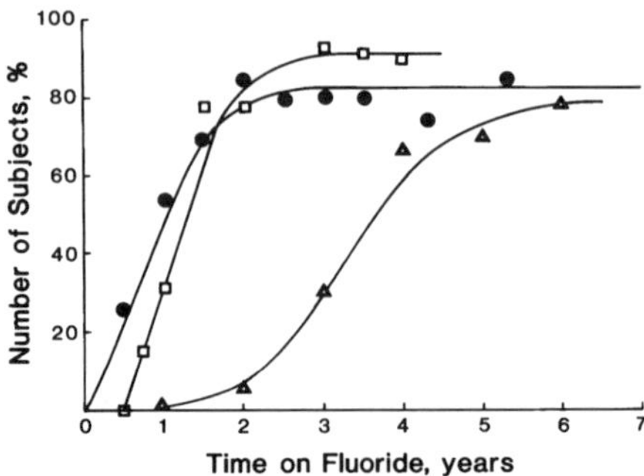

Figure 9.5
The time-dependent effects of fluoride therapy on skeletal alkaline phosphatase (solid circles), decreased back pain (open squares), and fluoridic changes on vertebral X-rays (open triangles) in osteoporotic patients. (From Farley, S. M. G., Wergedal, J. E., Smith, L. C., Lundy, M. W., Farley, J. R., and Baylink, D. J., Fluoride therapy for osteoporosis: characterization of the skeletal response by serial measurements of serum alkaline phosphatase activity, *Metabolism,* 36, 211, 1987. With permission.)

1. Biochemical Bone Formation Markers

Serial serum alkaline phosphatase measurements are often used as a quantitative index of the skeletal response to fluoride.[187] (Serum alkaline phosphatase is a biochemical marker of bone formation.)[188] Increases in serum alkaline phosphatase activity precede and predict the bone density gains (Figure 9.5).[187] Serum alkaline phosphatase activity also correlates to the fluoride-dependent increase in histomorphometric bone biopsy measures of bone formation.[187] Thus, serum alkaline phosphatase activity may be a useful early indicator of the osteogenic response to fluoride in humans. Unfortunately, fluoride therapy can also cause osteomalacia, which is associated with an increase in serum alkaline phosphatase activity. Hence, a rise in serum alkaline phosphatase measurement alone does not allow the distinction of the two potential causes of elevated values, namely increased bone formation or defective mineralization. Other biochemical markers may be needed to assist in distinguishing between these two causes of the rise in serum alkaline phosphatase. Accordingly, when the increase in alkaline phosphatase is associated with calcium deficiency and osteomalacia, the biochemical marker changes are typically those seen in secondary hyperparathyroidism, which include a decrease in urine calcium, an increase in serum PTH, and an increase in urine bone resorption markers.

A potential alternative approach can be used to determine whether the increase in skeletal alkaline phosphatase represents increased bone formation or a mineralization defect. Typically, in vitamin D deficiency-associated osteomalacia, there is an increase in skeletal alkaline phosphatase but not an increase in serum procollagen peptide. Thus, one might use serum procollagen peptide either to evaluate bone formation or as a means of determining whether the increase in skeletal alkaline phos-

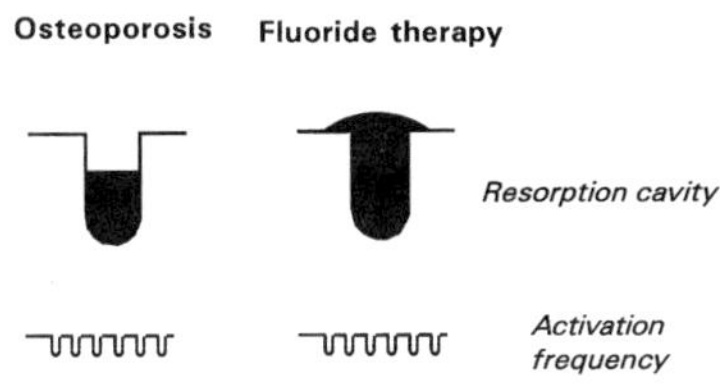

Figure 9.6
Model of the effect of fluoride on bone formation. In osteoporosis, the resorption cavities are underfilled, due to impaired bone formation. As a consequence, bone density decreases at a given site with each cycle of bone remodeling. Fluoride corrects this deficit by promoting an overfilling of the resorptive cavity (and thereby increasing mean wall thickness). The activation frequency (the number of active resorptive sites created per unit of bone surface/unit of time in a given unit of bone) is not affected by fluoride. (From Libanati, C., Lau, K.-H. W., and Baylink, D., Fluoride therapy for osteoporosis, in *Osteoporosis,* Marcus, R., Feldman, D., and Kelsey, J., Eds., Academic Press, San Diego, 1996, 1259. With permission.)

phatase indicates a mineralization defect. Further work will be needed in the future to establish that, in the case of fluoride-induced osteomalacia, procollagen peptide remains an accurate measurement of bone formation.

2. *Bone Histomorphometry*

Bone histomorphometric data, which have been derived almost exclusively from iliac crest biopsies, reveal that fluoride therapy causes large increases in osteoblast number,[7,8] which are due to increased osteoblast proliferation. This leads to increased bone formation, and subsequently results in an overfilling of the resorption excavation cavity (Figure 9.6), which, in turn, leads to an increase in trabecular bone volume with trabecular thickening and an increase in osteoid volume.[189] The increase in osteoid volume is due in large part to an increase in osteoid surface and, to a lesser extent, to an increase in osteoid thickness.[8,190-194] Consistent with the interpretation that fluoride therapy increases trabecular bone volume, lateral lumbar spine X-ray analysis (Figure 9.7) shows that coarsening of vertebral trabeculae and increased prominence of the vertebral end plates are observed after 3.5 years of fluoride (30 mg/day elemental fluoride) and calcium carbonate (1500 mg/day) therapy. Accordingly, these data provide the unambiguous evidence for an osteogenic effect of fluoride therapy in humans.

Loss of trabecular connectivity is a known characteristic of established osteoporosis. Thus, the question as to whether fluoride therapy would restore the trabecular connectivity is a relevant issue. Despite the positive findings of two recent reports,[195,196] the conclusion that fluoride therapy enhances trabecular connectivity has not been universally accepted. Accordingly, while fluoride treatment significantly increases trabecular thickness and volume, it is not yet settled that the therapy can restore the microarchitecture of trabeculae that have been disrupted during the development of osteoporosis.

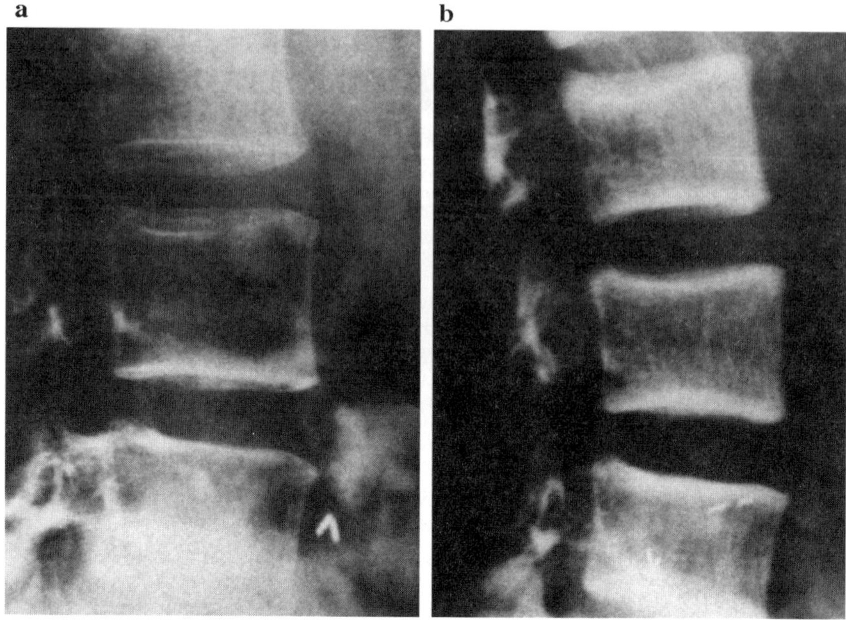

Figure 9.7
Lateral lumbar spine X-rays of a 60-year-old postmenopausal woman before (panel a) and after (panel b) 3.5 years of fluoride (30 mg/day elemental fluoride) and calcium carbonate (1500 mg/day) therapy. Note the remarkable thickening of the trabeculae and the coarsening of the end plates. This patient had two spinal fractures before treatment with fluoride, but none in the subsequent 10 years of follow-up. (From Libanati, C., Lau, K.-H. W., and Baylink, D. J., Fluoride therapy for osteoporosis, in *Osteoporosis*, Marcus, R., Feldman, D., and Kelsey, J., Eds., Academic Press, San Diego, 1996, 1259. With permission.)

A negative aspect of fluoride is that the therapy is frequently associated with a delay in mineralizing newly synthesized osteoid.[118,139,193,197] This effect may relate to the fluoride dose and the availability of calcium to adequately mineralize the osteoid matrix.[7,191,193,198] The calcium insufficiency due to rapid and large increase in bone formation in response to fluoride therapy would probably be more evident in the elderly osteoporotic patients, because they have a reduced efficiency of calcium absorption. Accordingly, large and rapid fluoride-induced increases in bone formation are likely associated with the mineralization defect than smaller and slower increases.

The fluoride-associated osteomalacia may be related to the fluoride-induced calcium deficiency. However, it is also possible that fluoride incorporation into bone minerals may be directly responsible for at least part of the mineralization delay. Accordingly, the possibility that fluoride ion may act through physicochemical interactions with bone minerals to directly retard the mineralization process *per se* cannot be ruled out. Nevertheless, it is clear that fluoride-induced osteomalacia, along with high fluoride incorporation, could significantly impair the biomechanical properties of bone, which, in turn, increase fracture risks. Thus, it can be speculated that the greater the incidence of fluoride-associated osteomalacia, the greater would be the incidence of deleterious side effects. If this speculation is valid, the calcium deficiency-associated osteomalacia could explain, to some extent, the lack of positive results in some past fracture studies. Consequently, it would be essential to avoid or correct osteomalacia and calcium deficiency during fluoride therapy with adequate supplements of calcium and/or 1α,25-dihydroxy vitamin D_3 (calcitriol).

3. *Bone Density*

An end point of the osteogenic effect of fluoride therapy is to increase bone mineral mass and density. Bone density can be evaluated with high precision and accuracy in both axial and the appendicular skeletal sites by noninvasive methods, *viz.* quantitative computed tomography (QCT) and dual energy X-ray absorptiometry (DEXA). It has been known for a number of years that not all parts of the skeleton respond in a similar manner to pathogenic events or therapeutic maneuvers. In this regard, there is evidence that fluoride preferentially affects axial more than appendicular skeletal sites.

a. Axial Bone Mass

Fluoride therapy has consistently been shown to increase axial trabecular (lumbar spine) bone mass in osteoporotic patients. The increase in spinal bone density induced by fluoride therapy is progressive with time for as long as six years (Figure 9.8).[180,199-201] Even though there is some suggestion that there is a dose-response increase in bone density between 5 and 30 mg/day of elemental fluoride,[199,202] this issue has not been examined in prospective studies.

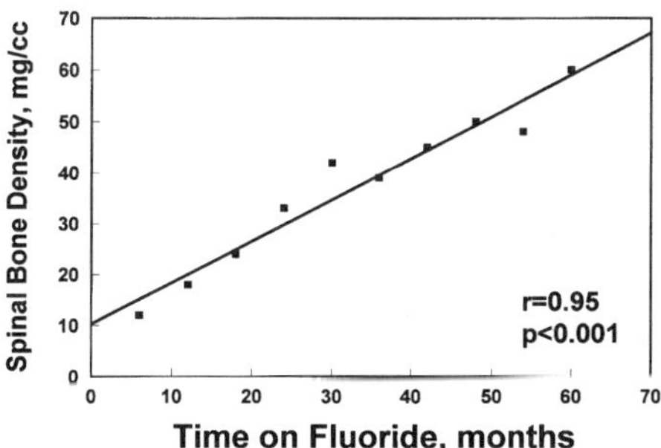

Figure 9.8
The fluoride-dependent increase in spinal bone density as measured by quantitative computed tomography, as a function of time in 389 osteoporotic patients treated with fluoride (30 ± 8 mg/day elemental fluoride) and calcium carbonate (1500 mg/day) for up to six years. Note the apparent linear increase in spinal bone density with fluoride treatment time for up to 6 years.

Depending on the dose and the regimen, the annual increase in axial bone density has been reported to be 10 to 30% with QCT, or 4 to 20% with DEXA. (A larger percentage increase can be seen with QCT because this method, unlike DEXA, measures trabecular bones exclusively, and because fluoride therapy preferentially increases trabecular bone mass.) The increase in spinal bone density is not related to the severity of osteoporosis, the age of the patient, or the cause of the disease.[33] However, it is important to note that not all patients respond to fluoride therapy with an increase in spinal bone density, because 20 to 25% of the osteoporotic patients fail to manifest an increase in spinal bone density, and are considered nonresponders.[7,192,203] The causes of the nonresponsiveness and the individual variability in response to fluoride therapy have not been determined.

b. Appendicular Bone Mass

Total body bone scintigrams (Figure 9.9) suggest that increased bone formation can be detected in both the appendicular and axial skeleton after eleven months of fluoride therapy. Thus, fluoride therapy may also have an anabolic effect on the appendicular skeleton.

There is radiological[204] and bone density[205] evidence supporting the contention that fluoride therapy induces new bone formation in several appendicular skeletal sites which contain a large amount of cancellous bones, e.g., knee, ankle, foot, hips, diaphysis of tibia, and femoral condyle. The magnitude of the effects on these appendicular skeletal sites is much smaller than those on the axial trabecular skeleton (Figure 9.10). Measurements in regions of the appendicular skeleton rich in trabecular bone, such as the proximal tibia,[206] the femoral condyle,[205] or the femoral neck,[180] are consistent with the contention that fluoride acts on the entire skeleton, but preferably on trabecular bone sites.

At one site in the peripheral skeleton, a statistically significant decrease in bone density was observed in one well-controlled prospective study. Accordingly, in the Mayo Clinic study, there was a 7.7% per year decrease in forearm bone density in fluoride-treated patients, despite the fact that the same patients showed an increase in spinal bone density.[180] The investigators postulated that the increase in axial bone density occurs at the expense of the appendicular skeleton. This possibility is further supported by the finding in the same study that significant osteomalacia was present, raising the possibility that calcium deficiency and secondary hyperparathyroidism existed and contributed to this peripheral bone loss.[118]

The effect of fluoride on the appendicular skeleton appears to be influenced by mechanical loading, as fluoride appears to increase bone formation of weight-bearing bones preferentially over non-weight-bearing bones. It is speculated that the more significant increase in the weight-bearing bones may be the result of a synergism between mechanical

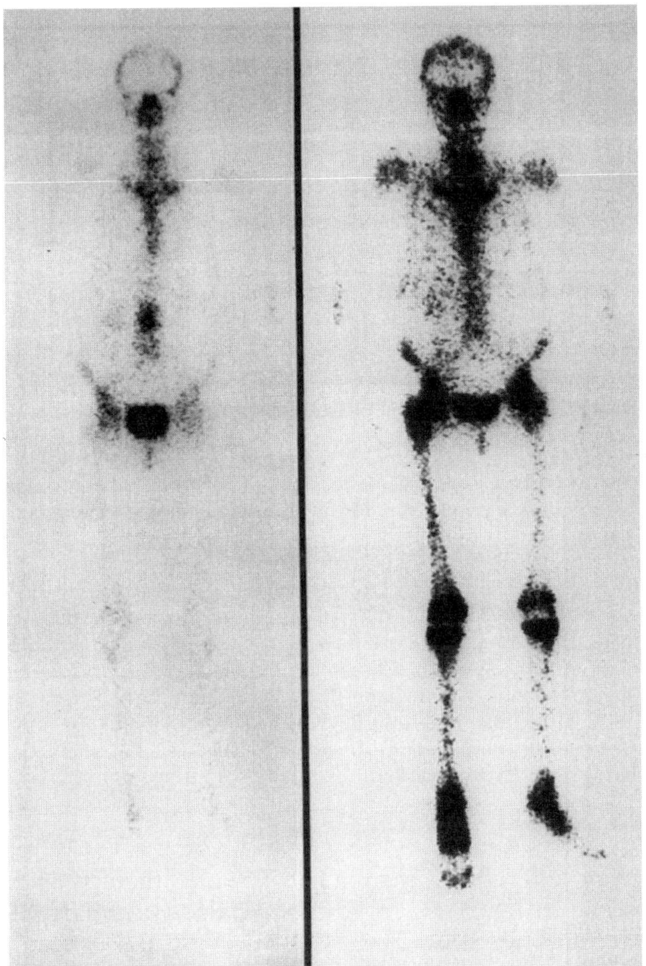

Figure 9.9
Skeletal scintigram (Tc-99m methylene diphosphonate) before (left panel) and 11 months after (right panel) fluoride therapy. Note the marked increased activity in metaphyseal regions of the weight-bearing peripheral skeleton which are rich in trabecular bone. These scintigraphic findings are consistent with an increase in bone formation and are associated with increases in bone density. The increased scintigraphic uptake was probably also exaggerated by calcium deficiency. (From Schulz, E. E., Libanati, C. R., Farley, S. M., Kirk, G. A., and Baylink, D. J., Skeletal scintigraphic changes in osteoporosis treated with sodium fluoride, *J. Nucl. Med.*, 25, 651, 1984. With permission of the Society of Nuclear Medicine.)

loading and fluoride action.[207] This potential synergy is consistent with the proposed mechanism of fluoride action (described in Section II.D.), since mechanical loading may increase production of growth factors in bone cells,[208] the effect of which is potentiated by the osteogenic effect of fluoride.

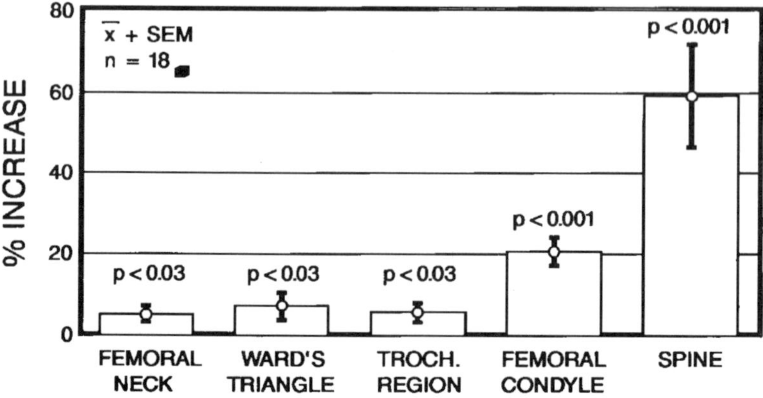

Figure 9.10
Site-specific increases in bone density in osteoporotic patients in response to fluoride therapy. Increases in bone density were measured by quantitative computed tomography in the spine and femoral condyle and by dual X-ray absorptiometry in the hip. Note that only trabecular bone density was measured by quantitative computed tomography in the spine and femoral condyle, whereas cortical and trabecular bone density was measured by dual energy X-ray absorptiometry in the hip. Thus, the different responses in spine and hip are, in part, due to different measuring techniques. Bone density increases associated with fluoride therapy are typically larger in the spine than in the axial skeleton and are also typically larger in trabecular bone compared to cortical bone. (From Dure-Smith, B. A., Kraenzlin, M. E., Farley, S. M., Libanati, C. R., Schulz, E. E., and Baylink, D. J., Fluoride therapy for osteoporosis: a review of dose response, duration of treatment, and skeletal sites of action, *Calcif. Tissue Int.*, 49 (Suppl.), S64, 1991. With permission.)

E. Side Effects

The major side effects ascribed to fluoride therapy in humans are gastrointestinal irritation, peripheral joint pain, calcium deficiency, stress fractures, and hip fractures.

1. Gastrointestinal Irritation

In the past, when plain NaF was used, gastrointestinal irritation was a common side effect, occurring in 25% or more of patients who received the therapy.[173] The most common symptoms are epigastric pain, nausea, and vomiting, which can be effectively treated with antacids or H_2 blockers. The gastrointestinal irritation side effect is dose dependent. In rare cases, patients who were treated with large doses of plain NaF developed duodenal ulceration and bleeding. However, the recent use of slow-release preparations of NaF or MFP has virtually eliminated the incidence of gastrointestinal irritation and related side effects.

2. Peripheral Pain Syndrome

Pain, sometimes severe, develops at peripheral joints (e.g., knees, ankles, or feet) in 10 to 40% of patients receiving the fluoride therapy.[173,209]

This effect is related to dose and is less frequent at low doses (i.e., <20 mg/day elemental fluoride), especially so when the drug is given cyclically.[210] The pain subsides within a few days when the fluoride therapy is discontinued or when the fluoride dosage is reduced.[210]

The etiology of this side effect is controversial. While some investigators suggest that the peripheral joint pain may stem from stress fracture,[211-213] others have argued that the pain may be related to a marked increase in bone formation locally by the fluoride therapy.[33,214,215] This type of pain may be analogous to the bone pain in rapidly growing children. That the total body bone scintigram shown in Figure 9.9, which demonstrates that increased uptake is primarily localized in trabecular-rich weight-bearing areas in the lower skeleton, such as ankles and femoral condyles, and that the increases are bilaterally symmetrical, provides circumstantial evidence for the latter possibility. It has been reported that radiological changes indicative of new bone formation were frequently associated with painful episodes in some patients.[204] Accordingly, the majority of the peripheral joint pain in the lower extremities during fluoride therapy is probably due to a local rapid increase in periosteal bone formation. While fluoride therapy can also cause stress fractures,[180,189] this is probably a minor contributing factor of the peripheral pain syndrome.

3. Calcium Deficiency

A serious concern with fluoride therapy is that patients with very rapid and large increases in bone formation may develop a calcium deficiency, which would lead to secondary hyperparathyroidism, increased bone resorption, and perhaps peripheral bone loss and osteomalacia.[216,217] Accordingly, early studies with fluoride therapy have included the daily supplementation of a large dose of calcium in the hope that this would ensure the availability of sufficient calcium for adequate mineralization of the newly formed bone matrix to avoid osteomalacia. However, despite calcium supplementation, there is unambiguous histomorphometric evidence confirming the development of osteomalacia in some fluoride-treated patients.[118] This is probably because elderly osteoporotic patients have a limited efficiency of calcium absorption, and calcium supplementation alone (without calcitriol to increase calcium absorption) may not be able to prevent calcium deficiency in patients with exuberant bone formation.

Because the fluoride-induced calcium deficiency appears to be corrected by calcitriol and calcium, it would be important to identify patients with calcium deficiency during the fluoride therapy to avoid this side effect. One means by which calcium deficiency can be detected is by measuring serum skeletal alkaline phosphatase, serum PTH, and 24-hour urine calcium before fluoride therapy and at six-month intervals thereafter. Large increases in skeletal alkaline phosphatase and PTH with decreases in 24-hour urine calcium typify the patient who becomes calcium deficient on fluoride therapy. In addition, those patients who develop calcium deficiency are likely to show large increases in bone density.

4. *Stress Fractures*

It has been reported that fluoride therapy increases prevalence of stress fractures in the weight-bearing appendicular skeleton (mainly legs) of fluoride-treated osteoporotic patients.[180,189] The stress fractures that have been attributed to fluoride therapy are predominantly incomplete stress fractures.[199] Whether these stress fractures are due to accelerated bone loss, excessive osteoid accumulation, or poor bone material quality is unknown.

Calcium deficiency could contribute to stress fractures by causing cortical bone loss (because of secondary hyperparathyroidism) and by producing osteomalacia. The loss of cortical bone reduces the biomechanical strength of the bone, and osteomalacia impairs microdamage healing in the skeleton. Accumulation of microdamage would increase the risk of stress fractures. In accordance with this speculation, the histomorphometric evaluation of the bone biopsy samples obtained from the Mayo Clinic trial demonstrates that some of the patients developed osteomalacia.[118]

Another contributor to stress fracturing in fluoride-treated patients is the improved ability to engage in physical activity that results from fluoride therapy. Thus, in patients who respond to fluoride therapy with large increases in spinal bone density, there is decreased back pain, which allows the patient to engage in increased amounts of physical activity. This increase in activity, coupled with the above-described skeletal changes which attend calcium deficiency, may be responsible for the increased incidence of stress fractures in fluoride-treated patients.

5. *Hip Fractures*

The most disconcerting of all side effects of fluoride therapy is the possible increase in the incidence of hip fractures. A high incidence of spontaneous hip fractures has been reported in severely osteoporotic patients who were on fluoride therapy.[218-220] Subsequent studies by the same investigators have suggested that fluoride caused the hip fractures.[218,220] Because the number of patients in these studies was relatively small, and because of the serious nature of hip fractures, a multicenter retrospective analysis was undertaken of more than 1000 patient-years of fluoride treatment by five international medical centers who have extensive experience in the use of fluoride therapy.[221] The analysis did not confirm that fluoride causes hip fractures but, instead, indicated that hip fracture risk is increased in the osteoporotic population because of the bone deficit, and that the risk was unaffected by the fluoride therapy. However, because this was not a prospective study, the issue as to whether fluoride therapy would result in increased risk of hip fractures is not resolved. Additional studies are required to address this very important issue.

F. Efficacy

The ultimate assessment of the efficacy of fluoride therapy of established osteoporosis is reduction of vertebral fracture rate. Because severe back pain is a serious complication of osteoporosis, a secondary index of efficacy is its ability to ease back pain.

1. *Vertebral Fracture Rates*

Several past studies have shown a strong inverse relationship between spinal bone density and vertebral fracture rate.[222,223] A comparison evaluation between trabecular vertebral body density measured by QCT and spinal fracture rate has provided a putative "fracture threshold" of 100 mg/cm^3 for females and 132 mg/cm^3 for males.[223] Because there is unambiguous evidence that fluoride therapy increases axial bone density, it would be reasonable to expect a reduced vertebral fracture rate in those patients who respond to fluoride therapy with an increase in bone density.

There is a general agreement that fluoride therapy increases axial bone density. However, several past uncontrolled studies showed a significant reduction in vertebral fracture rate associated with increased spinal bone density in osteoporotic patients.[7,210,222,224-229] For instance, in a retrospective study wherein 510 osteoporotic patients were treated with an average dose of 30 mg/day of elemental fluoride for five years, there was a marked, highly significant, and progressive increase in spinal bone density and an exponential decrease in the vertebral fracture rate as a function of the increase in spinal bone density (Figure 9.11).[222] When the fracture rate of the fluoride responders (i.e., those who responded with a statistical significant increase in spinal bone density) was compared to that of nonresponders, there was a 76% reduction in vertebral fracture rate in the responders.[230] On the other hand, a placebo-controlled trial failed to produce a significant reduction of vertebral fracture rate in spite of a significant increase in spinal bone density.[206] The controversy is further intensified because of the conflicting results of three recent randomized, placebo-controlled, prospective clinical trials of fluoride therapy.[180-184] Accordingly, in one of two NIH-sponsored clinical trials,[180,181] fluoride therapy did not significantly reduce spinal fracture, but the intermittent low doses of slow-release fluoride in the other trial impressively reduced the spinal fracture rate.[183,184] To add to the controversy, a follow-up report from the Mayo Clinic group who performed one of the NIH-sponsored clinical trials acknowledged that, upon extended observation and reanalysis of their data, those fluoride-treated patients with a relatively low

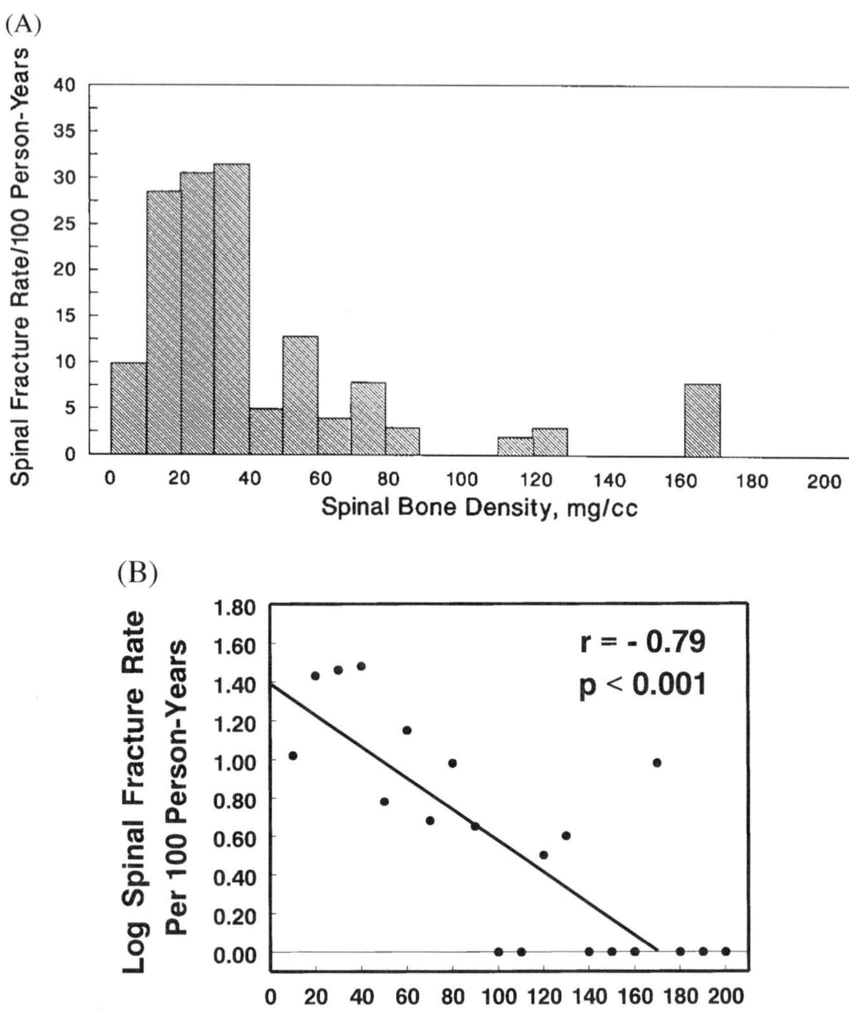

Figure 9.11
Relationship between spinal fracture rate and bone density, both assessed at T12 through L4, during fluoride therapy in 389 patients. Top panel shows the incidence of spinal fractures in T12 through L4 at given levels of bone density, measured by quantitative computed tomography, during fluoride therapy for osteoporosis. Bottom panel shows the plot of log spinal fracture rate/100 patient-years against spinal bone density. The plot has been shifted by adding 1 to all fracture rate data shown in top panel, so that the log of all data, including that of no fracture, could be included in the plot. Note that the spinal fracture rate decreases as a function of increasing bone density during fluoride therapy, suggesting that the bone accumulated during fluoride therapy increases vertebral mechanical strength *in vivo*. (From Farley, S. M., Wergedal, J. E., Farley, J. R., Javier, G. N., Schulz, E. E., Talbot, J. R., Libanati, C. R., Lindegren, L., Bock, M., Goette, M. M., Mohan, S. S., Kimball-Johnson, P., Perkel, V. S., Cruise, R. J., and Baylink, D. J., Spinal fractures during fluoride therapy for osteoporosis: relationship to spinal bone density, *Osteoporosis Int.*, 2, 213, 1992. With permission.)

serum fluoride level had an unequivocally reduced vertebral fracture rate.[182] Thus, the efficacy of fluoride therapy with respect to reduction of spinal fracture rate remains an unsettled issue.[231,232] The following considerations may provide some insights into this controversy.

a. Loss of Trabecular Connectivity and Number

Osteoporosis is characterized by the loss of trabecular number and connectivity, which leads to reduction of biomechanical strength of the skeleton. To fully restore the biomechanical integrity and strength of the skeleton of osteoporotic patients, it may be necessary to regain the number and connectivity of trabeculae. There is no convincing evidence that fluoride therapy could restore the number and connectivity of trabeculae. Accordingly, inasmuch as fluoride treatment increases trabecular bone volume by thickening the remaining trabeculae, this effect alone may not be sufficient to re-establish the biomechanical integrity of the skeleton. In other words, the thickened but less connected trabeculae in the fluoride-treated skeleton may increase the biomechanical strength compared to osteoporotic trabeculae, but the bone strength per unit of bone density may be less than normal. If this speculation is correct, any agent that only increases bone density without restoring the number and connectivity of trabeculae in osteoporotic patients may not correct the biomechanical deficit of the skeleton, unless the bone density is increased above the putative fracture threshold. Therefore, the number and connectivity of the trabeculae existing in the patient before initiation of therapy may be a significant variable in determining the efficacy of fluoride therapy on reduction of fracture risks: the more severe the disease, the less likely fluoride would be to completely correct the fracture risk. In this regard, patients enrolled in the intermittent slow-release NaF trial appear to have less severe osteoporosis than those in the two NIH sponsored studies.[180-184]

It should, however, be emphasized that there is evidence for an inverse relationship between spinal fracture rate and spinal bone density (with an intercept of zero fractures at a QCT bone density of 140 mg/cc) in fluoride-treated patients.[199,201] These observations would be consistent with the concept that the increase in trabecular thickness that occurs in response to fluoride therapy may compensate for the decrease in trabecular number and connectivity during the development of osteoporosis.

b. Fluoride-Induced Calcium Deficiency

As indicated earlier, fluoride-treated patients, especially those who show a rapid and large increase in bone density, are susceptible to calcium deficiency, secondary hyperparathyroidism, and the consequent osteomalacia (see Section IV.D). While many patients in the NIH-sponsored study developed osteomalacia, which may be associated with calcium deficiency,[118] there is no evidence that the patients enrolled in the study at Southwestern University had developed secondary hyperparathyroidism or osteomalacia.[183,184] The lack of development of osteomalacia in the latter study may be due to the use of different fluoride salts (plain NaF vs. slow-release NaF), a lower fluoride dose, an intermittent vs. continuous regimen, and a more readily absorptible calcium salt (i.e., calcium citrate). Accordingly, these differences with respect to reduction in spinal fracture rates could be in part due to whether or not the patients developed calcium deficiency and/or osteomalacia.

2. *Bone Quality and Strength*

A general conclusion from studies with laboratory animal models is that the incorporation of a large amount of fluoride into bone mineral reduces bone quality and strength (see Section III.D). Fluoride therapy in osteoporotic patients significantly increased bone fluoride content in cancellous bone.[171] It is likely that accumulation of a high level of fluoride in bone may also reduce bone quality and strength in humans.

Theoretical considerations suggest that fluoride incorporation into bone may act through the following three means to reduce bone strength and quality:

1. Fluoride therapy may produce bone of histologically abnormal appearance and structure, i.e., "woven bone."[232] Accordingly, formation of bone with an abnormal structure would lead to increased fragility and increased fracture risk. Although bone of woven appearance can be seen in patients with endemic fluorosis, woven bone is not detected in iliac crest bone biopsies from fluoride-treated osteoporotic patients — even with relatively high doses, as in the Mayo Clinic study.[118] Accordingly, there is no compelling evidence to support the contention that poorly organized bone matrix is a significant problem in fluoride-treated patients;
2. Fluoride therapy causes calcium deficiency and osteomalacia. It is possible that uncorrected fluoride-induced calcium deficiency and osteomalacia would impair bone strength in at least two ways:
   a. Ca^{2+} deficiency would cause secondary hyperparathyroidism, which in turn would increase bone resorption and promote trabecular perforation, which leads to deterioration of trabecular microarchitecture; and
   b. osteomalacia, which would impair the repair of microdamage, the accumulation of which will further corrupt the trabecular integrity
3. Fluoride increases bone material density, which may diminish bone quality. This is associated with the mineral crystals in fluoride-treated bone that are larger and denser than those of normal bone (because fluorohydroxyapatite crystals are denser than hydroxyapatite). The increased bone mineral density would be expected to produce an increased compressive strength but a reduced bending strength.

The existing data regarding cancellous bone quality and strength are largely contradictory. Richards and co-workers[233] examined the effects of normal age-related accumulation of fluoride in bone matrix on vertebral trabecular bone quality by biomechanical testing of iliac crest bone biopsies in 73 normal individuals and found that fluoride did not significantly affect bone quality. The same group also reported that there was a significant 45% reduction of trabecular bone strength and a 58% decrease in trabecular bone quality in 12 osteoporotic patients after five years therapy with NaF.[234] In contrast, Antich et al.,[235] with the noninvasive reflection ultrasound technique, determined that the intermittent slow-release fluoride therapy with calcium citrate significantly improved the bone quality in 14 osteoporotic patients. The observation of a positive effect on bone quality is somewhat surprising in light of a vast body of evidence in the literature supporting a deleterious effect on bone quality and strength (see Section III.D). The reason for the lack of a deleterious effect on bone quality in this study is unclear. In addition to the use of different treatment regimens and analytical methods to determine bone quality, the number of patients in the studies was small. Therefore, it is difficult to draw definitive conclusions regarding the improvement of bone quality and strength in osteoporotic patients by fluoride therapy. Further studies are required to settle this issue.

3. Back Pain

Back pain is a frequent symptom of osteoporosis. A major symptomatic change in response to fluoride therapy is a feeling of increased strength, a feeling that the patient can perform tasks that she could not perform before therapy. There are at least three studies which show a significant reduction of back pain as a result of fluoride therapy.[7,187,236] This is a very important benefit of any osteoporosis therapy because it enables the patient to become more active and participate in physical therapy and exercise programs, and thus significantly improve the quality of life.

V. CONCLUDING REMARKS

Despite intense investigations during the past three decades, there is no consensus regarding the suitability of fluoride therapy for treating established osteoporosis. However, it is now clear that fluoride therapy can have several side effects, as well as several significant advantages as an anabolic agent for established osteoporosis (Table 9.1).

Most of the side effects of fluoride therapy appear to be manageable. For example, all of the side effects shown in Table 9.1 (i.e., gastrointestinal irritation, peripheral bone pain, calcium deficiency and osteomalacia, stress fracture, and reduced bone quality and strength) appear to be dose

TABLE 9.1

Advantages and Disadvantages of Fluoride Therapy of Established Osteoporosis

Advantages	Disadvantages
1. Oral administration	1. Gastrointestinal irritation
2. Large increases in bone density	2. Peripheral bone pain
3. Increases in trabecular and cortical–endosteal bone sites	3. Calcium deficiency
	4. Osteomalacia
4. No increase in bone resorption	5. Stress fractures
5. Specific for bone	6. Decreased bone material quality and strength
6. Unique mechanism of action	

related. Accordingly, the use of a lower but effective dose of fluoride can significantly reduce most of these adverse side effects. In addition, the gastrointestinal irritation side effect can virtually be eliminated with the use of newly developed enteric-coated, sustained-release fluoride preparations. The fluoride-induced calcium deficiency and osteomalacia appear to be corrected with calcitriol and calcium supplementation. The fluoride-associated stress fractures may be related to the complication of calcium deficiency. The most significant adverse side effect, reduction of bone quality and strength, seems to be associated with the amount of fluoride incorporated into bone. Thus, this side effect may be alleviated by limiting the amount of fluoride deposited in bone, which may be achieved by using a low dose of fluoride, given cyclically.

The advantages of fluoride therapy are as follows: fluoride is currently the only orally active bone formation agent in clinical trials; fluoride therapy causes a large increase in bone density, which is needed to restore bone density to normal for many patients with established osteoporosis within a reasonable time frame; fluoride increases bone formation at trabecular, as well as cortical–endosteal, bone sites, which are sites of bone loss in osteoporosis; fluoride treatment does not increase bone resorption. Unlike many other potential therapies, the anabolic action of fluoride is specific for bone; and finally, fluoride acts through a unique mechanism — it inhibits a specific osteoblastic fluoride-sensitive PTPP, which leads to a potentiation of the osteogenic actions of endogenous bone cell growth factors. Accordingly, fluoride, in effect, is an inexpensive, orally active, bone-specific growth factor therapy.

In light of these advantages and the manageability of the side effects, fluoride therapy remains a viable anabolic treatment of established osteoporosis. In addition, on the basis of the positive findings of fluoride therapy in several clinical studies, including those of Pak and co-workers,[183,184] the extended analysis of Rigg's study,[182] and others,[7,210,222,224-229] we feel that further studies to optimize fluoride therapy are warranted.

ACKNOWLEDGMENTS

This work was supported in part by research grants from the National Institutes of Health (DE08681) and the Veterans Administration. The authors wish to thank the Medical Media Staff of the Jerry L. Pettis Memorial Veterans Administration Medical Center for assistance in the preparation of the chapter.

REFERENCES

1. Whitford, G. M., *The Mechanism and Toxicity of Fluoride*, Basel, Karger, 1989, 1.
2. Moller, P. F. and Gudjonsson, S. V., Massive fluorosis of bones and ligaments, *Acta Radiol. (Stockh.)*, 13, 269, 1932.
3. Roholm, K., *Fluorine Intoxication: A Clinical Hygienic Study.* H. K. Lewis, Co. Ltd., London, 1937.
4. Rich, C. and Ensinck, J., Effect of sodium fluoride on calcium metabolism of human beings, *Nature (London)*, 191, 184, 1961.
5. Rich C. and Ensinck, J., Effect of sodium fluoride in subjects with metabolic bone disease, *Clin. Res.*, 10, 118, 1962.
6. Rich, C., Ensinck, J., and Ivanovich, P., The effects of sodium fluoride on calcium metabolism of subjects with metabolic bone diseases, *J. Clin. Invest.*, 43, 545, 1964.
7. Briancon, D. and Meunier, P. J., Treatment of osteoporosis with fluoride, calcium, and vitamin D, *Orthop. Clin. North Am.*, 12, 629, 1981.
8. Harrison, J. E., McNeill, K. G., Sturtridge, W. C., Bayley, T. A., Murray, T. M., Williams, C., Tam, C., and Fornasier, V., Three-year changes in bone mineral mass of osteoporotic patients based on neutron activation analysis of the central third of the skeleton, *J. Clin. Endocrinol. Metabol.*, 52, 751, 1981.
9. Odvina, C. V., Wergedal, J. E., Libanati, C. R., Schulz, E. E., and Baylink, D. J., Relationship between trabecular body density and fractures: a quantitative definition of spinal osteoporosis, *Metabolism*, 37, 221, 1988.
10. Parfitt, A. M., Bone remodelling: relationship to the amount and structure of bone, and the pathogenesis and prevention of fractures, in *Osteoporosis: Etiology, Diagnosis, and Management*, Riggs, B. L. and Melton, L. J., Eds., Raven Press, New York, 1988, 45.
11. Farley, J. R., Wergedal, J. E., and Baylink, D. J., Fluoride directly stimulates proliferation and alkaline phosphatase activity of bone forming cells, *Science*, 222, 330, 1983.
12. Wergedal, J. E., Lau, K.-H. W., and Baylink, D. J., Fluoride and bovine bone extract influence cell proliferation and phosphatase activities in human bone cell cultures, *Clin. Orthop. Rel. Res.*, 233, 274, 1988.
13. Lau, K.-H. W., Yoo, A., and Wang, S. P., Aluminum stimulates the proliferation and differentiation of osteoblasts in vitro by a mechanism that is different from fluoride, *Mol. Cell. Biochem.*, 105, 93, 1991.
14. Bellows, C. G., Aubin, J. E., and Heersche, J. N. M., Differential effects of fluoride during initiation and progression of mineralization of osteoid nodules formed *in vitro*, *J. Bone Min. Res.*, 8, 1357, 1993.
15. Bellows, C. G., Heersche, J. N. M., and Aubin, J. E., The effects of fluoride on osteoblast progenitors in vitro, *J. Bone Min. Res.* 5, S101, 1990.

16. Hall, B. K., Sodium fluoride as an initiator of osteogenesis from embryonic mesenchyme in vitro, *Bone* 8, 111, 1987.
17. Reed, B. Y., Zerwekh, J. E., Antich, P. P., and Pak, C. Y. C., Fluoride-stimulated [^{3}H]thymidine uptake in a human osteoblastic osteosarcoma cell line is dependent on transforming growth factor β, *J. Bone Min. Res.*, 8, 19, 1993.
18. Modrowski, D., Miravet, L., Feuga, M., Bannie, F., and Marie, P. J., Effect of fluoride on bone and bone cells in ovariectomized rats, *J. Bone Min. Res.*, 7, 961, 1992.
19. Kassem, M., Mosekilde, L., and Eriksen, E. F., 1,25-Dihydroxyvitamin D_3 potentiates fluoride-stimulated collagen type I production in cultures on human bone marrow stromal osteoblast-like cells, *J. Bone Min. Res.*, 8, 1453, 1993.
20. Kassem, M., Mosekilde, L., and Eriksen, E. F., Effects of fluoride on human bone cells in vitro: differences in responsiveness between stromal osteoblast precursors and mature osteoblasts, *Acta Endocrinol.*, 130, 381, 1994.
21. Khokher, M. A. and Dandona, P., Fluoride stimulates ^{3}H-thymidine incorporation and alkaline phosphatase production by human osteoblasts, *Metabolism*, 39, 1118, 1990.
22. Burgener, D., Bonjour, J.-P., and Caverzasio, J., Fluoride increases tyrosine kinase activity in osteoblast-like cells: regulatory role for the stimulation of cell proliferation and Pi transport across the plasma membrane, *J. Bone Min. Res.*, 10, 164, 1995.
23. Simmons, D. J., Seitz, P., Kidder, L., Klein, G. L., Waeltz, M., Gundberg, C. M., Tabuchi, C., Yang, C., and Zhang, R. W., Partial characterization of rat marrow stromal cells, *Calcif. Tissue Int.*, 48, 326, 1991.
24. Baylink, D. J., Serum fluoride levels, in *Primers on the Metabolic Bone Diseases and Disorders of Mineral Metabolism*, 2nd Ed., Favus, M. J., Ed., Raven Press, New York, 1993, 262.
25. Farley, J. R., Hall, S. L., Herring, S., and Tanner, M. A., Fluoride increases net ^{45}Ca uptake by SaOS-2 cells: the effect is phosphate dependent, *Calcif. Tissue Int.*, 53, 187, 1993.
26. Zerwekh, J., Morris, A., Padalino, P., Gottschalk, F., and Pak, C. Y. C., Fluoride rapidly and transiently raises intracellular Ca in human osteoblasts, *J. Bone Min. Res.*, 5 (Suppl. 1), S131, 1990.
27. Selz, T., Caverzasio, J., and Bonjour, J.-P., Fluoride selectively stimulates Na-dependent phosphate transport in osteoblast-like cells, *Am. J. Physiol.*, 260, E833, 1991.
28. Farley, J. R., Tarbaux, N., Hall, S., and Baylink, D. J., Mitogenic action(s) of fluoride on osteoblast line cells: determinants of the response in vitro, *J. Bone Min. Res.*, 5 (Suppl. 1), S107, 1990.
29. Lau, K.-H. W., Tanimoto, H., and Baylink, D. J., Vanadate stimulates bone cell proliferation and bone collagen synthesis in vitro, *Endocrinology*, 123, 2858, 1988.
30. Weischer, C. H., Krisinger, J., and Karzel, K., Effects of mellitic acid (MA) and sodium fluoride (NaF) on the histological appearance of murine fetal tibiae cultured in vitro, *Histology Histopath.*, 1, 303, 1986.
31. Lau, K.-H. W., Farley, J. R., Freeman, T. K., and Baylink, D. J., A proposed mechanism of the mitogenic action of fluoride on bone cells: inhibition of the activity of an osteoblastic acid phosphatase, *Metabolism*, 38, 858, 1989.
32. Farley, J. R., Tarbaux, N., Hall, S., and Baylink, D. J., Evidence that fluoride-stimulated [^{3}H]thymidine incorporation in embryonic chick calvarial cell cultures is dependent on the presence of a bone cell mitogen, sensitive to changes in the phosphate concentration, and modulated by systemic skeletal effectors, *Metabolism*, 37, 988, 1988.
33. Libanati, C., Lau, K.-H. W., and Baylink, D. J., Fluoride therapy for osteoporosis, in *Osteoporosis*, Marcus, R., Feldman, D., and Kelsey, J., Eds., Academic Press, San Diego, 1996, 1259.
34. Ullrich, A. and Schlessinger, J., Signal transduction by receptors with tyrosine kinase activity, *Cell*, 61, 203, 1990.
35. Fantl, W. J., Johnson, D. E., and Williams, L. T., Signalling by receptor tyrosine kinases, *Annu. Rev. Biochem.*, 62, 453, 1993.

36. Rozakis-Adcock, M., McGlade, J., Mbamalu, G, Pelicci, G., Daly, R., Li, W., Batzer, A., Thomas, S., Brugge, J., and Pelicci, P. G., Association of shc and Grbs/Sem5 SH2-containing proteins is implicated in activation of the Ras pathway by tyrosine kinases, *Nature*, 360, 689, 1992.
37. Haubruck, H. and McCormick, F., Ras p21: effects and regulation, *Biochim. Biophys. Acta*, 1072, 215, 1991.
38. Morrison, D. K., Kaplan, D. R., Rapp, U., and Roberts, T. M., Signal transduction from membrane to cytoplasm: growth factors and membrane-bound oncogene products increase Raf-1 phosphorylation and associated protein kinase activity, *Proc. Natl. Acad. Sci. USA*, 85, 8855, 1988.
39. Ellis, C., Moran, M., McCormick, F., and Pawson, T., Phosphorylation of GAP and GAP-associated proteins by transforming and mitogenic tyrosine kinases, *Nature (London)*, 343, 377, 1990.
40. Manser, E., Leung, T., Salihuddlin, H., Tan, L., and Lim, L., A non-receptor tyrosine kinase that inhibits the GTPase activity of $p21^{cdc42}$, *Nature (London)*, 363, 364, 1993.
41. Lange-Carter, C. A., Pleiman, C. M., Gardner, A. M., Blumer, K. J., and Johnson, G. L., A divergence in the MAP kinase regulatory network defined by MEK kinase and Raf, *Science*, 260, 315, 1993.
42. Pouyssegur, J. and Seuwen, K., Transmembrane receptors and intracellular pathways that control cell proliferation, *Annu. Rev. Physiol.*, 54, 195, 1992.
43. Pulverer, B. J., Kyriakis, J. M., Avruch, J., Nikolakaki, E., and Woodgett, J. R., Phosphorylation of c-jun mediated by MAP kinases, *Nature (London)*, 353, 216, 1991.
44. Gille, H., Sharrocks, A. D., and Shaw, P. E., Phosphorylation of transcription factor $p62^{TCF}$ by MAP kinase stimulates ternary complex formation at c-fos promoter, *Nature (London)*, 358, 414, 1992.
45. Kawase, T. and Suzuki, A., Studies on the transmembrane migration of fluoride and its effects on proliferation of L-929 fibroblasts (L cells) in vitro, *Archs. Oral Biol.*, 34, 103, 1989.
46. Cerklewski, F. L., Enhancement of fluoride retention by low dietary chloride without manifestation of chloride deficiency in the rat, *J. Nutrition*, 116, 1752, 1986.
47. Antonny, B., Bigay, J., and Chabre, M., A novel magnesium-dependent mechanism for the activation of transduction by fluoride, *FEBS Lett.*, 268, 277, 1990.
48. Lau, K.-H. W., Wu, L.-W., and Baylink, D. J., Mitogenic action of fluoride on human bone cells is mediated through a sustained activation of the Ras-Raf-MAPK signal transduction pathway by inhibition of phosphotyrosyl phosphatase activities, *FASEB J.*, 10, A1519, 1996.
49. Lau, K.-H. W., Farley, J. R., and Baylink, D. J., Phosphotyrosyl specific protein phosphatase activity of a bovine skeletal acid phosphatase isoenzyme: comparison with the phosphotyrosyl protein phosphatase activity of skeletal alkaline phosphatase, *J. Biol. Chem.*, 260, 4653, 1985.
50. Lau, K.-H. W., Freeman, T. K., and Baylink, D. J., Purification and characterization of a tartrate-resistant acid phosphatase that displays phosphotyrosyl protein phosphatase activity from bovine cortical bone matrix, *J. Biol. Chem.*, 262, 1389, 1987.
51. Wergedal, J. E. and Lau, K.-H. W., Human bone cells contain a fluoride sensitive acid phosphatase: evidence that this enzyme functions at neutral pH as a phosphotyrosyl protein phosphatase, *Clin. Biochem.*, 25, 47, 1992.
52. Thomas, A. B., Hashimoto, H., Baylink, D. J., and Lau, K.-H. W., Fluoride at mitogenic concentrations increases the steady state phosphotyrosyl phosphorylation level of cellular proteins in human bone cells, *J. Clin. Endocrin. Metabol.*, 81, 2570, 1996.
53. Lau, K.-H. W., Wu, L.-W., Yoon, H.-K., and Baylink, D. J., Inhibition of phosphotyrosine dephosphorylation leads to increased phosphotyrosine phosphorylation of MAP kinase, MAP kinase activity, and human bone cell proliferation, *Bone*, 16 (Suppl.), 96S, 1995.

54. Caverzasio, J., Imai, T., Ammann, P., Burgener, D., and Bonjour, J.-P., Aluminum potentiates the effect of fluoride on tyrosine phosphorylation and osteoblast replication in vitro and bone mass in vivo, *J. Bone Min. Res.*, 11, 46, 1996.
55. Vinals, F., Testar, X., Palacin, M., and Zorzano, A., Inhibitory effect of fluoride on insulin receptor autophosphorylation and tyrosine kinase activity, *Biochem. J.*, 291, 615, 1993.
56. Lau, K.-H. W., Yoo, A., and Wang, S. P., Aluminum stimulates the proliferation and differentiation of osteoblasts in vitro by a mechanism that is different from fluoride, *Mol. Cell. Biochem.*, 105, 93, 1991.
57. Turner, C. H., Akhter, M. P., and Heaney, R. P., The effects of fluoridated water on bone strength, *J. Orthop. Res.*, 10, 581, 1992.
58. Baylink, D., Wergedal, J., Stauffer, M., and Rich, C., Effects of fluoride on bone formation, mineralization, and resorption in the rat, in *Fluorine in Medicine*, Vischer, T. L., Ed., Hans Huber, Bern, 37, 1970.
59. Turner, R. T., Francis, R., Brown, D., Garand, J., Hannon, K. S., and Bell, N. H., The effects of fluoride on bone and implant histomorphometry in growing rats, *J. Bone Min. Res.*, 4, 477, 1989.
60. Cheng, P.-T., and Bader, S. M., Effects of fluoride on rat cancellous bone, *Bone Miner.*, 11, 153, 1990.
61. Mizohata, M., and Kameyama, Y., Histological, histometrical and fluoride electrode studies of the effects of fluoride on the mandibular condyles in growing newborn rats, *Acta Anatomica*, 133, 134, 1988.
62. Ekstrand, J., Lange, A., Ekberg, O., and Hammarstrom, L., Relationship between plasma, dentin and bone fluoride concentrations in rats following long-term fluoride administration, *Acta Pharmacol. Toxicol.*, 48, 433, 1981.
63. Whitford, G. M., Effects of plasma fluoride and dietary calcium concentrations on GI absorption and secretion of fluoride in the rat, *Calcif. Tissue Int.*, 54, 421, 1994.
64. Rigalli, A., Ballina, J. C., Beinlich, A. D., Alloatti, R., and Puche, R. C., Pharmacokinetic differences between sodium fluoride and sodium monofluorophosphate and comparative bone mass increasing activity of both compounds in the rat, *Arzneimittel-Forschung.*, 44, 762, 1994.
65. Rigalli, A., Cabrerizo, M. A., Beinlich, A. D., and Ouche, R. C., Gastric and intestinal absorption of monofluorophosphate and fluoride in the rat, *Arzneimittel-Forschung.*, 44, 651, 1994.
66. Rao, H. V., Beliles, R. P., Whitford, G. M., and Turner, C. H., A physiologically based pharmacokinetic model for fluoride uptake by bone, *Reg. Tox. Pharm.*, 22, 30, 1995.
67. Richards, A., Fejerskov, O., and Ekstrand, J., Fluoride pharmacokinetics in the domestic pig, *J. Dent. Res.*, 61, 1099, 1982.
68. Richards, A., Kragstrup. J., and Nielsen-Kudsk, F., Pharmacokinetics of chronic fluoride ingestion in growing pigs, *J. Dent., Res.*, 64, 425, 1985.
69. Whitford, G. M., Biles, E. D., and Birdsong-Whitford, N. L., A comparative study of fluoride pharmacokinetics in five species, *J. Dent. Res.*, 70, 948, 1991.
70. Whitford, G. M., Intake and metabolism of fluoride, *Adv. Dent. Res.*, 8, 5, 1994.
71. Whitford, G. M., Pashley, D. H., and Stringer, G. I., Fluoride renal clearance: a pH-dependent event, *Am. J. Physiol.*, 230, 527, 1976.
72. Whitford, G. M., The mechanism and toxicity of fluoride, in: *Monographs in Oral Science 13*, Myers, H. M., Ed., Basel, Karger, 1989, 60.
73. Whitford, G. M. and Angmar-Mansson, B., Fluorosis-like effects of acidosis, but not NH_4^+, on rat incisor enamel, *Caries Res.*, 129, 20, 1995.
74. Cerklewski, F. L., Influence of dietary magnesium on fluoride bioavailability in the rat, *J. Nutrition*, 117, 496, 1987.
75. Charkes, N. D., Brookes, M., and Makler, P. T., Studies of skeletal tracer kinetics. II. Evaluation of a five-compartment model of [^{18}F]fluoride kinetics in rats, *J. Nucl. Med.*, 20, 1150, 1979.

76. Hall, L. L., Kilpper, R. W., Smith, F. A., Morken, D. A., and Hodge, H. C., Kinetic model of fluoride metabolism in the rabbit, *Environ. Res.*, 13, 285, 1977.
77. Kessabi, M., Braun, J. P., Benard, P., Burgat-Sacaze, V., and Rico, A. G., Acute kidney toxicity of sodium fluoride in the rat, *Toxicology Lett.*, 5, 169, 1980.
78. Kessabi, M., Braun, J. P., Burgat-Sacaze, V., Benard, P., and Rico, A. G., Comparison of sodium and stannous fluoride nephrotoxicity, *Toxicology Lett.*, 7, 463, 1981.
79. Takagi, M. and Shiraki, S., Acute sodium fluoride toxicity in the rat kidney, *Bull. Tokyo Med. Dent. Univ.*, 29, 123, 1982.
80. Willinger, C. C., Moschen, I., Kulmer, S., and Pfaller, W., The effect of sodium fluoride at prophylactic and toxic doses on renal structure and function in the isolated perfused rat kidney, *Toxicology*, 95, 55, 1995.
81. Shashi, Thapar, S. P., and Singh, J. P., Pulmonary damage caused by fluoride in rabbits during experimental fluorosis, *APMIS*, 96, 333, 1988.
82. Gaugl, J. F. and Wooldridge, B., Cardiopulmonary response to sodium fluoride infusion in the dog, *J. Toxicol. Environ. Health*, 11, 765, 1983.
83. Rigalli, A., Ballina, J. C., Roveri, E., and Puche, R. C., Inhibitory effect of fluoride on the secretion of insulin, *Calcif. Tissue Int.*, 46, 333, 1990.
84. Fujii, A. and Tamura, T., Deleterious effect of sodium fluoride on gastrointestinal tract, *Gen. Pharmacol.*, 20, 705, 1989.
85. Easmann, R. P., Pashley, D. H., Birdsong, N. L., McKinney, R. V., Jr., and Whitford, G. M., Recovery of rat gastric mucosa following single fluoride dosing, *J. Oral Pathol.*, 14, 779, 1985.
86. Das, T. K. and Susheela, A. K., Effect of long-term administration of sodium fluoride on plasma calcium level in relation to intestinal absorption and urinary excretion in rabbits, *Environ. Res.*, 62, 14, 1993.
87. Appleton, J., Changes in the plasma electrolytes and metabolites of the rat following acute exposure to sodium fluoride and strontium chloride, *Archs. Oral Biol.*, 40, 265, 1995.
88. Smith, F. A. and Hodge, H. C., Toxicology of monofluoro phosphate, *Caries Res.*, 17 [Suppl. 1], 36, 1983.
89. Tsutsui, T., Suzuki, N., Ohmori, M., and Maizumi, H., Cytotoxicity, chromosome aberrations and unscheduled DNA synthesis in cultured human diploid fibroblasts induced by sodium fluoride, *Mutation Res.*, 139, 193, 1984.
90. Caspary, W. J., Myhr, B., Bowers, L., McGregor, D., Riach, C., and Brown, A., Mutagenic activity of fluorides in mouse lymphoma cells, *Mutation Res.*, 187, 165, 1987.
91. Aaremia, M. J., Gibson, D. P., and LeBoeuf, R. A., Sodium fluoride-induced chromosome aberrations in different stages of the cell cycle: a proposed mechanism, *Mutation Res.*, 223, 191, 1989.
92. Skare, J. A., Schrotel, K. R., and Nixon, G. A., Lack of DNA-strand breaks in rat testicular cells after in vivo treatment with sodium fluoride, *Mutation Res.*, 170, 85, 1986.
93. Tong, C. C., McQueen, C. A., Brat, S. V., and Williams, G. M., The lack of genotoxicity of sodium fluoride in a battery of cellular tests, *Cell Biol. Toxicol.*, 4, 173, 1988.
94. Li, Y. M., Zhang, W., Noblitt, T. W., Dunipace, A. J., and Stookey, G. K., Genotoxic evaluation of chronic fluoride exposure sister-chromatid exchange study, *Mutation Res.*, 227, 159, 1989.
95. Slamenova, D., Gabelova, A., and Ruppova, K., Cytotoxicity and genotoxicity testing of sodium fluoride on Chinese hamster V79 cells and human EUE cells, *Mutation Res.*, 279, 109, 1992.
96. Collins, T. F. X., Sprando, R. L., Sharkelford, M. E., Black, T. N., Ames, M. J., Welsh, J. J., Balmer, M. F., Olejnik, N., and Ruggles, D. I., Developmental toxicity of sodium fluoride in rats, *Food Chem. Toxicol.*, 33, 951, 1995.
97. Maurer, J. K., Cheng, K. C., Boysen, B. G., and Anderson, R. L., Two-year carcinogenicity study of sodium fluoride in rats, *J. Natl. Cancer Inst.*, 82, 1118, 1990.

98. Martin, G. R., Brown, K. S., Matheson, D. W., Lebowitz, H., Singer, L., and Ophaug, R., Lack of cytogenetic effects in mice or mutations in salmonella receiving sodium fluoride, *Mutation Res.*, 66, 159, 1979.
99. Dunipace, A. J., Wilson, C. A., Wilson, M. E., Zhang, W., Kafrawy, A. H., Brizendine, E. J., Miller, L. L., Katz, B. P., Warrick, J. M., and Stookey, G. K., Absence of detrimental effects of fluoride exposure in diabetic rats, *Archs. Oral Biol.*, 41, 191, 1996.
100. Dunipace, A. J., Brizendine, E. J., Zhang, W., Wilson, M. E., Miller, L. L., Katz, B. P., Warrick, J. M., and Stookey, G. K., Effect of aging on animal response to chronic fluoride exposure, *J. Dent. Res.*, 74, 358, 1995.
101. Chavassieux, P., Bone effects of fluoride in animal models in vivo. A review and a recent study, *J. Bone Min. Res.*, 5 (Suppl. 1), S95, 1990.
102. Chang, P.-T., Bader, S. M., and Grynpas, M. D., Biphasic sodium fluoride effects on bone and bone mineral: a review, *Cells Materials*, 5, 271, 1995.
103. Burkhart, J. M., and Jowsey, J., Effect of variations in calcium intake on the skeleton of fluoride-fed kittens, *J. Lab. Clin. Med.*, 72, 943, 1968.
104. Wenzel, A., Kragstrup, J., and Richards, A., Radiologic assessment of bone maturity and cortical thickness in experimental osteofluorosis in the young pig, *Archs. Oral Biol.*, 29, 745, 1984.
105. Kessabi, M., Hamliri, A., and Braun, J. P., Experimental fluorosis in sheep: alleviating effects of aluminum, *Vet. Hum. Toxicol.*, 28, 300, 1986.
106. Ream, L. J., The effect of short-term fluoride ingestion on bone formation and resorption in the rat femur, *Cell Tissue Res.*, 221, 421, 1981.
107. Marie, P. J., and Hott, M., Short-term effects of fluoride and strontium on bone formation and resorption in mouse, *Metabolism*, 35, 547, 1986.
108. Liu, C. C. and Baylink, D. J., Stimulation of bone formation and bone resorption by fluoride in thyroparathyroidectomized rats, *J. Dent. Res.*, 56, 304, 1977.
109. Kragstrup, J., Richards, A., and Fejerskov, O., Experimental osteofluorosis in the domestic pig: a histomorphometric study of vertebral trabecular bone, *J. Dent. Res.*, 63, 885, 1984.
110. Mosekilde, L., Kragstrup, J., and Richards, A., Compressive strength, ash weight, and volume of vertebral trabecular bone in experimental fluorosis in pigs, *Calcif. Tissue Int.*, 40, 318, 1987.
111. Chavassieux, P., Pastoureau, P., Boivin, G., Chapuy, M. C., Delmas, P. D., and Meunier, P. J., Dose effects on ewe bone remodeling of short-term sodium fluoride administration — a histomorphometric and biochemical study, *Bone*, 12, 421, 1991.
112. Chavassieux, P., Pastoureau, P., Boivin, G., Delmas, P. D., Milhaud, G., and Meunier, P. J., Fluoride-induced bone changes in lambs during and after exposure to sodium fluoride, *Osteoporosis Int.*, 2, 26, 1991.
113. Lundy, M. W., Farley, J. R., and Baylink, D. J., Characterization of a rapidly responding animal model for fluoride-stimulated bone formation, *Bone*, 7, 289, 1986.
114. Snow, G. R. and Anderson, C., Short-term chronic fluoride administration in beagles: a pilot study, *Bone*, 6, 365, 1985.
115. Einhorn, T. A., Wakley, G. K., Linkhart, S., Rush, E. B., Maloney, S., Faierman, E., and Baylink, D. J., Incorporation of sodium fluoride into cortical bone does not impair the mechanical properties of the appendicular skeleton in rats, *Calcif. Tissue Int.*, 51, 127, 1992.
116. Cheng, P.-T. and Bader, S. M., Biphasic effect of fluoride on mineral apposition rates in canine ribs, in *Osteoporosis 1990*, Christiansen, C., and Overgaard, K., eds., Osteopress, Copenhagen, 1990, 1474.
117. Kragstrup, J., Richards, A., and Fejetskov, O., Effects of fluoride on cortical bone remodeling in the growing domestic pig, *Bone*, 10, 421, 1989.
118. Lundy, M. W., Stauffer, M., Wergedal, J. E., Baylink, D. J., Featherstone, J. D., Hodgson, S. F., and Riggs, B. L., Histomorphometric analysis of iliac crest bone biopsies in placebo-treated versus fluoride-treated subjects, *Osteoporosis Int.*, 5, 115, 1995.

119. Snow, G. R. and Anderson, C., Short-term chronic fluoride administration and trabecular bone remodeling in beagles: a pilot study, *Calcif. Tissue Int.*, 38, 217, 1986.
120. Spencer, G. R., El-Sayed, F., Kroening, G. H., Pell, K. L., Shoup, N., Adams, D. F., Franke, M., and Alexander, J. E., Effects of fluoride, calcium and phosphorus on porcine bone, *Am. J. Vet. Res.*, 32, 1751, 1971.
121. Prince, C. W. and Navia, J. M., Glycosaminoglycan alterations in rat bone due to growth and fluorosis, *J. Nutrition*, 113, 1576, 1983.
122. Gedalia, I., Hodge, H. C., Anaise, J., White, W. E., and Menczel, J., The effect of sodium monofluorophosphate and sodium fluoride on bone immobilization in rats, *Calcif. Tissue Res.*, 5, 146, 1970.
123. Ohta, T., Wergedal, J. E., Matsuyama, T., Baylink, D. J., and Lau, K.-H. W., Phenytoin and fluoride act in concert to stimulate bone formation and to increase bone volume in adult male rats, *Calcif. Tissue Int.*, 56, 390, 1995.
124. Faccini, J. M., Inhibition of bone resorption in the rabbit by fluoride, *Nature*, 214, 1269, 1967.
125. Faccini, J. M. and Care, A. D., Effect of sodium fluoride on the ultrastructure of the parathyroid glands of the sheep, *Nature*, 207, 1399, 1965.
126. Spiers, R. L., The relationship between fluoride concentrations in serum and in mineralized tissues in the rat, *Archs. Oral Biol.*, 31, 373, 1986.
127. Søgaard, C. H., Mosekilde, L., Schwartz, W., Leidig, G., Minne, H. W., and Ziegler, R., Effects of fluoride on rat vertebral body biomechanical competence and bone mass, *Bone*, 16, 163, 1995.
128. Eanes, E. D. and Reddi, A. H., The effect of fluoride on bone mineral apatite, *Metab. Bone Dis.*, 2, 3, 1979.
129. Singer, L., Armstrong, W. D., Zipkin, I., and Frazier, P. D., Chemical composition and structure of fluorotic bone, *Clin. Orthop. Rel. Res.*, 99, 303, 1974.
130. Schraer, H., Posner, A. S., Schraer, R., and Zipkin, I., Effect of fluoride on bone minerals, *Clin. Orthop.*, 86, 260, 1972.
131. Baud, C. A. and Bang, S., Biophysical study of the bone tissue of fluoride-treated mice, *J. Dent. Res.*, 52, 589, 1973.
132. Grynpas, M. D., Fluoride effects on bone crystals, *J. Bone Min. Res.*, 5, S169, 1990.
133. Franke, J., Runge, H., Grau, P., Fengler, F., Wanka, C., and Rempel, H., Physical properties of fluorosis bone, *Acta Orthop. Scand.*, 47, 20, 1976.
134. Yamamoto, K., Wergedal, J. E., and Baylink, D. J., Increased bone microhardness in fluoride treated rats, *Calcif. Tissue Res.*, 15, 45, 1974.
135. Lundy, M. W., Russell, J. E., Avery, J., Wergedal, J. E., and Baylink, D. J., Effect of sodium fluoride on bone density in chickens, *Calcif. Tissue Int.*, 50, 420, 1992.
136. Lees, S., Hanson, D., Page, E., and Mook, H. A., Comparison of dosage-dependent effects of β-aminoproprionitrile, sodium fluoride, and hydrocortisone on selected physical properties of cortical bone, *J. Bone Min. Res.*, 9, 1377, 1994.
137. Lundy, M. W., Wergedal, J. E., Teubner, E., Burnell, J., Sherrard, D. J., and Baylink, D. J., The effect of prolonged fluoride therapy for osteoporosis: bone composition and histology, *Bone*, 10, 321, 1989.
138. Boivin, G., Chavassieux, P., Chapuy, M. C., Baud, C. A., and Meunier, P. J., Skeletal fluorosis: histomorphometric analysis of bone changes and bone fluoride content in 29 patients, *Bone*, 10, 89, 1989.
139. Baylink, D. J. and Bernstein, D. S., The effects of fluoride therapy on metabolic bone disease, *Clin. Orthop.*, 55, 51, 1967.
140. Fratzl, P., Roschger, P., Eschberger, J., Abendroth, B., and Klaushofer, K., Abnormal bone mineralization after fluoride treatment in osteoporosis: a small-angle X-ray scattering study, *J. Bone Min. Res.*, 9, 1541, 1994.
141. Wiers, B. H., Francis, M. D., Hovanick, K., Ritchie, C. K., and Baylink, D. J., Theoretical physical chemical studies of the cause of fluoride-induced osteomalacia, *J. Bone Min. Res.*, 5, S63, 1990.

142. Carter, D. R. and Beaupre, G. S., Effects of fluoride treatment on bone strength, *J. Bone Min. Res.*, 5, S177, 1990.
143. Wolinsky, I., Simkin, A., and Guggenheim, K., Effects of fluoride on metabolism and mechanical properties of rat bone, *Am. J. Physiology*, 223, 46, 1972.
144. Turner, C. H., Hasegawa, K., Zhang, W., Wilson, M., Li, Y., and Dunipace, A. J., Fluoride reduces bone strength in older rats, *J. Dent. Res.*, 78, 1475, 1995.
145. Jiang, Y., Zhao, J., Van Audekercke, R., Dequeker, J., and Geusens, P., Effects of low-dose long-term sodium fluoride preventive treatment on rat bone mass and biomechanical properties, *Calcif. Tissue Int.*, 58, 30, 1996.
146. Saville, P. D., Water fluoridation: effect on bone fragility and skeletal calcium content in the rat, *J. Nutr.*, 91, 353, 1967.
147. Riggins, R. S., Zeman, F., and Moon, D., The effects of sodium fluoride on bone breaking strength, *Calcif. Tissue Int.*, 14, 283, 1974.
148. Riggins, R. S., Rucker, R. C., Chan, M. M., Zeman, F., and Beljan, J. R., The effect of fluoride supplementation on the strength of osteopenic bone, *Clin. Orthop. Rel. Res.*, 114, 352, 1976.
149. Kanwar, K. C. and Dhar, S., Bone strength and fluoride supplementation, *Zool. J. Physiol.*, 93, 145, 1989.
150. Lees, S. and Hanson, D. B., Effect of fluoride dosage on bone density, sonic velocity, and longitudinal modulus of rabbit femurs, *Calcif. Tissue Int.*, 50, 88, 1992.
151. Li, J., Nakagaki, H., Kato, K., Tsuboi, S., Kato, S., Morita, I., Ohno, N., Kameyama, Y., Chen, R., and Robinson, C., Effect of stopping fluoride administration on the distribution profiles of fluoride in three different kinds of rat bones, *Calcif. Tissue Int.*, 56, 292, 1995.
152. Merkley, J. W., The effect of sodium fluoride on egg production, egg quality, and bone strength of caged layers, *Poultry Sci.*, 60, 771, 1981.
153. Merkley, J. W., Increased bone strength in coop-reared broilers provided fluoridated water, *Poultry Sci.*, 55, 1313, 1976.
154. Merkley, J. W. and Miller, E. R., The effect of sodium fluoride and sodium silicate on growth and bone strength of broilers, *Poultry Sci.*, 62, 798, 1983.
155. Chan, M. M., Riggins, R. S., and Rucker, R. B., Effect of ethane-1-hydroxy-1,1-diphosphonate (EHDP) and dietary fluoride on biomechanical and morphological changes in chick bones, *J. Nutrition*, 107, 1747, 1977.
156. Suttie, J. W., Kolstad, D. L., and Sunde, M. L., Fluoride tolerance of the young chick and turkey poult, *Poultry Sci.*, 63, 738, 1984.
157. Rahn, K. A., Vanderby, R., Kohles, S. S., Kiratli, B. J., Thielke, R. J., Clay, A. B., and Suttie, J. W., Mechanical effects of sodium fluoride on bovine cortical bone, *Clin. Biomech.*, 6, 185, 1991.
158. Henrikson, P., Lutwak, L., Krook, L., Skogerboe, R., Kallfelz, F., Belanger, L. F., Marier, J. R., Sheffy, B. E., Romanus, B., and Hirsch, C., Fluoride and nutritional osteoporosis: physiochemical data on bones from an experimental study in dogs, *J. Nutrition*, 100, 631, 1970.
159. Kraenzlin, M. E., Kraenzlin, C., Farley, S. M. G., Fitzsimmons, R. J., and Baylink, D. J., Fluoride pharmacokinetics in good and poor responders to fluoride therapy, *J. Bone Min. Res.*, 5 (Suppl. 1), 49, 1990.
160. Duursma, S. A., Raymakers, J. A., de Raadt, M. E., Karsdorp, N. J. G. H., van Dijk, A., and Glerum, J., Urinary fluoride excretion in responders and nonresponders after fluoride therapy in osteoporosis, *J. Bone Min. Res.*, 5 (Suppl. 1), 43, 1990.
161. Murray, T. M., Harrison, J. E., Bayley, T. A., Josse, R. G., Sturtridge, W. C., Chow, R., Budden, F., Laurier, L., Pritzker, K. P. H., Kandel, R., Vieth, R., Strauss, A., and Goodwin, S., Fluoride treatment of postmenopausal osteoporosis: age, renal function, and other clinical factors in osteogenic response, *J. Bone Min. Res.*, 5 (Suppl. 1), 27, 1990.
162. Farley, J. R., Tarbaux, N. M., Lau, K.-H. W., and Baylink, D. J., Monofluorophosphate is hydrolyzed by alkaline phosphatase and mimics the actions of NaF on skeletal tissues in vitro, *Calcif. Tissue Int.*, 40, 35, 1987.

163. Sebert, J. L., Richard, P., Mennecier, I., Bisset, J. P., and Loeb, G., Monofluorophosphate increases lumbar bone density in osteopenic patients: a double-masked randomized study, *Osteoporosis Int.*, 5, 108, 1995.
164. Delmas, P. D., Dupuis, J., Duboeuf, F., Chapuy, M. C., and Meunier, P. J., Treatment of vertebral osteoporosis with disodium monofluorophosphate: comparison with sodium fluoride, *J. Bone Min. Res.*, 5 (Suppl. 1), S143, 1990.
165. Liote, F., Bardin, C., Liou, A., Brouard, A., Terrier, J. L., and Kuntz, D., Bioavailability of fluoride in postmenopausal women: comparative study between sodium fluoride and disodium monofluorophosphate-calcium carbonate, *Calcif. Tissue Int.*, 50, 209, 1992.
166. Jowsey, J. and Riggs, B. L., Effect of concurrent calcium ingestion on intestinal absorption of fluoride, *Metabolism*, 27, 971, 1978.
167. Ericsson, Y., Monofluorophosphate physiology: general considerations, *Caries Res.*, 17 (Suppl. 1), 46, 1983.
168. Dustin, J.-P., Monitoring of fluoride dosage during treatment of bone disease, in *Fluoride in Medicine*, Vischer, T. L., Ed., Bern, Switzerland, Hans Huber, 1970, 178.
169. Cremer, H. D. and Butner, W., Absorption of fluorides, in *Fluorides and Human Health*, World Health Organization Monograph Series, Geneva, 1970, 75.
170. Rao, G. S., Dietary intake and bioavailability of fluoride, *Annu. Rev. Nutri.*, 4, 115, 1984.
171. Boivin, G., Chapuy, M. C., Baud, C. A., and Meunier, P. J., Fluoride content in the human iliac bone, results in controls, patients with fluorosis, and osteoporotic patients treated with fluoride, *J. Bone Min. Res.*, 3, 497, 1988.
172. Gabovich, R. D. and Ovrutsky, G. D., Fluorine in stomatology and hygiene, *NIH Publ. 78-785*, National Institutes of Health, Bethesda, Maryland, 1977, 1.
173. Pak, C. Y. C., Fluoride and osteoporosis, *Proc. Soc. Exp. Biol. Med.*, 191, 278, 1989.
174. Ekstrand, J. and Spak, C.-J., Fluoride pharmacokinetics: its implications in the fluoride treatment of osteoporosis, *J. Bone Min. Res.*, 5 (Suppl. 1), 43, 1990.
175. Spencer, H., Kramer, L., Gatza, C., Norris, C., Wiatrowski, E., and Gandhi, V. C., Fluoride metabolism in patients with chronic renal failure, *Arch. Intern. Med.*, 140, 1331, 1980.
176. Kanis, J. A. and Meunier, P. J., Should we use fluoride to treat osteoporosis? A review, *Q. J. Med.*, 210, 145, 1984.
177. Ekstrand, J., Ehrnebo, M., and Boreus, L. O., Fluoride bioavailability after intravenous and oral administration: importance of renal clearance and urine flow, *Clin. Pharmacol. Ther.*, 23, 329, 1978.
178. Taves, D. R., New approach to the treatment of bone disease with fluoride, *Fed. Proc.*, 29, 1185, 1970.
179. Van Kesteren, R. G., Duursma, S. A., Visser, W. J., van der Sluys, V., and Backer Dirks, O., Fluoride in serum and bone during treatment of osteoporosis with sodium fluoride, calcium, and vitamin D, *Metab. Bone Dis. Rel. Res.*, 4, 31, 1982.
180. Riggs, B. L., Hodgson, S. F., O'Fallon, W. M., Chao, E. Y., Wahner, H. W., Muhs, J. M., Cedel, S. L., and Melton, L. J., III, Effect of fluoride treatment on the fracture rate in postmenopausal women with osteoporosis, *N. Engl. J. Med.*, 322, 802, 1990.
181. Kleerekoper, M., Peterson, E. L., Nelson, D. A., Phillips, E., Schork, M. A., Tilley, B. C., and Parfitt, A. M., A randomized trial of sodium fluoride as a treatment for postmenopausal osteoporosis, *Osteoporosis Int.*, 1, 155, 1991.
182. Riggs, B. L., O'Fallon, W. M., Lane, A., Hodgson, S. F., Wahner, H. W., Muhs, J., Chao, E., and Melton, L. J., III, Clinical trial of fluoride therapy in postmenopausal osteoporotic women: extended observations and additional analysis, *J. Bone Min. Res.*, 9, 265, 1994.
183. Pak C. Y. C., Sakhaee, K., Piziak, V., Peterson, R. D., Breslau, N. A., Boyd, P., Poindexter, J. R., Herzog, J., Heard-Sakhaee, A., Haynes, S., Adams-Huet, B., and Reisch, J. S., Slow-release sodium fluoride in the management of postmenopausal osteoporosis. A randomized controlled trial, *Ann. Intern. Med.*, 120, 625, 1994.

184. Pak C. Y. C., Sakhaee, K., Adams-Huet, B., Piziak, V., Peterson, R. D., and Poindexter, J. R., Treatment of postmenopausal osteoporosis with slow-release sodium fluoride. Final report of a randomized controlled trial, *Ann. Intern. Med.*, 123, 401, 1995.
185. Pak, C. Y. C., Sakhaee, K., Parcel, C., Poindexter, J., Adams, B., Bahar, A., and Beckley, R., Fluoride bioavailability from slow-release sodium fluoride given with calcium citrate, *J. Bone Min. Res.*, 5, 857, 1990.
186. Murray, T. M., Harrison, J. E., Bayley, T. A., Josse, R. G., Sturtridge, W. C., Chow, R., Budden, F., Laurier, L., Pritzker, K. P. H., Kandel, R., Vieth, R., Strauss, A., and Goodwin, S., Fluoride treatment of postmenopausal osteoporosis: age, renal function, and other clinical factors in osteogenic response, *J. Bone Min. Res.*, 5 (Suppl. 1), S27, 1990.
187. Farley, S. M. G., Wergedal, J. E., Smith, L. C., Lundy, M. W., Farley, J. R., and Baylink, D. J., Fluoride therapy for osteoporosis: characterization of the skeletal response by serial measurements of serum alkaline phosphatase activity, *Metabolism*, 36, 211, 1987.
188. Farley, J. R. and Baylink, D. J., Skeletal alkaline phosphatase activity as a bone formation index in vitro, *Metabolism*, 35, 563, 1986.
189. Boivin, G., Dupuis, J., and Meunier, P. J., Fluoride and osteoporosis, in *Osteoporosis: nutritional aspects, World Rev. Nutr. Dict.*, Simopoulos, A. P. and Galli, C., Eds., Karger, Basel, 1993, Vol. 73, 80.
190. Kuntz, D., Marie, P., Naveau, B., Maziere, B., Tubiana, M., and Ryckewaert, A., Extended treatment of primary osteoporosis by sodium fluoride combined with 25 hydroxycholecalciferol, *Clin. Rheumatol.*, 3, 145, 1984.
191. Eriksen, E. F., Mosekilde, L., Melsen, F., Effects of sodium fluoride, calcium, phosphate, and vitamin D_2 on trabecular bone balance and remodeling in osteoporosis, *Bone*, 6, 381, 1985.
192. Harrison, J. E., Bayley, T. A., Josse, R. G., Murray, T.M., Sturtridge, W., Williams, C., Goodwin, S., Tam, C., and Fornasier, V., The relationship between fluoride effects on bone histology and on bone mass in patients with postmenopausal osteoporosis, *Bone Miner.*, 1, 321, 1986.
193. Olah, A. J., Reutter, F. W., and Dambacher, M. A., Effects of combined therapy with sodium fluoride and high doses of vitamin D in osteoporosis. A histomorphometric study in the iliac crest, in *Fluoride and Bone*, Courvoisier, B., Donath, A., and Baud, C. A., Eds., Bern, Huber, 1978, 242.
194. Vigorita, V. J. and Suda, M. K., The microscopic morphology of fluoride-induced bone, *Clin. Orthop.*, 177, 274, 1983.
195. Vesterby, A., Gundersen, H. J. G., Melsen, F., and Mosekilde, L., Marrow space star volume in the iliac crest decreases in osteoporotic patients after continuous treatment with fluoride, calcium, and vitamin D_2 for five year, *Bone*, 12, 33, 1991.
196. Zerwekh, J. E., Hagler, H. K., Sakhaee, K., Gottschalk, F., Peterson, R. D., and Pak, C. Y. C., Effect of slow-release sodium fluoride on cancellous bone histology and connectivity in osteoporosis, *Bone*, 15, 691, 1994.
197. Compston, J. E., Chadha, S., and Merrett, A. L., Osteomalacia developing during treatment of osteoporosis with sodium fluoride and vitamin D, *Br. Med. J.*, 281, 910, 1980.
198. Jowsey, J., Riggs, B. L., Kelly, P. J., and Hoffmann, D. L., Effect of combined therapy with sodium fluoride, vitamin D and calcium in osteoporosis, *Am. J. Med.*, 53, 43, 1972.
199. Kleerekoper, M., Fluoride and the skeleton, *Crit. Rev. Clin. Lab. Sci.*, 33, 139, 1996.
200. Kleerekoper, M. and Balena, R., Fluorides and osteoporosis, *Annu. Rev. Nutri.*, 11, 309, 1991.
201. Farley, S. M. G., Libanati, C. R., Mariano-Menez, M. R., Tudtud-Hans, L. A., Schulz, E. E., and Baylink, D. J., Fluoride therapy for osteoporosis promotes a progressive increase in spinal bone density, *J. Bone Min. Res.*, 5 (Suppl. 1), S37, 1990.
202. Hansson, T. and Roos, B., The effect of fluoride and calcium on spinal bone mineral content: a controlled, prospective (3 years) study, *Calcif. Tissue Int.*, 40, 315, 1987.

203. Budden, F. H., Bayley, T. A., Harrison, J. E., Josse, R. G., Murray, T. M., Sturtridge, W. C., Kandel, R., Vieth, R., Strauss, A. L., and Goodwin, S., The effect of fluoride on bone histology depends on adequate fluoride absorption and retention, *J. Bone Min. Res.*, 3, 127, 1988.
204. Schulz, E. E., Engstrom, H., Sauser, D. D., and Baylink, D. J., Osteoporosis: radiographic detection of fluoride-induced extra-axial bone formation, *Radiology*, 159, 457, 1986.
205. Resch, H., Libanati, C., Farley, S., Bettica, P., Schulz, E., and Baylink, D. J., Evidence that fluoride therapy increases trabecular bone density in a peripheral skeletal site, *J. Clin. Endocrin. Metabol.*, 76, 1622, 1993.
206. Dambacher, M. A., Ittner, J., and Ruegsegger, P., Long-term fluoride therapy of postmenopausal osteoporosis, *Bone*, 7, 199, 1986.
207. Farley, S. M., Libanati, C. R., Schulz E. E. Kirk, G. A., and Baylink, D. J., Fluoride stimulates bone formation in the peripheral skeleton particularly at weight-bearing sites, *Clin. Res.*, 32, 394A, 1984.
208. Rawlinson, S. C., Mohan, S., Baylink, D. J., and Lanyon, L. E., Exogenous prostacyclin, but not prostaglandin E2, produces similar responses in both G6PD activity and RNA production as mechanical loading, and increases IGF-II release, in adult cancellous bone in culture, *Calcif. Tissue Int.*, 53, 324, 1993.
209. Riggs, B., Treatment of osteoporosis with sodium fluoride: an appraisal, in *Bone and Mineral Research*, Peck, W. A., Ed., Annu. 2, 366, Elsevier Science Publ., Amsterdam, 1983.
210. Pak, C. Y. C., Sakjaee, K., Zerwekh, J. E., Parcel, C., Peterson, R., and Johnson, K., Safe and effective treatment of osteoporosis with intermittent slow-release sodium fluoride: argumentation of vertebral bone mass and inhibition of fractures, *J. Clin. Endocrinol. Metabol.*, 68, 150, 1989.
211. O'Duffy, J. D., Wahner, H. W., O'Fallon, W. M., Johnson, K. A., Muhs, J. M., Beabout, J. W., Hodgson, S. F., and Riggs, B. L., Mechanism of acute lower extremity pain syndrome in fluoride-treated osteoporotic patients, *Am. J. Med.*, 80, 561, 1986.
212. Schnitzler, C. M. and Solomon, L., Trabecular stress fractures during fluoride therapy for osteoporosis, *Skeletal Radiol.*, 14, 276, 1985.
213. Bayley, T. A., Harrison, J. E., Murray, T. M., Josse, R. G., Sturtridge, W., Pritzker, K. P., Strauss, A., Vieth, R., and Goodwin, S., Fluoride induced fractures: relation to osteogenic effect, *J. Bone Min. Res.*, 5 (Suppl. 1), 217, 1990.
214. Gruber, H. E. and Baylink, D. J., The effects of fluoride on bone, *Clin. Orthopaed. Rel. Res.*, 267, 264, 1991.
215. Kleerekoper, M. and Mendlovic, D. B., Sodium fluoride therapy of postmenopausal osteoporosis, *Endocr. Rev.*, 14, 312, 1993.
216. Duursma, S. A., Glerum, J. H., van Dijk, A., Bosch, R., Kerkhoff, H., van Putten, J., and Raymakers, J. A., Responders and non-responders after fluoride therapy in osteoporosis, *Bone*, 8, 131, 1987.
217. Dure-Smith, B. A., Farley, S. M., Linkhart, S. G., Farley, J. R., and Baylink, D. J., Calcium deficiency in fluoride-treated osteoporotic patients despite calcium supplementation, *J. Clin. Endocrin. Metabol.*, 81, 269, 1996.
218. Gutteridge, D. H., Price, R. I., Nicholson, G. C., Kent, G. N., Retallack, R. W., Devlin, R. D., Worth, G. K., Glancy, J. J., Michell, P., and Gruber, H., Fluoride in osteoporotic vertebral fractures — trabecular increase, vertebral protection, femoral fractures, in *Osteoporosis: Proceedings of the Copenhagen International Symposium on Osteoporosis*, Christiansen, C., Arnaud, C. D., Nordin, B. E. C., Parfitt, A. M., Peck, W. A., and Riggs, B. L., Eds., Aalborg Stiftsbogtrykkeri, Denmark, 1984, 705.
219. Hedlund, L. R. and Gallagher, J. C., Increased incidence of hip fracture in osteoporotic women treated with sodium fluoride, *J. Bone Min. Res.*, 4, 223, 1989.
220. Gutteridge, D. H., Price, R. I., Kent, G. N., Prince, R. L., and Michell, P. A., Spontaneous hip fractures in fluoride-treated patients: potential causative factors, *J. Bone Min. Res.*, 5 (Suppl. 1), 205, 1990.

221. Riggs, B. L., Baylink, D. J., Kleerekoper, M., Lane, J. M., Melton, L. J., and Meunier, P. J., Incidence of hip fractures in osteoporotic women treated with sodium fluoride, *J. Bone Min. Res.*, 2, 123, 1987.
222. Farley, S. M., Wergedal, J. E., Farley, J. R., Javier, G. N., Schulz, E. E., Talbot, J. R., Libanati, C. R., Lindegren, L., Bock, M., Goette, M. M., Mohan, S. S., Kimball-Johnson, P., Perkel, V. S., Cruise, R. J., and Baylink, D. J., Spinal fractures during fluoride therapy for osteoporosis: relationship to spinal bone density, *Osteoporosis Int.*, 2, 213, 1992.
223. Odvina, C. V., Wergedal, J. R., Libanati, C. R., Schulz, E. E., and Baylink, D. J., Relationship between trabecular body density and fractures: a quantitative definition of spinal osteoporosis, *Metabolism*, 37, 221, 1988.
224. Mamelle, N., Meunier, P. J., Dusan, R., Guillaume, M., Martin, J. L., Gaucher, A., Prost, A., Zeigler, G., and Netter, P., Risk benefit of sodium fluoride treatment in primary vertebral osteoporosis, *Lancet*, 2, 361, 1988.
225. Riggs, B. L., Hodgson, S. F., Hoffman, D. L., Kelly, P. J., Johnson, K. A., and Taves, D., Treatment of primary osteoporosis with fluoride and calcium. Clinical tolerance and fracture occurrence, *J. Am. Med. Assoc.*, 243, 446, 1980.
226. Heaney, R. P., Baylink, D. J., Johnson, C. C., Melton, L. J., III, Meunier, P. J., Murray, T. M., and Nagant de Deuxchaisnes, C., Fluoride therapy for the vertebral crush fracture syndrome (a status report), *Ann. Intern. Med.*, 111, 687, 1989.
227. Nagant de Deuxchaisnes, C., Devogelaer, J. P., Depresseux, G., Malghem, J., and Maldague, B., Treatment of the vertebral crush fracture syndrome with enteric-coated sodium fluoride tablets and calcium supplements, *J. Bone Miner. Res.*, 5 (Suppl. 1), S5, 1990.
228. Riggs, B. L., Seeman, E., Hodgson, S. F., Taves, D. R., and O'Fallon, W. M., Effect of fluoride/calcium regimen on vertebral fracture occurrence in postmenopausal osteoporosis: comparison with conventional therapy, *N. Engl. J. Med.*, 306, 446, 1982.
229. Lane, J. M., Healey, J. H., Schwartz, E., Vigorita, V. J., Schneider, R., Einhorn, T. A., Suda, M., and Robbins, W. C., Treatment of osteoporosis with sodium fluoride and calcium: effects on vertebral fracture incidence and bone histomorphometry, *Orthop. Clin. North Am.*, 15, 728, 1984.
230. Fratzl, P., Roschger, P., Eschberger, J., Abendroth, B., and Klaushofer, K., Abnormal bone mineralization after fluoride treatment in osteoporosis: a small-angle X-ray-scattering study, *J. Bone Min. Res.*, 9, 1541, 1994.
231. Pak, C. Y. C., Zerwekh, J. E., Antich, P. P., Bell, N. H., and Singer, F. R., Slow-release sodium fluoride in osteoporosis, *J. Bone Min. Res.*, 11, 561, 1996.
232. Kleerekoper, M., Fluoride: the verdict is in, but the controversy lingers, *J. Bone Min. Res.*, 11, 565, 1996.
233. Richards, A., Mosekilde, L., and Søgaard, C. H., Normal age-related changes in fluoride content of vertebral trabecular bone — relation to bone quality, *Bone*, 15, 21, 1994.
234. Søgaard, C. H., Mosekilde, L., Richards, A., and Mosekilde, L., Marked decrease in trabecular bone quality after five years of sodium fluoride therapy — assessed by biomechanical testing of iliac crest bone biopsies in osteoporotic patients, *Bone*, 15, 393, 1994.
235. Antich, P. P., Pak, C. Y., Gonzales, J., Anderson, J., Sakhaee, K., and Rubin, C., Measurement of intrinsic bone quality in vivo by reflection ultrasound: correction of impaired quality with slow-release sodium fluoride and calcium citrate, *J. Bone Min. Res.*, 8, 301, 1993.
236. Bernstein, D. S. and Cohen, P., Use of sodium fluoride in the treatment of osteoporosis, *J. Clin. Endocrinol.*, 27, 197, 1967.

INDEX

B

C

D

E

F

I

L

M

O

P

Q

R

U

V

W